THE LIFE AN
OF A VICT
COUNTRY DOCTOR

A PORTRAIT OF REGINALD GROVE

VOLUME I

LIFE AT HOME

THE LIFE AND TIMES OF A VICTORIAN COUNTRY DOCTOR

A PORTRAIT OF REGINALD GROVE

VOLUME I

LIFE AT HOME

PETER FLOWER

BROWN DOG BOOKS

First published 2021

Published under licence by Brown Dog Books and
The Self-Publishing Partnership, 7 Green Park Station, Bath BA1 1JB

www.selfpublishingpartnership.co.uk

ISBN printed book: 978-1-83952-207-9

Cover design by Kevin Rylands
Internal design by Tim Jollands

Printed and bound in the UK
This book is printed on FSC certified paper

MIX
Paper from responsible sources
FSC® C013604
FSC www.fsc.org

All proceeds from the sale of this book, after publishing costs, will be donated to The British Thyroid Foundation (Charity Number 1006391) which helps and supports those suffering from thyroid disorders and supports research into the causes and possible cures for this disease – one of which is Grave's Disease. This was a condition from which Hilda, Reginald Grove's wife, suffered.

DEDICATION

Jane Grove (1909–1985)

Reginald Grove's fifth daughter
and my aunt, godmother, mentor and friend.

One in our faith, and one our longing
To make the world within our reach
Somewhat the better for our living,
And gladder for our human speech.

All hearts grew warmer in the presence
Of one who, seeking not his own,
Gave freely for the love of giving,
Nor reaped for self the harvest sown.

Thy greeting smile was pledge and prelude
of generous deeds and kindly words:
In thy large heart were fair guest-chambers,
open to sunrise and the birds.

The task was thine to mould and fashion
Life's plastic newness into grace;
To make the boyish heart heroic,
And light with thought the maiden's face.

Volume IV Personal Poems by John Greenleaf Whittier,
the 19th century American poet.[1]

---

[1] From 'A Memorial' to Moses Austin Cartland, a dear friend who led a faithful life as a teacher and died in the summer of 1863. Cited by Horatia Katharine Frances Gatty in *Juliana Horatia Ewing and Her Books* (Society for Promoting Christian Knowledge, 1885).

Contents

Preface

'The child is father of the man.'
William Wordsworth

Reginald Grove was my grandfather. He practised as a family doctor for 53 years and lived most of his life in the Huntingdonshire market town of St Ives. He died aged 79 in 1948 just after the start of the National Health Service. In many respects he was a Victorian, shaped by the family and society he was brought up in.

Those who recalled him after his death spoke with great affection and respect about him, especially his patients who knew him as a reassuring family doctor.[2] Indeed, his obituary in the *British Medical Journal* stated that he

> made personal friends of his patients and knew their past history and domestic troubles. He always emphasised the fact that doctors have to deal with human beings, with troubles mental and physical, and not with diseases. Acute observations of his patients and a keenness to absorb and try out new ideas in medicine were characteristic of him, but always with the belief that the latest cure-alls have their day and vanish.

I was educated at King's College Choir School and Uppingham School, both of which he attended. Although nearly 80 years separated my schooldays from his, most of the buildings at King's and Uppingham remained much the same as in his day. His experience and mine at boarding school have helped me enormously in writing his story. I was brought up in a rural medical practice where, like Reginald, my father ran his general medical practice surgery from home.

But what began as a short biographical account of his life soon developed into a much more comprehensive social history of the last three decades of the 19th century presented as a trilogy. Volume 1 covers his life as a boy at home in St Ives, Volume 2 his life at boarding school at King's Cambridge

[2] One of the staff at the Norris Museum in St Ives told me that he remembered his grandmother, Sarah Ann Walker, who died in 1969, talking about 'old Doctor Grove' with great affection (conversation 9 November 2017 & 10 October 2018 with Richard Carter).

and Uppingham, and Volume 3 his life at Sidney Sussex, Cambridge, as a medical student at Guy's Hospital, London, and as a young doctor in St Ives up to the First World War. Aspects of his life naturally overlap across the volumes as it is impossible to compartmentalise Reginald's Christian faith, and relationships with his family and friends, to take two examples.

Reginald grew up in a world that was changing relentlessly. John Galsworthy's character, Soames Forsyte, depicted in his novel *In Chancery*, probably voiced the views of many of his generation when he said in 1901 that 'well-nigh two generations had slipped by, of steam boats, railways, telegraphs, bicycles, electric light, telephones, and now these motor cars…'[3]

Society was transformed in countless and profound ways during the course of the mid- to late-19th century; this was in stark contrast to the centuries which preceded it. By the time of Queen Victoria's death, the population of Great Britain had grown to 37 million[4] and extraordinary technical innovation had occurred in engineering, industry, trade, travel, communications, medicine, leisure and education. These changed the face of the country. It was also a period of rapid colonial expansion with the 'Scramble for Africa'. By the turn of the century, the British Empire comprised 450 million subjects over 14 million square miles.

In his preface to *Eminent Victorians*[5] Lytton Strachey writes that 'the history of the Victorian Age will never be written: we know too much about it'.[6] With the passing of over one hundred years since he wrote this, a vast array of new material has come to light, including Reginald Grove's diaries and letters.

Strachey went on to suggest that the historian of the period should 'row out over that great ocean of material, and lower down into it, here and there, a little bucket, which will bring up to the light of day some characteristic specimen, from those far depths, to be examined with a careful curiosity'. This is what I have done. Various diaries, letters and other family papers have been handed down by Reginald's children to the next generation. And these became the basis of my research.

---

[3] Galswothy, John *In Chancery*, (1920) Penguin Edition reprinted 1967, Part 3, Chapter 10, p. 267.

[4] Walvin, James, *Victorian Values* (1987) André Deutsch p. 7.

[5] Strachey, Lytton *Eminent Victorians* (1918) Folio Press. From the Preface.

[6] Strachey was one of the Bloomsbury Set which included Virginia Woolf. John Maynard Keynes and E. M. Forster lived, worked or studied together in the Bloomsbury area, close to the British Museum in London. Born in 1880, his boyhood was a Victorian one. He died in 1932.

Besides his diaries from 1881 to 1893 and letters written to and from his wife, Hilda, I have used other written contemporary material extensively – in biographies, diaries, letters and newspaper reports. I have quoted verbatim from them as the language used vividly conveys life in late-19th-century England.

However, there are gaps in his diaries and gaps, too in his story.

According to Professor John Carey,[7] all exploration of the past is 'part fact and part imagination'.[8] While Carey is no historian there is some truth in his assertion, and this portrait reflects both fact and imagination on my part. But equally, the role of a historian is storytelling. As Professor William Cronon of the American Historical Society[9] says, it 'is through storytelling that the past is brought alive.[10] And in weaving together Reginald's story I have placed it firmly in the context of the era when Great Britain was approaching the height of its international influence and power: an era of massive upheaval and change.

His was an ordinary life but he met or was connected with some extraordinary Victorians. They range from eminent educationalists like Edward Thring of Uppingham and George Howson of Gresham's, to medical authorities like Sir James Paget, Surgeon to Queen Victoria, and Sir Thomas Stevenson, an expert in forensics.

He met the Test cricketer A. P. 'Bunny' Lucas, knew Luke Paget, later Bishop of Chester, and artists like the Fraser brothers. He was taught by the artist Charles Rossiter, his art master at Uppingham, as well as by Howard Hinton, the mathematician. Through his father he had connections with the poet Algernon Swinburne and possibly the naturalist Charles Darwin.

He was taught by two eminent Cambridge men – Arthur Mann, the King's College Chapel Organist, and the King's Vice Provost Augustus Austen Leigh. Reginald also heard renowned musicians play at concerts on a number of occasions – Joseph Joachim, the violinist, and Julius Klengel,

---

[7] John Carey is a British literary critic and Merton Professor of English Literature at the University of Oxford.

[8] Carey wrote this in reviewing a biography *Lost Girls* by D. J. Taylor in *The Sunday Times* 18 August 2019.

[9] Presidential address delivered at the 127th annual meeting of the American Historical Association, held in New Orleans in 2013.

[10] Professor Cronon said that the core task of the historian is 'resurrection: helping the dead past live again. We forget this most basic task at our peril, for there is no deeper betrayal of the historical imagination than to leave the past inertly, boringly forgettable.'

the cellist. As a conductor and composer Joachim worked closely with Johannes Brahms. Many of these names are to be found in the pages of the *Dictionary of National Biography*.[11]

Towards the end of his life, reflecting on the past, he wrote that he had been 'born in a country practice and destined from my earliest years for a medical career'.[12]

As Wordsworth wrote: 'The child is Father of the Man'.[13]

Whether you read just one volume or all of the trilogy, my hope is that you will get a flavour of what it was like to be a boy and young man in the latter stages of the Victorian period.

***

Note: I have included the approximate value in today's decimal currency of figures from this period using data from the Office for National Statistics' composite price index, where £100 in 1886 represents approximately £12,651 in today's prices. However, relative values have changed substantially over time and the comparisons should be treated with caution. Pre-decimal currency was expressed in pounds, shillings and pence, with one shilling being made up of 12 pence, and one pound of 20 shillings.

[11] The *Dictionary of National Biography* is a standard work of reference on notable figures from British history, published since 1885. The updated *Oxford Dictionary of National Biography* was published in 2004 in 60 volumes and online, with 50,113 biographical articles covering 54,922 lives.

[12] Undated typed memoir (probably 1947) deposited by his daughter Mary Grove in the Huntingdon County Archives.

[13] 'My Heart Leaps Up when I Behold', William Wordsworth (1802).

Prologue

'I was born in a country practice and destined from my earliest years for a medical career' [14]

Reginald Grove

The reporter from *The Hunts Post* made a difficult visit to Tenterleas. It was a detached house, built 11 years previously in 1937, and stood in an acre of ground half a mile from the town centre of St Ives, a small market town in the county of Huntingdonshire. Called 'Tenterleas' after the road it was built in, it was the home of a family mourning the sudden death of a well-known and respected local doctor. He had run his rural medical practice for 53 years in St Ives and died of a heart attack[15] aged 79, five months after the launch of the National Health Service in July 1948. His name was Reginald Grove.

The reporter spoke with the doctor's second son, David Grove, who had hurried to be with his mother, Hilda Grove from Woodford, North London, where he lived. David registered his father's death the following day on Monday 29 November 1948, having given the reporter additional information for inclusion in the newspaper article being written. The reporter knew the local townspeople well, but wanted to make sure that he got his facts right.

He headed the front-page article 'Friend of Two Generations'.[16] The report gave a résumé of the doctor's life; from his schooldays at King's College Choir School, Cambridge, to Uppingham School in Rutland. Then his time at Sidney Sussex College,[17] Cambridge, reading Medicine, his training at Guy's Hospital in London, before returning to St Ives to help run his father's practice in 1893 when his father, Dr William Richard

[14] Undated typed memoir (probably 1947) deposited by his daughter Mary Grove in the Huntingdon County Archives.

[15] Death certificate 1948.

[16] *Hunts Post* 2 December 1948.

[17] Where Oliver Cromwell, another son of St Ives, had also studied in 1616–17.

Grove,[18] was in ill health.

On his father's early death at 57, Reginald took over the practice and later succeeded his father as the Medical Officer of Health for the borough; holding this office for 50 years he was also the Medical Officer for St Ives Rural District Council for 20 years. The report went on to mention him being on the staff of the Huntingdon County Hospital – again following in his father's footsteps; his father had trained at the hospital before moving into practice in St Ives in 1863. This was six years before Reginald was born.

He had married Hilda Clara Stevenson,[19] the daughter of a distinguished professor of forensic medicine,[20] when he was 28. He and his wife had ten children. *The Hunts Post* report continued by saying he was 'an enthusiastic rowing man … a keen photographer … and one of the first motorists in the county…' The newspaper article concluded by describing how he and his wife took an active part in the work of the parish church and he had been the Diocesan Chairman of the Church of England's Men Society. While mentioning his interest in photography, it omitted to mention that he was President of the Stereoscopic Society from 1925 to 1948.

An obituary,[21] which appeared in the *British Medical Journal* a few days later, provided details of his medical career. It is likely that the information which was printed was provided by his eldest son, Dr William Stevenson Grove, who had been in practice with him in St Ives since 1937, living above the surgery of Slepe House, a large, end-of-terrace house in Cromwell Terrace, a stone's throw from Market Place in the town.

He loved his wife with deep devotion; their love letters written in the 1890s show the intensity of their relationship before their marriage. Both were convinced it was God's will they had been brought together. Their relationship matured through their 51 years together through her

---

[18] The name William was used in the Grove family through six generations: William Grove (1810–41); his son Dr William Richard Grove (1838–95); his son Dr William Reginald Grove (1869–1948); his son Dr William Stevenson Grove (1902–79); his son William Baird Andrew Grove (born 1943); and his son William Roy Grove (born 1974).

[19] The correspondence between Reginald and Hilda before the marriage provides an intimate insight into their relationship. Writing every couple of days, they clearly loved each other deeply. In their letters they constantly encouraged each other with expressions of their love.

[20] Sir Thomas Stevenson, Professor of Forensic Medicine at Guy's Hospital. Reginald trained under him after he had finished his medical studies at the University of Cambridge.

[21] *British Medical Journal* 12 December 1948.

continuing illness,[22] as well as the death of their youngest son, John, at the early age of 19.[23]

His children remembered him as a kind man, a loving father. The earliest recollections of Jane, one of his seven daughters, was of him in 1912 when she was three being held up in his arms so that she could touch a rabbit carved in the stone of one of the spandrels in the porch of the parish church at St Ives.[24]

Those who recalled him in the years after his death spoke with great affection and respect about him, especially his patients who knew him as a reassuring family doctor. Indeed, his obituary in the *British Medical Journal*, quoted in the preface, stated as much.

He was born at a time of immense change in Victorian England, demographic, social, economic, educational, leisure, commercial, religious and medical. Research carried out in 2019 by Warwick and Glasgow universities[25] into the happiness across four countries – Great Britain, the United States, Italy and Germany – over the last 200 years concluded that the 1880s saw the rise of national optimism, when the British Empire was approaching its peak.[26] It was the most content that Britain has been.

On 22 June 1887, when Reginald was 18 and in his last year of school, Queen Victoria's Golden Jubilee was held. *The Times* reported that 26,000 children had 'disported themselves from noon to dewy eve' in Hyde Park, London, to celebrate this unique event. The children were fed in tents, 250 at a time, on meat pies, cakes, buns and oranges. There were Punch and Judy shows, performing dogs, monkeys and ponies. The Queen joined them in a carriage accompanied by the Life Guards. Reginald celebrated with the school and town in Uppingham on the day

---

[22] Reginald's wife, Hilda, had Graves' disease.

[23] John George Stevenson Grove died of tuberculous in 1932.

[24] From a eulogy spoken at Jane Grove's funeral in Norwich Cathedral in 1985 by her friends Betty Brady and Rachel Young. The full eulogy manuscript is in the Grove Family Archive.

[25] Nature Human Behaviour: *Historical Analysis of National Subjective Wellbeing* (2019) co-written by Prof. Thomas Hills, Prof. Eugenio Proto, Prof. Daniel Sgroi, and Dr Chanuki Seresinhe.

[26] This research analysed 8 million books and 65 million newspaper articles from 1820 to the present day. The researchers found that data collected from books and newspapers is a reliable guide to the national mood. They did acknowledge that the era was notable for high rates of disease, child labour, poor housing and poverty, but found that the national mood among the reading classes was exceptionally high.

before[27] (see Volume 2). There was a special service in the school chapel, followed by a procession through the town which included an old man and his wife who had taken part in George III's Jubilee held in 1809, 78 years previously.

Reginald's early years shaped his life. As Wordsworth wrote in 'My heart leaps up when I behold': 'The child is Father of the Man'.

This is the story of his life as a boy living in St Ives.

[27] Diary 21.06.87.

Part 1

Life in St Ives

***

CHAPTER 1

St Ives

'The town has many delightful old-fashioned houses, and a great open space where in those days a very important cattle market was held.'

Revd Luke Paget, Vicar of All Saints Parish Church, St Ives

THE NEW GROVE FAMILY

On 13 January 1869 a baby boy was born to a young couple living in the small market town of St Ives in Huntingdonshire.

The father waited outside the second-floor bedroom of their home anxiously, as first-time fathers do, for the news of the birth. His concern was heightened because he knew full well the dangers of labour and childbirth as a doctor.

Reginald's parents were William Richard and Maria Grove. They named their son William Reginald. Maria (née Long) was 24 and Richard was 30 when they had married the year before. Richard Grove was a Staffordshire man who, after his medical training at Guy's Hospital in London, and a short spell at Huntingdon Hospital, moved into general practice in St Ives in 1863, working for a Dr Girling. On the marriage certificate Richard was entered as 'MD'.[28] His bride was called a 'gentlewoman'.

Maria's father, Hanslip Long, farmed at Carleton Grange in the small village of Carlton in North Cambridgeshire where Maria grew up. But he also farmed in Swavesey, a few miles south east of St Ives. It was here that Richard had met her on his medical rounds visiting patients. Two years before their marriage in 1868,[29] Richard had been appointed the first Medical Officer of Health for St Ives, and he had also set up practice on his own. It was common for a man from the newly emerging middle classes to get married at a later age; it meant that he was established in his chosen profession and able to support a wife as well as a suitable household.

[28] Doctor of Medicine (abbreviated MD from the Latin, Medicinae Doctor).

[29] They were married by Revd John Wilder on 20 February 1868 at St Peter's Parish Church, Carlton-cum-Willingham. The village is ten miles south-east of Cambridge near the Suffolk border.

In asking Maria's father, a wealthy tenant farmer, he had been able to demonstrate his suitability of being her husband. Within two months of their marriage, Maria was pregnant.

There is no record who delivered young Reginald, but besides a midwife it is likely that Girling, who lived a few doors away, was in attendance. Very probably Maria took chloroform to ease the pain. Its use was became widespread after Queen Victoria had first been given it 16 years before at the birth of her eighth child.[30] The most common birthing position used at this time was the Sims position which preserved the mother's modesty when a male doctor was present.[31] Middle-class women were expected to stay in bed after a birth for at least nine days and often for longer to regain their strength. If anything, a prolonged lying in often left women weaken at the end of the enforced period.

Whether he was breastfed or bottle-fed is not recorded. The use of wet-nurses was common, although the risk of infection was recognised (see Volume 3). Equally, the use of bottle-feeding grew with the manufacture of cheaper glass bottles (with a rubber teat) and prepared food. Bottles were more convenient in many ways, but sterilisation of the teats only became widespread in the 1890s, long after Maria had finished child-rearing.

The month after his birth, Reginald was christened at All Saints Parish Church which was just a few hundred yards away from the Groves' home. Besides Richard and Maria, there were Hanslip Long, Maria's brother, and Martha Long, her sister, as his godparents, together with Joseph Francis (Frank) Grove, who was Richard's only brother. The Longs had travelled from North Cambridgeshire, while Frank had come down from the Midlands where he practised as a solicitor.

Reginald was their first child – four other siblings were to follow over the next five years: Ernest in 1870, Mabel in 1871, Edward (Ted) in 1872, and finally Richard (known as Tom, after his middle name Thomas) in 1874.

---

[30] When chloroform was found to have anaesthetic qualities, Queen Victoria's doctors cautioned her against using it during childbirth, the main objection being that pain relief would slow the progress of labour. But before the birth of her eighth child in 1853 she was allowed to try it for 53 minutes from a handkerchief. She described 'blessed chloroform, soothing, quieting and delightful beyond measure'. The procedure became known as 'chloroform à la reine'.

[31] This involved lying on the left side with knees bent and drawn up into the abdomen which prevented the doctor and patient from seeing each other. With chloroform becoming widely used in childbirth, doctors became much more present at a birth than before.

ST IVES – REGINALD'S HOME

Reginald spent his childhood up to the age of eight living in the prosperous market town of St Ives situated on the north bank of the Great Ouse. The town was five miles east of the county town of Huntingdon and 59 miles from London. For ten years afterwards he lived in two other market towns in Cambridge and Uppingham, apart from his school holidays when he returned home.

The Revd Luke Paget, a friend of the Groves', who was the vicar of All Saints Parish Church from 1886 to 1887, writing later about St Ives, said that

> it is a town of about 3,000 set in the flat country near Ely and Cambridge. The Ouse flows broad and smoothly past it, and under one of the most beautiful ancient bridges in England. The town has many delightful old-fashioned houses, and a great open space where in those days a very important cattle market was held.[32]

The area around St Ives was sometimes called 'Cowslip Country' or 'Buttercup Land',[33] and was a peaceful, rural setting in which to grow up. The poet William Cowper lived in Huntingdon a hundred years before Reginald was born and wrote with great affection on leaving the town:

> Here Ouse, slow winding through level plain
> Of spacious meads with cattle sprinkled o'er,
> Conducts the eye along its sinuous course
> Delighted. There fast rooted in his bank,
> Stand, never overlooked, our favourite elms,
> That screen the herdsman's solitary hut;
> While far beyond, and overthwart the stream
> That as with molten glass inlays the vale,
> The sloping land recedes into the clouds;
> Displaying on its varied side the grace
> Of hedge-row beauties numberless, square tow'r,
> Tall spire, from which the sound of cheerful bells
> Just undulates upon the list'ning ear,
> Groves, heaths, and smoking villages remote.[34]

---

[32] Cited in *Henry Luke Paget: Portrait and Frame* by Elma K. Paget, his wife. 1939 Longmans Green.

[33] Douglas, James, *Theodore Watts-Dunton* (1904) p. 27.

[34] Cowper, William, 'The Task, Book I: The Sofa' from *Poems of William Cowper* (1794).

This peaceful scene was transformed five miles downstream when the bustling livestock market in St Ives was held every Monday. There were also two annual fairs held on Whit Monday and 11 October, which meant that St Ives was a thriving hub for the local rural economy. With its railway station built in 1847, served by the Great Eastern Railway and the East Anglian Line, as well as the Midland Line, its rail network supported the market, as well as providing easy passenger travel for East Anglia, the Midlands, and London and the South.

The *Harrod's Directory*[35] of 1877 stated that the population was 3,800, up from the 3,500 who were recorded as living there in the 1851 National Census. Incorporated in 1874 as a municipal borough, Dr Grove had acted as the deputy to the electoral officer (a solicitor) when the councillors were first elected. There was a town council with four Aldermen, 12 councillors, and a town clerk who was also a local solicitor. All these officers were well known to the Grove family. There was a union or workhouse which could house over 300 inmates whose medical officer later became young Dr Grove. There was a grammar school in Cromwell Place (near Slepe House where the Groves were later to live after moving from where Reginald was born), a National School in Station Road, again near the Groves' second home, and a British School in Globe Place. The National School was run by the Church of England, while the British School was established under the auspices of the British Society founded in 1816.

The Magistrates' Bench sat on Monday each week. St Ives had a Post and Telegraphic Office in Bridge Street, branches of Prescott & Co, Barclays and the London and County banks.

As mentioned, the parish church was All Saints where the Groves were to worship as a family, and with the town's strong Dissention history, there were a variety of Non-conformist chapels – Independent Free Church (Congregational), Wesleyan,[36] Particular Baptist,[37] Primitive Methodist,[38]

[35] Harrod, J. G., *Royal County Directory of Huntingdonshire 1877.*

[36] This was a branch of the Methodist tradition which also accepted the teachings of the 16th-century Dutch Reformed theologian Jacobus Arminius.

[37] This was a branch of the Baptist tradition who believed in the teachings of the 16th-century John Calvin.

[38] This was a branch of the Methodist tradition, which began in England in the early 19th century with the teaching of the American evangelist Lorenzo Dow.

Quaker, and a 'New Jerusalem' Church.[39]

St Ives had then, and still has, a unique medieval bridge over the Great Ouse with a distinctive chapel dedicated to St Leger.[40] Once travellers had crossed over the bridge from the south they came to a 'T' junction after about 50 yards. To the left was the Bullock Market (now called the Broadway), and to the right was Market Hill. Both streets in Reginald's time had a large number of public houses where the huge crowds, who came to the weekly livestock market, quenched their thirst. Westwards the road led to Godmanchester, crossing the Great Ouse into the county town of Huntingdon. Eastwards, the road out of St Ives led towards the village of Earith, Ely and the heart of the Fens.

A PROSPEROUS MARKET TOWN

The town had been commercially important for hundreds of years before the Grove family arrived. The market in St Ives had been set up by Royal Charter by King John around 1200, and by the middle of the 19th century it was said to be the second most important livestock market in England, after Smithfield Market in London. Cattle, sheep, pigs, goats and horses were sold in the streets. Cattle were sold right outside Dr Grove's front door on Mondays in what was then known as the Bullock Market. This was a cobbled area, elliptical in shape, perhaps 80 feet wide at its widest point, which ran from Crown Street to The Waits by the river.

Thomas Carlyle, the renowned Scottish essayist and historian, wrote[41] after his visit to St Ives in 1845 that 'the little town of somewhat dingy aspect and very acquiescent except on market days runs parallel to the shore of the Ouyse [sic], a short furlong in length'. His comments stung the townsfolk long afterwards. Herbert Norris, writing at the end of the century, said that he must have been suffering from an attack of bile. He had 'belied the country and blasphemed the river'.[42] Carlyle's comments were in contrast to another well-known writer, Daniel Defoe, a century earlier who said:

---

[39] This was a church that based its beliefs on the Bible and of writings of the 18th-century theologian Emanuel Swedenborg.

[40] There are only three other medieval bridges in England which have a chapel incorporated into their design – Rotherham, Wakefield and Bradford on Avon.

[41] *Letters and Speeches of Oliver Cromwell.*

[42] Norris, Herbert, *A History of St Ives* (1889), p. 1.

> Here are the most beautiful meadows on the banks of the river Ouse, that I think are to be seen in any part of England; and to see them in the summer season, covered with such innumerable stocks of cattle and sheep, is one of the most agreeable sights of its kind in the whole world.[43]

Like Cowper, he was actually speaking of the river downstream of Huntingdon, but the bucolic scene he described extended down to St Ives and beyond.

James Douglas, also writing at the end of the century, reckoned that Carlyle had been disparaging because he had only spent about an hour in the town, having ridden 17 miles by horse from Ely. From the bridge Carlyle saw an enormous fleet of barges which were frequently then moored at the quay and it was

> from the newly tarred keels of this fleet of barges that came the oily exudation which Carlyle, in his ignorance of the physical sciences and his contempt for them, believed to arise from a greasy river-bottom. And so, the misconception prevailed. And this is what makes strangers, walking along the tow-path of Hemingford meadow, express so much surprise when, instead of seeing the oily scum they expected, they see a broad mirror as clear as glass whose iridescence is caused by the reflection of the clouds overhead and by the gold and white water lilies on the surface of the stream.[44]

But both Norris and Douglas really missed the point. Once the railway came to St Ives two years after Carlyle's visit, the town became rapidly transformed. With its new borough status in 1874 the town thrived; but this change was at the expense of the river traffic which was Carlyle's centre of attention.

ST IVES' CLAIMS TO FAME

Now a dormitory town for Cambridge with a population of 16,000[45] and a tourist attraction for its picturesque river frontage, it had in the 19th century, as today, two well-known claims to fame.

The first was with Oliver Cromwell, Lord Protector during the brief period in the 17th century when England was a republic. Cromwell farmed in St Ives from 1631 to 1636 before moving to Ely. It was popularly

---

[43] Defoe, Daniel, *A Tour Through the Whole Island of Great Britain*, edited by P. N. Furbank and W. R. Owens, Yale University Press (1991), p. 225.

[44] Douglas, James, *Theodore Watts-Dunton* (1904), p. 28.

[45] National Census Information 2011.

believed, incorrectly, that his farm was on land that was built to erect Cromwell Place and Terrace where Reginald and his family moved to in 1881. Cromwell was elected MP for Huntingdon in 1628 and was Lord Protector during the period of the English republic, 1653–58, before his death. His impressive statue, similar in design to that of the one outside the Houses of Parliament in London, was erected in 1901 in Market Hill. In the parish church records was a parish book with his signature, dated 1634.

The other claim to fame was the well-known children's rhyme and riddle:

> As I was going to St Ives,
> I met a man with seven wives,
> Every wife had seven sacks,
> Every sack had seven kits,
> Kits, cats, sacks and wives,
> How many were going to St Ives?

Both St Ives in Cornwall and St Ives in Huntingdonshire lay claim to be the town named. The former because years ago it was a fishing village which had many cats to keep the rodent population down attracted by the fish stored for curing; the latter because of the large, international medieval fairs held in the town from the 12th century onwards. They drew traders from Italy, France and the Low Countries, together with wool merchants from across England. Merchants, servants, peasants and nobles travelled to St Ives, hence the rhyme reflecting the traders visiting the fair each year for six weeks or so after Easter.[46] However, new scholarly research by a local author, Bridget Flanagan, has cast doubt on this claim.[47]

Two further allusions to the town were made. The first was in the 17th century when on the flyleaf of a copy of Chaucer's *Canterbury Tales*, dated

---

[46] Mary Grove, one of Reginald's seven daughters who lived much of her life in St Ives, certainly thought the town of the rhyme was the Huntingdonshire one. Interviewed on BBC Radio's *Down Your Way* by the presenter Brian Johnston on 10 February 1980, she stoutly declared that the rhyme featured her town. A recording of her reciting the rhyme in the medieval chapel on the bridge was played during her interview. *Down Your Way* was one of the most popular programmes on BBC Radio from 1946 until 1992. Every week the presenter would visit a different city, town or village and interview six local people about its history, traditions and customs. Brian Johnston presented the series for 15 years.

[47] Flanagan, Bridget, *The St Ives Problem: A 4000 Year Old Nursery Rhyme?* (2003).

1602, a Gulielmus Nelson[48] wrote rather salaciously:

> … of Cambridge was this clerk, not Oxenford. Well know of Stilton, Stowboy, and Stamford. He haunted Fenny Staunton and St Ives and faire could glaze among ye country wives.[49]

Then in the 20th century Rupert Brooke, the First World War poet, made a waspish aside in his poem 'The Old Vicarage, Grantchester' that 'strong men have blanched and shot their wives, rather than send them to St. Ives'.[50] What he meant is unclear, but he must have been alluding to the rhyme in some obscure way.

THE OLD LIVESTOCK MARKET

When Dr Grove set up home with his new bride in a house in the Bullock Market, drovers continued to bring their lean cattle from Scotland down the Great North Road, grazing as they went, for sale at St Ives Market; fattened on the local pastures around the town and held in paddocks, they were then sold at the St Ives fat stock sales, held each Monday. Sometimes livestock cattle came from Wales. The drovers arrived on Sundays and the Census figures showed as many as 15 drovers lodging in the many pubs around the town on a Sunday night. Cattle, sheep and other animals arrived early on Monday morning market days well before daylight; the livestock was led down to the river at The Waits 30 yards from the Groves' front door. There they were washed by the drovers before being encouraged to drink and then driven and kept in pens made from wooden hurdles in the Bullock Market and on Market Hill, a few hundred yards to the east. The whole town was taken over by the livestock each Monday. Three years after Reginald was born, at a public meeting held in St Ives to discuss the granting of borough status for the town, at which his father spoke, it was stated that at some of the Monday markets there were 7,000 head of cattle, 3,000 sheep besides 'a large number of horses and swine'. Crammed into the Bullock Market, Market Hill and the surrounding streets and alleys,

---

[48] This was William Nelson (1565–1633) who was at St John's College, Cambridge, and was Chaplain to Sir John Stanhope, Treasurer to Queen Elizabeth. He was vicar of Holy Trinity, Cambridge, from 1593 to 1598 before becoming Rector of Little Peatling in Leicestershire where he wrote in his copy of *The Canterbury Tales.*

[49] *Huntingdon and the Great Ouse Handbook* (1905) cited on p. 91.

[50] Brooke, Rupert, *Collected Poems*, 1916 (The Old Vicarage, Grantchester 1914).

this was a huge number.[51]

The Scottish cattle trade began to be affected in the 1820s when steamships began transporting cattle by sea to London, and the advent of the railways eventually ended droving live cattle as they were sent to Smithfield direct. But cattle kept pouring into St Ives as steamships and the railway opened up new trade to St Ives from Ireland. By 1850 the main north-south line from London was built with a station at Huntingdon, and a link was made to St Ives on the East Anglian Line for both freight and passenger travel. Thousands of cattle were transported via the ports of Bristol and Liverpool, with the new station at St Ives being the end of the line for the sale. On Mondays St Ives resembled a Wild West cattle town with livestock thronging the streets. The station became the hub of the town's commercial prosperity.

OUTSIDE THEIR FRONT DOOR

Reginald's first home, which doubled as his father's surgery, was on the south side of what was then called the Bullock Market.[52] As its name suggests, it was here that livestock was bought and sold every Monday. His father spent much of his time visiting patients at their homes, but it was customary for doctors to use their home as their surgery well into the middle of the next century. The Monday market made it impossible for patients to visit his surgery and pretty nigh impossible for Dr Grove to go out on his rounds, except mounted on a horse to enable him to weave his way out of town on the Ramsey Road, avoiding the herds of livestock.

Reginald and his family went to sleep on Sunday evenings to the sound of lowing cattle across the river waiting being moved to market very early the next morning. There was excitement for the Grove children when the household woke up very early on Mondays to the deafening noise of bleating sheep, pigs, sheep and poultry and the cries of drovers, graziers and farmers as their stock was driven past their house. The Bullock Market was paved with large cobbles[53] and lined with wooden rails to keep the cattle off the pavement. There were openings in the rails to allow pedestrians to cross the road. Added to this cacophony were the shouts of the owners

---

[51] Cambridge Independent Press 27.12.1873.

[52] After a new livestock market was built to the east of the town in 1886 the name of the Bullock Market was changed to The Broadway.

[53] Known to the townsfolk as 'petrified kidneys'.

hawking their stock, and livestock buyers bargaining over the price.

In winter, sales began by torchlight and fat stock sales were completed by 6.00am! The beasts were herded off by 7.00 to Cambridge, St Neots and other local towns. English 'store' cattle were brought to market at 8.00, and Irish stock by 9.00. It was reported that some cattle salesmen would show more than 1,000 beasts in a day, while droves of 600–800 were common.[54]

Cattle were sold in the Bullock Market, pigs behind the White Hart, off Market Hill, and sheep in the Market Hill between the Robin Hood and White Hart pubs. Horses were sold in Oliver Road and East Street, and poultry was sold in Crown Yard. Other traders set up stalls – basket dealers at the top of Bridge Street, dairy farmers with cheese and milk in Free Church Lane, and other stalls selling china, knives, razors and agricultural tools where space could be found. The pubs and inns did a roaring trade, with the Unicorn and the Golden Lion being the most popular. From 1850 until it was closed in 1871 the chapel on the bridge was used as a pub. It had a notorious reputation and became known as 'Little Hell': 'Pigs were kept in the cellar. During a drunken brawl on a Fair day, a man was thrown over the balcony into the river and almost drowned.'[55]

St Ives on market day was mayhem.

Crossing the street was a hazardous occupation, and trying to walk along the narrow pavement, which was protected by wooden railings, was difficult. Newspaper reports at the time described the alleys and roads leading to the market as 'crowded with beasts unable to get in to the bullock market until afternoon'.[56] Shopkeepers had to guard their premises against cattle breaking shop windows. On one occasion two 'beasts while being driven through the streets, quietly walked into the shop of Messrs Hankin and Son, stationers. One of them took up its position behind the counter, the other satisfied himself with standing in the shop.'[57] Thankfully, they were persuaded to leave without causing any damage.

On another occasion three beasts were seen swimming down the river. One of the newly appointed 'Water Bailiffs', albeit with a wooden leg, 'put off in a boat and with considerable difficulty and personal danger, directed

[54] Hudson, Noel, *St Ives: Slepe by the Ouse* (1989), p. 89.

[55] Carter, Mary, *19th Century St Ives* (2010), p. 64.

[56] Hudson, Noel, *St Ives: Slepe by the Ouse* (1989), p. 86.

[57] *Hunts County News*, date unknown.

the course of the animals, turning two of them into "The White Horse" yard and the other he succeeded in landing at Ballard's Yard. The owner of the animals rewarded him with two pence [£1.04].'[58] A pastime of the local boys was 'bullock walloping' which involved sneaking up on unsuspecting cattle and seeing their reaction to a hard slap on their hindquarters![59]

The stench on market day was foul: the dung spread across the roads and a huge clean-up was needed as the evening drew in and the day's business came to an end; this was when the inns and public houses nearby did good business as the traders relaxed after a busy day.

And then, twice a year, the town became transformed as traders and visitors flooded in for the two fair days of Whitsun (in April) and Michaelmas (in October). Dating back hundreds of years, these markets attracted merchants, hucksters, livestock dealers and a huge throng of street traders. In Reginald's time, mechanised fairground attractions became popular, with steam engines powering roundabouts and music. Stalls spread across the town, and the noise of the cries of vendors and carts and traps passing over the cobblestones outside their front door rose to a crescendo from dawn to dusk during the days that the fairs ran.[60] It could be a dangerous place, too. In October 1884, for instance, a Mr Hight was knocked down by one of the fairground 'swinging boats' on Market Hill due to some horses taking fright, as described in Chapter 9.

As the new Medical Officer of Health, Reginald's father wrote a report in 1867 to the Improvement Commissioners about the insanitary conditions of the market. Two years later the first suggestion was made about erecting a new, purpose-built market. Nothing came of this idea initially, but it was put to the Duke of Manchester, who owned the market tolls, in 1874. Negotiations between the Borough Council and the Duke dragged on but eventually were resolved.

---

[58] *Hunts County News*, 02.04.87.

[59] This is recounted in an undated talk about St Ives given by Jane Grove, called 'Old St Ives'. She said that 'bullock walloping was always a sport of the boys of the town and I know my brothers used to disappear on Mondays to indulge in this absorbing pastime'. The manuscript of the talk is in the Grove Family Archive.

[60] In the 1950s the fairs were quite large affairs still and I remember the fairground attractions, as well as snake oil salesmen persuading gullible villagers to buy bottles of medicine that cured anything from warts to lumbago. The fairs are still held now but have shrunk to fairground attractions with Ferris wheels, dodgem cars, merry-go-rounds, ghost trains and the like, with some stalls held in the Broadway and Market Hill (visit made to the fair on 10.10.2018).

THEIR NEIGHBOURS IN THE BULLOCK MARKET

Their neighbours were a social mix in their first home. Some were professionals like themselves, but there were also tradespeople with businesses fronting the market, as well as skilled workers involved in the river trade or local manufacturing. It was a busy, bustling area.

There were three public houses on the Groves' side of the street, the Eagle Tavern and the King's Arms to the east, and the Queen Victoria[61] to the west. Nearly opposite their house was the George Inn, then further along the Unicorn and the Woolpack – all catering for the visitors to the livestock market and river port traders. Additionally, their neighbours included a boatwright and his family, a waterman's widow, a solicitor's clerk and a Dr Deane. St Ives had a number of doctors at this time, some qualified like Reginald's father, and others without qualifications (see Volume 3).

The medical practice was well established by the early 1880s and with the size of the growing family, it was time for larger premises to be acquired. Apart from poor hygiene from dung and flies in the hot summer months, a surgery fronting a busy cattle market did not convey the right image to private patients. By this period, medical professionals were establishing their surgeries in the better areas of towns and cities, and the Groves moved to a larger home in Cromwell Place ¾ mile away in the summer of 1881. Richard was 43 and Maria was 37. A Charles Northrop moved into their old house.[62] His father was a well-known local livestock dealer.

Their new house had been built on the site of an 18th-century house which had been pulled down in 1848. The streets that replaced the old house were the first examples in St Ives of street planning.[63] Two new streets were built – the first being Cromwell Place where the houses were built into a terrace, which still stands today. Another terrace was constructed that was at right angles called Cromwell Terrace. Besides 'Slepe House', there were five other homes in Cromwell Terrace. These stand to this day.

Their new home was suitable for a larger family with servants, and had been owned by Mary Mumby who was 80 years old and a retired schoolmistress. She had lived there since the houses had been built over 33

---

[61] This site is now occupied by the Norris Museum.

[62] *Huntingdonshire Post*, 12.06.1909.

[63] Carter, Mary, *19th Century St Ives* (2010), p. 66.

years before and ran a school for young ladies from the premises.[64] These were day pupils rather than boarders.[65]

Reginald's parents called their new home Slepe House.[66] It was a fine, substantial building with an imposing front door and entrance hall.

THEIR NEIGHBOURS AT SLEPE HOUSE

Their new neighbours were all middle-class. One of the families in Cromwell Terrace were the Ulphs, with whom the Groves were good friends. Ulph senior owned an ironmongery shop in Bridge Street. Reginald was firm friends with Arnold (Arnie) Ulph who was the same age, and his diary contains many references to their friendship.

The 1862 *Cassey Directory for St Ives* and 1871 National Census, unusually for the period, showed house numbers in Cromwell Terrace, but no number was given in the next Census of 1881. There had been five separate houses (numbered 1 to 5),[67] but in 1881 the terrace was occupied by a larger number of middle-class individuals, or individuals and their servants. In addition to Miss Mumby, no less than 12 heads of households were listed, ranging from a retired businessman, a landowner, the daughter of a grocer, the widow of a corn factor, an insurance agent, an agricultural manufacturer, a cattle dealer, to a Wesleyan minister.

By the time of the First World War the terrace seems to have been subdivided into a number of homes. The *Kelly's Directory* shows the following homes – numbers 1, 2, 3, 4, 5, 6, 7, 8, 11, 12 and 13 – plus

---

[64] Edward Cassey & Co *History, Topography, & Directory of Bedfordshire and Huntingdonshire* (1862) p. 294 and J. G. Harrod's Directory (1877) p. 915.

[65] J. G. Harrod's *Directory* (1877) listed a grammar school in Cromwell Place (p. 911) with J. Honeybourne who, in the 1881 Census, was shown as running the grammar school at Manchester House in Ramsey Road near the parish church. The *Harrod's Directory* listed a Mr J. S. Bruce, at Manchester House, who was running the 'Commercial and Collegiate School'. Perhaps Bruce's school did not do very well and Honeybourne bought his property and moved the grammar school there.

[66] Slepe is the old name for St Ives, dating back to possible Saxon times. The name implies a muddy slipway coming up from a ford. The Ouse was much shallower then and the site of the ford, before the bridge was built, was upstream at the bottom of Church Street.

[67] The *Edward Cassey Directory* (1862) listed the following houses in Cromwell Terrace: No 10, Gentry: Mrs Ann Coles; No 6 John Johnson; No 3 George Seekings; and with no number Mrs Hannah Greene. Under Trades and Professions: 'Mary Mumby, No 7 (Ladies' School) and with no number Charles Culpin (Machine Maker), Richard Salmon (Plumber, Glazier and Painter) and Frederick Thorpe (Solicitor)'. The latter probably used one of the houses (No 8 or No 5) for their business while using a room each as an office.

a 'Cromwell House', as well as Slepe House and a Revd Wilkinson, a Wesleyan minister, without a house number.[68]

In nearby Cromwell Place there were other middle-class families: a solicitor, a land agent, an ironmonger, a wine merchant and a corn merchant.[69] John Birt Ulph, the ironmonger, was later to move to Cromwell Terrace near the Grove family. Robert Copley, another resident, was a 'bank agent'[70] who was a solicitor, too. It is possible that he was an agent for the London and County Bank. Copley had lived there with his wife Harriet, four children and two servants – a cook and a housemaid – for only a short time. Prior to moving there he had lived in the Bullock Market like Dr Grove, whom he knew well. It is an intriguing possibility that Copley arranged the mortgage for Reginald's father to buy Slepe House in 1881.

In their new home, the Groves had stepped up in St Ivian society.

THE NEW LIVESTOCK MARKET

As mentioned earlier, a new, much larger, purpose-built market, suitably equipped for the volume of increasing sales, was built by the Borough Council half a mile away to the west on vacant land in October 1886. It cost £15.000 (£1,897,650) It covered four acres and 'provides accommodation for about 100 fat bullocks, 2,500 store beasts (with pens), 600 fat sheep, and 3,000 sheep and lambs (all in pens)'.[71] It was an ambitious venture spurred on by the fact that Cambridge had built a new market in 1884 and this threatened the success of the one at St Ives.

Once built, the railway network to St Ives enabled the town to hold its own against the new market in Cambridge. A local newspaper recorded that 'St Ives now possesses one of the most compact, one of best appointed, one of the best built markets in England. It is fashioned after Leicester, but excellent as Leicester is, this marked by later improvements.'[72]

At the time of the market's move, the *Hunts County News* called the Bullock Market 'an eyesore to the reformer and a stain on the civic reputation of the town; holding in the streets 1,804 animals on one

---

[68] Kelly's *Directory for Huntingdonshire* (1914), pp. 61–62.

[69] National Census 1881.

[70] Harrod, J. G. Directory 1877.

[71] Cambridge Independent Press 09.1086.

[72] Hudson, Noel, *St Ives: Slepe by the Ouse* (1989), p. 83.

Monday in 1886 as against 1,062 at the same day the previous year'.[73]

On a long weekend trip from school at the end of November 1886, Reginald visited the new market. The pig market was privately owned. The pens were paved with blue bricks, the roads leading to the market were paved, and there was water supplied for livestock to be washed and troughs from which to drink.[74] As the livestock were moved out of the main streets of the town, stalls selling a variety of goods and produce became a regular feature in Market Hill. The livestock market boomed in the years immediately after opening, with dealers coming from far and wide. A newspaper report of 1889 noted that dealers had come from 43 towns, ranging from Birmingham, Burton-on-Trent, Bristol, Doncaster, Derby, Leicester, King's Lynn, Newark, Wakefield to York.[75] But the initial boom fell away and in 1891 business began to decline partly due to the Cambridge market attracting the Irish traders. This was a huge blow. Gradually, the livestock market declined into the 20th century, and finally closed in 1979.

THE DECLINING RIVER PORT

Behind their house in the Bullock Market lay the river. St Ives' prosperity had been built not only on its livestock and the two annual markets, but also on the river trade over the centuries, with its constant stream of boats offloading goods used for commercial purposes. From the 17th century the Great Ouse had become navigable upstream to Great Barford and later to Bedford, increasing the importance of St Ives as a trading port. Along the side of the Bullock Market were alleys leading down to the river; these housed numerous small businesses connected to the river freight business. The alleys were called by the name of the business owner, like Campion's Yard or Peak's Yard. Sometimes they were named after a public house like the Eagle Yard, and their large, arched doorways can still be seen today.

Despite competition upstream from the growing town of Bedford, when the Grand Union Canal was built in 1841, St Ives was still a lively river port until Reginald was ten or so, when the railway network killed off this type of transport. Vast quantities of coal, corn, timber, cattle food, stone and reeds were transported up and down the river. 15–20-tonne

---

73 Little, Bryan, and Werba, Herbert, *St Ives*, p. 43.

74 Hudson, Noel, *St Ives: Slepe by the Ouse* (1989), p. 88.

75 *St Ives Chronicle*, 01.06.89.

barges known as Fen Lighters transported the goods along the Great Ouse, which Reginald saw from the bank of the rear of his home or from his bedroom window.

Generally, seven to ten boats formed a small convoy, with the first boat called a fore-lighter which had the name of its owner painted on the front. Horses were often used to haul the boats, but if not in use at any time, they were kept in this lighter. The next barge had a cabin for the crew, with the remaining barges carrying cargo. Some of these might be covered, others open depending on the cargo. A small lighter brought up the rear and was often used to transport the horses from one side of the riverbank to the other. The towpath crossed from the south bank to the north near the Quay to offload the freight. The horses would then cross to the south, or Hemingford, side on the opposite bank from the Grove house, to follow the towpath upstream.

A stone's throw from the bottom of his garden in the Bullock Market, a hundred yards upstream, was Holt Island,[76] with its osier (willow) bed. This was an important part of the St Ives economy where willows were grown and then cut to be dried and used for basket-making. Barges moored alongside the island to transport the prepared willow to the workshops in Filbert's Walk, just downstream from the Groves' garden. As a young boy Reginald would often wander along the Bullock Market, down Merryland to Bridge Street, with its bustling array of shops to the bridge, before turning left onto the quay. There he would still be able to see goods being offloaded from the flat-bottomed barges. But by the late-1870s, the once-thriving river port was in gradual decline as the new railway network began to take the bulk of freight traffic. Like the canal network elsewhere, the use of freight transport by rail sounded the death knell for the river trade.

River navigation was still important, but less so as time went by and was hampered by winter floods, as well as the shoals and frequent low water which caused delays for the lighters travelling downstream to Earith; this was despite the rebuilding of the staunch between the town and Holywell, as well as the lock in 1835 next to the low road to the village of Fenstanton. The traffic in coal, malt, corn, timber, stones and reeds for thatching grew less. The need for boat builders, rope makers and boatwrights who lived around the Bullock Market diminished, too, as this form of transport

[76] The island is now a nature reserve.

became less used. By the mid-1880s there was very little commercial river traffic, and the river began to be used for leisure instead. The focus of the town's bustling economic activity moved completely from the quayside to the railway station.

The bridge and the river itself had made the town commercially important prior to the mid-19th century, but it was the advent of the railway that ensured the town's continued prosperity well into the mid-20th century.

The market provided employment and commercial opportunities for many businesses and skilled agricultural and trade workers until the livestock market began its slow decline in the 20th century. Ironically, while the rail link to St Ives saved the market initially, as time went by shipping livestock by rail direct to Smithfield made the St Ives market less and less relevant. The station closed in 1970 followed by the cattle market six years later. The Monday market selling fresh produce and a variety of wares continues in Market Hill to this day.

This was the town that was Reginald's home for most of his boyhood and adult life.

CHAPTER 2

A Tale of Two Houses

NO 33, THE BULLOCK MARKET (1868–81)

Reginald's first home, which doubled as his father's surgery, was on the south side of what was then called the Bullock Market in St Ives. As described in the last chapter, it was here that livestock was bought and sold every Monday.

The house was an early 19th-century red-bricked, double-fronted house rented by his father. Red brick had been fashionable then and the Oxford Clay was dug locally and the bricks fired in the brickworks at Green End, along the Needingworth Road and near How Lane (now The Thicket).[77] Facing out into the street there were iron railings at chest height at the front of the building to ensure that livestock from the market were kept away from the front door and windows. These have long since disappeared. Two steps up from the street level was the main entrance hall with rooms either side facing the Bullock Market. Despite the proliferation of mud and muck from the cobbled street, unlike some of the nearby houses, it did not have a boot-scraper.

The grounds backed down to the Great Ouse. Unlike many houses built during the 19th century it did not have a cellar due to the likelihood of flooding, which was common in St Ives. A young girl, Gwen Raverat, brought up in the 1880s in Cambridge in a middle-class family in a house whose garden swept down to the river Cam, recalled that from her nursery window she and her siblings 'could look right down on to the slow green river beneath us; and if a boat went by it was reflected upside down, as a patch of light moving across the ceiling; and the ripples always purled in a dancing rhythm there, when the sun shone'.[78] It must have been very similar for Reginald and his brothers and sister looking out from the

[77] It has been argued that red-brick construction in a number of the early houses in St Ives was due to the influence of Dutch design brought to England after the accession in 1688 of William and Mary. Bob Murdoch, *The Shaping of St Ives* (2009), p. 63.

[78] Raverat, Gwen, *Period Piece: A Cambridge Childhood* (Faber and Faber, 1952), p. 45.

windows at the back of the house onto the Ouse.

In the early days of the postal system houses were not numbered, as the occupants of those receiving mail were well known to the postmen and there is no record of the house in which the doctor and his young family lived. However, its location has been identified by comparing the returns of the 1861 and 1871 National Censuses against the existing houses. The Groves' home was what is now No 33. Designated as a Grade II listed building,[79] the house is now used as a shop with flats at the rear.

Compared to some of the buildings nearby, it was not substantial but was nevertheless still a good size, with four rooms facing the street on the first floor and a small lintel arch leading to stables, outbuildings and garden at the rear. While his father spent much of his time visiting patients at their homes, especially those who lived in outlying villages, it was also customary for doctors to use their home as their surgery for less wealthy patients, or for those living in St Ives who chose to visit him there.

Dr Grove's consulting room was on the first floor.[80] Given that in this period drawing rooms, where visitors were received in middle-class homes, were generally located on the first floor of Victorian houses, this is not surprising.

As the family grew in size, and Dr Grove's practice became established, the need to move into larger, more prestigious premises became more pressing. After 12 years renting the Bullock Market the family moved to their new home in the summer of 1881 when Reginald was 12.

SLEPE HOUSE, CROMWELL PLACE (1881 ONWARDS)

Dr and Mrs Grove called their new home 'Slepe House', a name that survives to this day. 'Slepe' was the old English name for St Ives up to AD c1000. Reginald went twice to have a look round this house during his half-term holiday from King's Choir School in June 1881. He had only known the Bullock Market as his home, so it is disappointing that he did

[79] The building is described being of 'gault stone cornice and brick blocking course. Square-headed recessed sash windows with stone architraves and original glazing bars. At left a carriage entrance with modern architrave; at right, modern shop front.' [1164424 National Heritage List for England]. The original house has been divided into two: numbers 33 and 33a at the rear.

[80] Just before the family moved to their new home the information in the National Census in April 1881 stated that the surgery was upstairs – but empty. It could well be that Dr Grove had already relocated his surgery to Slepe House in advance of the family's move.

not describe his new home at all in his diary. But at this age his thoughts were no doubt on cricket and going out on the river in his rowing boat

From other records we know that the house was part of a well-designed and substantial terrace built 33 years earlier as the first planned development in St Ives. All the houses were built with yellow gault brick[81] which over the years has darkened. The roof was constructed with grey slate.

The site had been occupied previously by the Old Slepe Hall[82] which had been pulled down in 1848. This had been the largest house in the town, dating from the 18th century. When the building was demolished it was discovered that it had been built on the foundations of a much older house whose cellars remained. It was thought at one time that Oliver Cromwell had lived there before he rose to fame and became the Lord Protector after the execution of King Charles I.[83]

This is now considered unlikely but for the residents of Cromwell Terrace and Cromwell Place it made for a good story. Rumours of the ghost of Cromwell persisted. Another local legend was that Cromwell had hidden his silver plate there before the Civil War began. As he was actually living in Ely when the Civil War broke out, the story is improbable. It is more likely that he lived at Green End Farm at the other end of the town. In any event, no plate was found, although in the cellars the workmen broke open and drank some old bottles of elderflower wine.[84]

Old Slepe Hall had been sold as the new railway line and station were constructed and encroached on its vast grounds. The White family, then owners of the Hall, sold the materials from the building when it was pulled down, and the site and grounds were then sold for building lots. Old Slepe Hall had been rented as a school for young ladies run by Revd Rugeley and his wife. The Rugeleys moved their school to Slepe Hall on the Ramsey Road. That building was demolished some years later, and the new building erected was again used as a girls' school, Slepe Hall School, run by Mrs Anna Lloyd, the wife of the Free Church Minister, as described

---

[81] These bricks are made with local thick, heavy clay mixed with soil and sand. The colour of the bricks is a shade between white and pale yellow, depending on the percentage of clay. With age, the colour darkens, as in the case of all the buildings in Cromwell Place and Cromwell Terrace.

[82] It had previously been called St Ives Hall according to the local author Mary Carter.

[83] The Lawrence family, who owned the Hall, were friends of Cromwell, but were not living there when Cromwell farmed in St Ives.

[84] Douglas, James, *Theodore Watts-Dunton* (1904), p. 37.

in a later chapter. The school took in both boarders and day girls. It closed in 1966.[85]

The Groves' new home fronted the end of an impressive row of six or so houses that was called Cromwell Terrace and was much larger than the other homes. The main entrance to Slepe House was actually in Cromwell Place through a high, pointed-arched porch. This was decorated with blue tiles with a tulip motif in yellow and brown, and there was a cast-iron boot-scraper set back into the wall which is still there today. It is oval-shaped with the head of an angel at the top, rather like a gargoyle. The road outside rumbled with horse traffic entering the town from the Earith and Ely direction and could be busy, especially on market day. As described in a later chapter, a two-year-old girl playing in the road outside in June 1887 was knocked down by a passing cart and seriously injured. Thankfully, under Dr Grove's care she recovered.

From maps of the period, it can be seen that the terrace was an inverted L shape, with Slepe House having a long yard which led onto the road to Needingworth. At the end of the yard was a stable block. This had stalls for a number of horses, a tack room, hayloft and a coach house for a trap and brougham. Across the road from the stable entrance was Darwoods Pond, in front of a large field called Darwood Place. The pond was useful for the horses to drink from after Dr Grove had returned from his patient rounds.[86]

Like the Bullock Market house, Slepe House is now designated as a Grade II listed building,[87] and is still used as a medical practice, called the Grove Medical Centre.[88] A large garden, shared with all the residents of the terrace, was situated opposite and had a tennis court on which Reginald

---

[85] My brother, John, was briefly a day pupil in the early 1950s when our family was living in St Ives.

[86] Sadly, the dew pond became an eyesore, covered with duckweed, and was used for dumped rubbish; it was filled in during the 1970s for use as a municipal car park.

[87] It is described as 'mid 19th century, with two stories, four windows with side entrance onto Cromwell Place. Slated roof with bracketed projected eaves. Gault brick. Gauged flat brick arches to recessed sash windows with original glazing bars.' [Ref 1128728 National Heritage List for England.]

[88] This name was chosen in 2020 when two medical practices merged: the Cromwell Place Surgery and the Old Exchange Surgery. The new name commemorated Reginald's father as one of the first qualified doctors in St Ives, and the town's first Medical Officer and the two other generations of Groves who practiced there until 1948. I had the privilege of being shown around the surgery building in June 2018 by the Practice Manager and seeing the rooms at the top of the building, originally used by the servants of the family.

and his family played regularly. A number of tall, mature trees planted when the terrace was built soar majestically skyward today. Ironically, five years after the Groves moved in, the new cattle market was built abutting the end of the garden of Slepe House. The Grove family knew before their move that there were plans for the old market to move to a new site near the new railway station, but clearly thought it was a better location than the Bullock Market.

The house plans from this period have not survived but it is likely that Dr Grove's surgery entrance and consulting room, with his small dispensary for making up tinctures and cough mixtures, were located to the left of the main entrance to the house itself. The stables at the rear were pulled down some years ago to build additional consulting rooms.

Apart from when he was away at school, Reginald spent his childhood within earshot of the weekly lowing of livestock and the stench of their manure in the old Bullock Market and the new one located within a stone's throw of Slepe House

HOME DECOR

Reginald left no diary record about the inside of either of his homes, so it is only possible to visualise them based on accounts of other Victorian middle-class homes and the trends of interior decor.

Discerning middle-class householders wanted to ensure that the interior of their homes, especially those rooms visited by their guests, such as the dining and withdrawing rooms, had the right 'look'. One guide that was very popular was Charles Eastlake's *Hints on Household Taste*,[89] published in 1868, the year that Richard and Maria were married.[90]

The bride and groom would not have been given a guide for their wedding as presents were generally useful, expensive household items. But it is likely that the new Mrs Grove bought a copy to help set up her home. Republished over the years, it became a standard reference book, with illustrations from Eastlake's own drawings on home interiors. It gave advice on dining tables, chairs, glassware, ceramics and cutlery. It had 12 chapters, starting with Street Architecture (the outside of the house) and

---

[89] Eastlake, Charles, *Hints on Household Taste in Furniture, Upholstery and Other Details* (1869), 2nd edition, Longmans, Green and Co.

[90] Charles Eastlake trained as an architect but moved into furniture design, making functional furniture with simple designs which contrasted with the trend of over-elaboration which had become widespread.

moving on to the Entrance Hall, the Dining Room, the Library, Drawing Room and Bedroom, together with others on wall coverings and floor coverings, and ending with dress and jewellery. Eastlake was critical of other furniture makers and upholsterers, saying that 'it is not sufficient for him to tell us that the dining-room table and sideboard should, on account of the use to which they are put, be made after a more solid fashion than the drawing room table and the cheffonier.[91] He is not content with informing his customers … that bookcases will be required for the library, and flower-stands are suitable for the boudoir; but he proceeds with great gravity to lay down a series of rules by which certain types of form and certain shades of color are to be, for some mysterious reason best known to himself, forever associated with certain apartments in the house.'[92]

Eastlake would have nothing of this.

FURNITURE

No photographs of the interior of Slepe House have survived.

Some furniture would have been bought locally, especially for those rooms not seen by visitors or guests. St Ives had one small shop, run by R. and G. Kiddle, in Bridge Street, which sold a small range of cabinet furniture and upholstery.[93] The shop was used for occasional furniture purchases. In the county town of Huntingdon, five miles away, there was a little more choice with an upholsterer, two cabinet makers and two furniture brokers (second-hand dealers).[94] In Cambridge there were also more shops[95] and on one occasion Reginald went on the train with his mother to Cambridge to help her chose a new rug for the house probably from either Eden Lilley or Robert Sayles which were two popular department stores in the town centre.

Customers who had a more discerning taste for a wider range of goods needed to look further afield. A number of furniture manufacturers became prominent as the century progressed and retailed their products in new, large shops drawing customers from across the country. Among them

---

91 A low cupboard.

92 Eastlake, pp. 64–5.

93 *St Ives Business Register 1885*.

94 J. Harrod's *Directory of Huntingdon* (1877).

95 There were eleven cabinet makers in Cambridge listed in the 1883 *Kelly's Directory of Cambridgeshire*. The main was Walter Stockbridge with an outlet in Sidney Street, near where Reginald was to live when he studied at Cambridge and the other in Green Street.

were Maple and Son Ltd, Heal and Son Ltd and James Shoolbred, all in Tottenham Court Road, London.[96] It was common for retailers to advertise their products far afield. The 1877 *Harrod's Directory for Huntingdonshire* had display advertisements from retailers in Maidenhead, Reading, Norwich and Northampton, with goods ranging from hosiery to pianos, all available for delivery. Blowers and Sons, for example, had a 'General Furnishing' shop in Reading, and advertised cabinet and upholstery goods specifically appealing to 'the Nobility, Clergy, and Gentry'.

Heal's took advantage of Dickens' novels to advertise their wares: *Bleak House* had a full-page advertisement for their bed and bedding products. They produced specific catalogues to market their products, and posted these free to customers,[97] with one in 1858 illustrated with pictures of entire rooms.[98] By 1895, line-drawn illustrations provided not just the items for sale, but also the layout of rooms and even ideas for where pictures could be displayed on walls, as well as the arrangement of tableware.[99] By then, Heal's was part of the Arts and Crafts movement, popularised by William Morris and his circle.[100] By the end of the 19th century it was one of the best-known furniture suppliers in London and shipped goods across the country by rail. Whether the Groves bought any Heal's furniture

---

[96] Of these, only Heal's has survived into the 21st century. I worked for 5 years at Heals at the start of my career when the founder's two great grandsons, Anthony and Christopher Heal were the Chairman and Design Director respectively. Oliver Heal, Anthony's son, was a colleague of mine.

[97] Mail order began in 1861 when a Welsh entrepreneur set up the first dedicated mail order business selling initially Welsh flannel but branching out to other products. By 1880 he had more than 100,000 customers. In the United States, the Montgomery Ward company produced its first mail order catalogue and Sears' first catalogue was launched in 1888. The rest is history.

[98] Adam, Mathew, *Heals Catalogues* 1844–1950. http://www.ampltd.co.uk/digital_guides/heals_catalogues_1844-1950/Publishers-Note.aspx.

[99] Their 1899 catalogue included an article on 'Simplicity of Design' by Gleason White with woodcut illustrations displaying simple, clean lines. White stated that 'Simplicity of design has been said to be the final refuge of the complex' and that 'to be simple in decoration is always in good taste'. By 1900, following the display of one of their rooms at the Paris Exhibition, they were described by a writer in *The Architectural Review* (June 1900) as 'Messrs Heal & Son, the well-known artistic furnishers'.

[100] The Arts and Crafts movement took its name from the Arts and Crafts Exhibition Society, a group founded in London in 1887. This group mounted its first annual exhibition in 1888, showing examples of work it hoped would help raise both the social and intellectual status of crafts including ceramics, textiles, metalwork and furniture. It was preceded by the Pre-Raphaelite Brotherhood (later known as the Pre-Raphaelites). This group of English painters, poets and art critics was founded in 1848.

is not recorded, but the move to the much larger Slepe House would have necessitated buying new furniture and furnishings.

Given the entertaining that was done at the Groves', Reginald's mother would have wanted to make sure that her home reflected her husband's rising standing in the town. Errors of judgement by the mistress of the house could lead to social disaster if, for instance, she chose the wrong interior decoration, even in a country town like St Ives.

In both the dining room as well as the withdrawing room (used after a formal meal had been finished to relax and chat) the furnishings needed to be in the correct style. A mirror over the fireplace, for instance, which was higher than it was wide, was deemed 'refined'. But a mirror width which was less than it was high was considered to be 'common' because it signified a low-ceilinged room. The advice given in the many magazines available for the aspiring middle classes gave clear instructions as to what was acceptable and what was not, much as interior design magazines do today.

The Hall

The entrance to Slepe House from Cromwell Place opened into a large, stone-paved hallway which had an imposing wood-panelled staircase leading to the first floor where the family bedrooms were located. A wrought-iron staircase with a mahogany rail snaked its way to the top of the stairs. The servants lived in small rooms on the upper floor under the sloping eaves of the roof.[101]

The hall and staircase was hung with portraits. One was a striking oil painting of Reginald's grandmother, the beautiful Georgiana Grove, displayed in a handsome gilt frame. It had been painted just after her wedding when she was 20. At her death in 1886, it was given to her eldest son, Dr Grove and then it was passed to his son, Reginald after his death.[102]

Two other portraits that hung in the hall or perhaps in the drawing room were those of Reginald's father and mother.[103] Painted by an unknown artist when they were in their late-forties, the portraits were designed to

---

[101] In some Victorian homes, the servants were not given their own rooms but slept where they worked – the scullery for a maid, the butler's pantry for the butler, and so on. (Flanders p. 2.) There is no evidence that this occurred in the Grove household.

[102] The painting is now in the possession of John Grove, one of his grandsons, and hangs in his house in Denver, Colorado, USA.

[103] These two paintings are now in the possession of Bill Grove, another grandson, and hang in his house in Berkshire.

hang next to each other. They depict a middle-class, middle-aged, well-matched couple.

Another portrait hanging in the hall or perhaps the drawing room was that of 'Master Bunbury'. This charming painting, oil on canvas,[104] was a copy of one executed by the well-known 18th-century painter Joshua Reynolds in 1781, eleven years before his death. The original painting hangs in the Philadelphia Museum of Art.[105] The boy was Reynolds' godson, Henry Edward Bunbury, who was three at the time that his portrait was painted. Reynolds kept the little boy still by telling him fairy stories. Young Bunbury became a distinguished soldier, appointed a Lieutenant General and Knight Commander of the Bath (KCB) in 1815.[106] He was High Sheriff of Suffolk in 1825 and the Member of Parliament for Suffolk from 1830 to 1832. Sir Henry died in 1860 when he was 72.[107] It is quite possible that some of Reginald's Long relatives, farming on the Suffolk border, knew Bunbury personally. Copies of Reynolds' portraits became popular in the Victorian period and this charming portrait of a young boy is a delightful replica. It became treasured by the Grove family and handed down through the generations.[108]

Dining and withdrawing rooms

To the right of the hallway were two large rooms,[109] with two sash windows apiece, facing the large garden. One was the dining room and the other probably a drawing room which, as its name implies, was a room for guests to be entertained after dinner. In large houses there would be a morning

---

[104] Engravings of the portrait were made by Francis Haward (1759–97), an accomplished 18th-century engraver, shortly after the painting was completed, and these became very popular. They were generally 14 x 16ins in size. His mezzotint of 'Master Bunbury' caused a sensation when it was published, and was widely admired for its 'stunning technical skill and dramatic intensity'. (https://www.donaldheald.com/pages/books/7399/francis-after-sir-joshua-reynolds-haward-1759-1797/master-bunbury.) On the reverse of the canvas of the painting is stencilled 'C. Davy, Artists Colourman, 83, Newman Street, Oxford St, London'. There is no date shown. This business was established in the 1790s and was based in Wardour Street, before moving nearby to Newman Street in 1822.

[105] Philadelphia Museum of Art Ref M1928-1-29.

[106] He had the responsibility of informing Napoleon of his sentence of deportation to St Helena in 1815.

[107] https://en.wikipedia.org/wiki/Sir_Henry_Bunbury,_7th_Baronet.

[108] The painting now hangs in my house.

[109] These have now been divided into consulting rooms used by a dental practice.

room which was for the exclusive use of women – where the mistress of the house spoke to the servants, wrote letters and kept her accounts, as well as a place to entertain close friends. However, both Grove houses were probably too small for this type of room. A passage from the hall led to the kitchen, pantry and other rooms used by the servants.

Bedrooms

These were always located upstairs – the family ones on the first floor at Slepe House, and those for servants on the top floor. These servant rooms were much smaller and utilitarian – garret-like under a sloping roof – with a single bed, and perhaps a simple chest of drawers and a chair. Reginald never wrote about what the bedrooms at the Bullock Market or Slepe House were like, but the walls for the family were likely to be covered with pale shades of distemper or light, delicately patterned wallpaper, both of which could be renewed easily.[110] The standard for servants' bedrooms was plain white, distempered walls, and furnished with second-hand furniture and rugs that had been worn bare elsewhere in the house. The children's rooms were painted white, too, which made an annual repaint easier.

The family bedrooms would be furnished with a table, chairs, a small bookcase and a washstand, with the bed likely to be made of cast iron or brass. Interestingly, bedside tables were not used and a chair beside the bed served this purpose. Most clothes were stored in trays and boxes, and hangers were not in general use until the 1900s when they were called 'shoulders'. Clothes were therefore hung from pegs or folded.

The two authors of *An Encyclopædia of Domestic Economy* believed that bedrooms should be 'neat and plain, and everything capable of collecting dust should be avoided as much as possible'.[111] This advice was endorsed by others. It was argued that bedroom furniture should be simple and kept to a minimum so as to be easy to clean, and not to collect dust. Plain, varnished floors for easy cleaning were preferred with a few scattered rugs, and window blinds favoured as being more hygienic than curtains.

Hygiene in bedrooms was a major concern, as babies were born, ill people nursed, and the very young and elderly died in them. Death was always faced at home in this period, which Reginald was well aware of as

[110] Guild, Robin, *The Victorian House Book.*

[111] Webster, Thomas, and Mrs Parkes, *An Encyclopaedia of Domestic Economy* (1884), Longmans, London.

the son of a doctor. But thankfully, during Reginald's boyhood none of his immediate family or any of the servants died in situ at the Bullock Market or Slepe House.

Bathrooms

Bathrooms, as a separate room with plumbed water and a fitted bath, began to be introduced towards the turn of the century; these were often put in dressing rooms but an alternative was building rear extensions, which was probably the case at Slepe House. Meanwhile, hip baths were used in bedrooms. These were made out of thin metal and supported on wooden cradles which were sometimes panelled. This was what was used by the Grove household at the Bullock Market. Hot water was brought up from the kitchen by the maid and then emptied out after use. Free-standing cast-iron bathtubs were not introduced until the 1880s and may well have been installed at Slepe House after the Groves moved in.

The classic reference book for the aspiring middle class, first published in German and called *Das Englische Haus*, was written by Hermann Muthesius in 1904, and described 'a well-equipped bathroom will contain a bath, shower bath, washbasin, hip bath, bidet, heated towel rail, mirror, clothes hooks, a shelf for towels, and a receptacle for used towels'. This development came after Reginald's wife, Hilda, went to live at Slepe House in 1897.

Kitchen

In some respects, the kitchen in a Victorian home was the most important room, as the impact on guests invited to dine was determined by the quality of the meal cooked and served. An effective and efficient kitchen was also essential in ensuring that the daily routine of a large household ran smoothly. A description of the kitchen of a provincial lower-middle-class home in the 1860s, given by the novelist Arnold Bennett in *The Old Wives' Tale*, illustrated what the newly married Mrs Grove might have found when she set up home: 'Forget-me-nots on a brown field ornamented the walls of the kitchen. Its ceiling was irregular and grimy, and a beam ran across it … A large range stood out from the wall between the stairs and the window.'

By the time the Grove household moved to Slepe House, cooking in the kitchen was carried out on a 'kitchener' [sic] range made of heavy, cast-iron plates with a single coal-burning firebox. The standard one was

12 inches deep and had a single oven on one side and a water boiler on the other. The base of the box had spaced iron bars so that the cinders and ash could fall into the tray below. Emptying this tray was a daily routine for the cook, having raked out the ashes from the night before and using black lead to burnish the whole range. This was a regular job, but a filthy and dangerous, one as black lead was highly poisonous but this was not known then. On the top was an iron cooking surface heated from the firebox. Flues would draw the gases and smoke from the fire up the chimney. The coal fire was used to boil hot water, as well as for cooking on the top and in the ovens.

The 1851 Great Exhibition held in Hyde Park enabled gas cookers to be showcased and sold in increasing numbers. But it was only towards the end of the century that gas came to be used in kitchen ranges in middle-class homes. By 1900, it has been estimated that 25% of urban households had a gas cooker.[112] Gas allowed a constant supply of energy as well as easy control of cooking temperatures, which enabled the number of dishes available to be extended; the popularity of the now traditional Sunday roast can be traced back to the innovation of the gas cooker. Reginald never mentioned how meals were cooked but it is probable that this type of cooker was not in use at Slepe House until the 1890s.

Bennett went on to say in his novel that

> The rest of the furniture comprised a table – against the wall opposite the range – a cupboard, and two Windsor chairs. Opposite the foot of the steps was a doorway, without a door, leading to two larders, dimmer even than the kitchen, vague retreats made visible by whitewash, where bowls of milk, dishes of cold bones, and remainders of fruit-pies, reposed on stillages;[113] the corner nearest the kitchen was a great steen[114] in which bread was kept.[115]

Victorian domestic cooking technology lagged behind that used in industry, but early food processors were in existence by the 1850s and other gadgets like apple corers, cherry pippers and knife polishers gradually came into use towards the end of the 19th century.

---

[112] Spours, Judy, *Cakes and Ale* (2006), National Archives, p. 144.

[113] A frame to keep an item off the ground or on a shelf.

[114] A large stone jar with a heavy lid.

[115] Bennett, Arnold, *The Old Wives' Tale* (1911), Chapman and Hall, Chapter 11.

Lavatories

While the 1848 Public Health Act made it obligatory for every household to have a fixed sanitary arrangement of some kind, it is unlikely that there were indoor toilets at either the Bullock Market or Slepe House. Few houses at this time had indoor facilities, so using the chamber pot at night was a universal alternative to tiptoeing to the outside privy with only a flickering candle to show the way.

Chamber pots were emptied in the outdoor privy but, to save many trips, slop buckets were used (with a lid to prevent the contents splashing out during transit). In her instructions on household management published in 1861,[116] Mrs Beeton advocated that housemaids should empty the chamber pots and jugs and basins daily, after breakfast had been served and the bedroom windows thrown open wide for fresh air. Having emptied the slops, her advice was that the pots should be cleaned by 'leaving a little scalding-hot water for a minute in vessels that require it; adding a drop of turpentine to the water, when that is not sufficient to cleanse them'.[117] Once the jugs and bowls had been emptied, rinsed and dried, the slop-pail was carried to the privy.

Florence Nightingale was keen to have pots individually removed and washed outside in the privy so that the faeces of a sick person were not brought into the bedrooms of others.[118] Chamber pots needed to be kept under the bed or a chair for easy location in the dark, but also to avoid unpleasant spillage accidents occurring. At a Coroner's inquest held in East Suffolk in 1891, it was found that a 60-year-old single woman called Ann Betts had fallen out of her bed onto an already broken chamber pot which caused a serious wound to her leg. Tragically, she bled to death alone.[119]

During the day the household would use the earth privy or closet. At no. 33 the Bullock Market it was located in an outhouse. Effectively it was

---

[116] Beeton's *Book of Household Management* was published in 1861 and became a bestseller in succeeding years. Section 2345 deals with the duties of the housemaid in the bedroom after breakfast described above. The first edition of the book did not use the title 'Mrs Beeton'.

[117] Beeton, Isabella, *The Book of Household Management* (1861) ISO-8859-1 www.gutenberg.net.

[118] In her *Notes on Nursing* published in 1859, Florence Nightingale wrote: 'The use of any chamber utensil without a lid should be utterly abolished, whether among sick or well. You can easily convince yourself of the necessity of this absolute rule, by taking one with a lid, and examining the under-side of that lid. It will be found always covered, whenever the utensil is not empty, by condensed offensive moisture. Where does that go, when there is no lid?' (p. 211.)

[119] Suffolk Record Office, Ipswich (SROi) EC5/34/13 Inquisition at the parish of Tuddenham on the body of Ann Betts, 22 July 1891.

merely a hole in the ground over which was a wooden seat. Whitewashed walls inside gave the appearance of hygiene, and the maids scrubbed the seat and floor daily. The ash from the grates was poured into it to act as an absorbent. The privy contents needed removing once in a while by specialists,[120] and often these were sold on and used to fertilise fields. The danger to public health became better known as medical science improved (see Volume 3). Cut-up newspaper was commonly used as toilet paper, threaded onto some string and hung up by the seat. Manufactured paper became widely used in middle-class households like the Groves' towards the 1880s.[121] The idea of special paper impregnated with a germ-killing agent – in other words, medicated paper – caught on. Dr Grove's knowledge as the Medical Officer of Health of the dangers of diseases carried by faeces meant that he would have seen the merits of using a medicated toilet paper.

With the advent of piped water, flush toilets began to be manufactured to replace the earth privy. The commonest was a funnel running or dropping into a sewer, but this resulted in a foul stench, especially in summer. A major incentive to the installation of flushing lavatories came as a result of Prince Albert's death from typhoid in 1861. Crapper and Humpherson were two major companies which manufactured these, and with the invention of the U-bend, preventing any smell coming up, the free-standing ceramic unit, called the water closet, became popular. Lavatories and bathrooms eventually became beautifully decorated with ornate tiles, but this innovation only became commonplace after Reginald became an adult.

Keeping clean and healthy

Before the mid-19th century water for the home was pumped up from wells; if one was located outside in the stable yard, then this saved a journey to the nearest common pump to collect pails of water. By the 1850s, before Dr Grove settled in St Ives, water began to be piped into middle-class homes. Besides making cooking and cleaning easier, it enabled purpose-built bathrooms to be built serviced by running water by the end of the century

[120] A long-handled shovel was used to remove the excrement into buckets which were taken away by the 'jakesman' in a cart for ultimate disposal. This practice was common until flush toilets and sewers replaced the earth closet.

[121] The British Perforated Paper Company began manufacturing medicated toilet paper in 1880. The paper was hard and shiny; the Bronco brand was later advertised using the slogan: 'Bronco, for the bigger wipe.' Another well-known brand, Izal continued production until 1981.

Until bathrooms were installed, washing for family and servants was carried out in bedrooms using a jug, water, soap and a towel. Soap, made with animal fats and caustic soda, was expensive but became more widely used as the century progressed. With industrialisation the price became cheaper and fresh water was brought daily up for the family by the general maid. The other servants would carry their own. The maid's job was also to remove the basin with its dirty water afterwards. Dr and Mrs Grove probably had hot water brought to them, but their children would have made do with cold water.

Frequent air changes were seen to be important for good sleep. Windows were often left open at home and at school throughout the year, and chimneys kept open when not being used, so the rooms did not become stuffy. There was a generally accepted view that it was preferable on health grounds to allow cool air to circulate.[122]

Bedlinen was changed weekly, but the top sheet moved to the bottom and the bottom sheet then taken for washing; the expression 'top to the bottom and bottom to the wash' summed up this approach and it continued to be used into the mid-20th century, especially at boarding schools.[123]

Keeping warm

Life in a middle-class home was comfortable compared to the working classes, but by today's standards it was spartan, with very little heating provided which was why many layers of thick clothing were worn. While the rooms on the ground floor had open fireplaces with a grate, as did the family bedrooms, fires were rarely lit upstairs unless the weather was very

[122] Dr Neil Arnott who died in 1874 was a Scottish scientist, and a member of the Royal Institution. Besides inventing a water bed and a smokeless grate, he was a well-known proponent of the health benefits of fresh air in homes. He believed that fresh air was one of four conditions leading to good health and a long life. The others were ' temperature, aliment, and exercise of the mind and of the body'. If an individual had access to all four of these items, while avoiding violence and poisons (items that Arnott believed caused disease and therefore were to be avoided), then the person would have no issues when it came to health throughout their life and would be able to live for as long as the body permitted.' By surrounding oneself with the four essential items, the human bodily makeup would slowly become modified by kindred circumstances not deemed diseases but called temperaments and varieties, compatible with health and long life.' https://en.wikipedia.org/wiki/Neil_Arnott

[123] I can attest to this being the case at King's Choir School and Uppingham School in the 1960s.

cold. It is unlikely that the servants' bedrooms had fireplaces at all

Thomas Carlyle's[124] wife, Jane, lived in a fashionable townhouse in London, but fires were only lit in bedrooms if someone was ill. While staying with a wealthy friend a fire was lit for her in her bedroom and she described this as 'a wanton luxury'.[125] Similarly, at both Reginald's boarding schools there was no heating in the dormitories apart from one small fireplace which was only used if the weather was very cold. When a fire was needed, it was the servants who carried out the task of lighting it. Remarkably Reginald never knew how it was done. Just before he went back to school after his 18th birthday he tried unsuccessfully to light his bedroom fire after he came home late one evening. He had to get the help of one of the servants, embarrassingly, as he could not master the art!

Hot water

Getting hot water for baths was solved when the geyser began to be manufactured from 1869 onwards, but a fixed bath and separate bathroom were needed; this was not possible in the Bullock Market as it was too small. When a geyser was installed at Slepe House is not known, but the gas-fired mechanism needed a huge machine which dominated the bathroom, if there was sufficient space. There were two dangers. Firstly, of asphyxiation, and secondly of being scalded as the water came out boiling hot. The dangers were demonstrated when Reginald's younger brother, Tom, burnt himself by pouring boiling water over his leg in March 1887 and 'scalded himself badly'. While this probably happened in the kitchen, rather than the bathroom, it illustrates the risk of this kind of accident at home.

Circulating hot-water systems were in their infancy until the late-1890s when they were introduced by the wealthy. The boiler was put at the back of the kitchen range which was used to send water through cast-iron pipes round the house. These tended to corrode, were liable to fracture, and turned the water red.[126]

124 His comments about St Ives when visiting the town in the early 1840s are noted in an earlier chapter.

125 Cited by Ruth Goodman, *How To Be a Victorian*, p. 5.

126 Marshall and Willox, *The Victorian House*, Sidgwick & Jackson (1986), pp. 77–78, 83–86.

Lighting

The mid-19th century saw the production of gas as a fuel, initially to light streets[127] but later to light homes, and much later to fuel stoves.[128] Gas was produced from coal being heated up, stored in local gasworks and then piped under existing roads. Its popularity grew after it was installed at Buckingham Palace in 1837, then at the Houses of Parliament in 1852. By the 1860s there were c.1000 gasworks[129] across the country, including one at Uppingham set up in 1839. The gasworks at St Ives were built in 1855 on the London Road.[130] In a directory of 1862, it was stated that in St Ives 'the streets are well paved and lighted [sic] with gas'[131]. The brighter lighting which gas provided allowed people to read more easily in their homes and for longer into the evening. There is no record of when gas was installed at the Bullock Market or Slepe House for lighting purposes but it is likely that after the Groves moved to Slepe House, it would have been installed. However, generally, gas fittings were only put into the ground-floor rooms rather than the bedrooms, due to the cost.

These were the houses in which Reginald lived as a boy.

---

[127] There are still 1,500 gas street lights in use in London today.

[128] By the 1860s gas lighting was to be found all over Britain and about a thousand gasworks had sprung up to meet the demand for the new fuel. The brighter lighting which gas provided allowed people to read more easily and for longer. There is no record of when gas was installed at Slepe House for lighting purposes.

[129] The Fakenham Museum of Gas and Local History in Fakenham, Norfolk, is the only surviving town gasworks in England and Wales. It displays the equipment used for the manufacture of gas from coal: retorts, condenser, purifiers, meter and gasholder. It is situated in the town's former gasworks, set up in 1846 which stopped production in 1965 after the discovery of natural gas in the North Sea

[130] Craven & Co's *Directory of Huntingdonshire* 1855 lists the gasworks in Fenstanton with Ulph and Browns as proprietors and Latchfield Joseph as manager.

[131] Cassey, Edward, *History, Topography, and Directory of Huntingdonshire* (1862), p. 290.

CHAPTER 3

Home, a Place of Peace

'This is the true nature of home – it is a place of Peace; the shelter, not only from injury, but from all terror, doubt and division. In so far as it is not this, it is not home.'[132]

John Ruskin

A PLACE OF PEACE

As depicted in many Victorian novels, especially those written by Dickens, home in middle-class households is shown as a special place of comfort and refuge. A cursory look at the titles of magazines aimed at middle-class female readers from the mid-19th century onwards points to the centrality of the home in Victorian life: *The Home Circle, The Home Companion, The Home Friend, Home Thoughts, Home Magazine, Family Record* and *Family Paper*, to name but a few.[133] Traditionally, it was where the husband, working hard in commerce, manufacturing, banking or increasingly in a profession, came home in the evening to his wife and family. She was the mistress of the household and had responsibility for the management of servants and children. There was a hierarchy which was clearly understood and accepted. As head of the household, authority for the family was given by God to the husband, and authority was then delegated by him to his wife for the upbringing of children and the management of domestic servants.

This principle of 'headship' was based on Scriptural teaching, particularly from the Apostle Paul's teaching to the Christians in Ephesus. Overall, this teaching emphasised submission by the individual. This was a universal principle and applied to everyone 'out of reverence to Christ'. Then within the home, husbands should love their wives sacrificially, as 'Christ loved the Church', and wives should submit to their husbands, 'as to the Lord', with children obeying their parents 'in the Lord'. Within the household, servants should obey their earthly masters with respect as

---

[132] Ruskin, John, *Sesame and Lilies* (1897), pp. 108–09.

[133] Flanders, Judith, *The Victorian House,* p. xx.

they would Christ.[134] In a popular book for women written by Marianne Farningham in 1889, at which many today would bridle, readers were advised that 'the most important person in the household is the head of the family – the father...though he may, perhaps, spend less time at home than any other member of the family – though he has scarcely a voice in family affairs – though the whole household machinery seems to go on without the assistance of his management – still it does depend entirely on that active brain and those busy hands'.[135]

In her study of the Victorian home Jenni Calder wrote that it was 'an environment maintained by women and controlled by men'.[136] The well-known Victorian philosopher, social thinker and philanthropist, John Ruskin, made his comments quoted at the beginning of this chapter three years before Reginald's father and mother got married. He saw women, as others did, presiding over the home as 'a place of peace' where the outside world was excluded. There is nothing to suggest that the home that Reginald grew up in at the Bullock Market and Slepe House was anything other than this.

For the Groves, of course, the world did intrude into their home, as patients visited Dr Grove for consultations and he was at their beck and call for night or weekend emergencies. But the essence of the home being a place of refuge and peace was at the heart of the Grove household. In his diaries Reginald depicted a loving, happy, and secure family environment. In short, a place of peace.

It is clear that Reginald enjoyed returning home at the end of each term and it was not because he disliked school. Home meant much to him and his siblings. It was a loving and hospitable place full of warmth, family fun and a vibrant social life as uncles, aunts and cousins regularly stayed for short periods.

As the children grew up, their dog, Charlie, was very much part of their lives, arriving as a puppy when Reginald was six or seven. As a farmer's daughter, his mother grew up with dogs kept in outside kennels and used for guard duty and ratting. Charlie's role in the stables was similar. And when the anxious relatives of a sick patient knocked on the door at Slepe

---

[134] Ephesians 5:21–25 and 33, and 6:1–5.

[135] Farningham, Marianne, *Home Life* (1889), pp. 10ff, cited by Flanders, Judith, *The Victorian House,* p. xxx.

[136] Calder, Jenni, *The Victorian Home* (1997), p. 9.

House in the middle of the night asking for Dr Grove for an emergency house call, Charlie's barking alerted the sleeping household quickly. No doubt Dr Grove also took him for company and protection in the horse and trap as he travelled along the pitch-black country lanes to see the patient.

Charlie died at a great age when Reginald was 18 and away at school. He had had a long life, and Reginald was pragmatic about his death: 'Had a letter from the Mater – Charlie is dead. Perhaps it was a mercy as the poor dog had been stone deaf for some time and literally, as well as in other respects, led a "dog's life".' Reginald's three brothers were all at school too when this happened, as was their 16-year-old sister, and many tears for faithful Charlie were shed. The large garden beside Slepe House was an obvious place for Charlie to be laid to rest.

A GROWING FAMILY AND HOUSEHOLD

Only a few years after Reginald's birth, there were seven living in their home in the Bullock Market in April 1871 at the time of the National Census. Besides Dr and Mrs Grove, Reginald and his brother Ernest, there was a general maid, 23-year-old Catherine Wilkinson, a nursemaid, Jane Bedford, aged 20, and William Brown, a 45-year-old groom.[137] Catherine was employed to help Mrs Grove clean the house and probably carry out some cooking. As Mrs Grove was four months pregnant with her third child, Mabel, Jane was needed to care for Reginald and Ernest. As groom, William, looked after the horse and trap stabled at the back of the building. The groom's role was essential in caring for the two or three horses needed for Dr Grove to visit his patients.

All the servants lived in and were born locally: Catherine in St Ives, Jane in the village of Warboys, and William in Newmarket, home of horse racing and rather appropriate for a groom. Horses were in his blood!

As the number of patients in the practice grew in the 1870s someone was needed to assist Reginald's father as a medical assistant. He employed a succession of these young men who were all newly qualified and needing practical training. The first that Reginald noted in his diary was Dr Bernard Guillemard, aged 26, who was appointed in 1881. By living in with the family he could take some of the night calls when an emergency arose. As living space was at a premium now, the groom did not live in.

[137] 1871 National Census.

The other occupants in 1881 were Lucy Mayhew, aged 21, employed as an under-governess with responsibility for the younger children; Maria Prior, aged 24, employed as a housemaid; and Annie King, aged 23, who was the cook. The Bullock Market could just about accommodate ten people, with the children now aged seven to 12; but with the children beginning to need their own rooms a move to a larger house became necessary.

Ten years on, at the next Census, when Reginald was carrying out his medical training in London, only Mabel, aged 19, and Richard, aged 16, were still living at home. The family now employed two live-in servants – Annie Barnham, aged 23, who was the cook as well as carrying out domestic duties, and Jemima Mansfield aged 24, who was the housemaid. There were two other residents who were brothers and listed in the National Census as 'boarders, Edward Sandys, aged 15, and Charles aged 12'.[138] They may have been attending the grammar school on the Ramsey Road; if so, they provided extra income for the Grove family when the older sons were away studying.

THE GROVE HOUSEHOLD

As mentioned earlier, a Victorian wife managed the running of the household and the domestic staff. Reginald's mother learnt the skills needed from her own mother who employed domestic staff, too in helping run the farm with her husband.

SERVANTS

Domestic servants were an integral part of a middle-class Victorian household. As more children arrived, the number of domestic servants increased. The duties of servants were described by Mrs Beeton in her *Book of Household Management*.[139] Mrs Beeton estimated that if a family's income was above £500 per annum, this was enough to employ a cook, housemaid and children's nurse. In country practices in East Anglia a good income was considered to be £600 pa (£76,000) at the turn of the century.[140] Dr Grove's gross income was probably more, but his running expenses, including employing a medical assistant, meant that his profit from the practice was much less. Mrs Beeton gave a range of salaries for

---

[138] 1891 National Census.

[139] Beeton, ibid.

[140] Reader, W. J., *Professional Men* (Weidenfeld & Nicolson, 1966), p. 192.

different posts for guidance, depending on the size of the household and whether the household was in London, another metropolitan city or the country. A cook might be paid £11–30 pa, a general maid £9–14,[141] a nursemaid, £9–14, and a groom £15–30, with rates of pay in rural areas like St Ives being at the bottom end of the range. Living expenses also had to be taken into account.

The work of domestic servants was hard, with long hours and little time off. They got up early in the morning, probably around 6.00 in the summer, and perhaps half an hour later in the winter. Grates were cleaned out, fires lit in the kitchen and dining room, and breakfast prepared. Often Reginald's father or his medical assistant would have been up during part of the night to visit a patient on an emergency call. The whole household was generally woken up, too, if this was the case, by the knocking at the front door. But on a normal day during the school holidays Reginald got up at about 7.30 and washed in cold water using a basin and jug in his bedroom. A quick wash kept him clean, although standing in a cold bedroom in a nightshirt would have been bracing at best.

Keeping the house clean was a high priority but was difficult with the smut from coal fires, dust from open windows and dirt brought in from outside. Lighting by oil was still used in parts of the home and heating by coal fires made the interior dirty. With poor street cleaning and the livestock market on their front doorstep, a great deal of dirt came into the house at number 33. At Slepe House, livestock were not penned in the street outside, but as the road in front of the entrance led to the new market, considerable dung was deposited along the route.

The groom's role

The most important and most highly paid servant in the household was the groom. Dr Grove's patients were scattered over an eight-mile radius outside St Ives itself and the better-off expected him to visit them at home. Horse transport was vital for Reginald's father to visit patients and the upkeep and care of his horses was essential. When a new horse was acquired it merited a diary entry by Reginald in January 1887: 'if it is as good as it looks, it will do for the Pater splendidly'.

It was generally considered that the maximum distance which a horse could be ridden was about 15 miles in a day, but the usual was perhaps six

[141] Reader, W. J., *Professional Men* (Weidenfeld & Nicolson, 1966), p. 192.

miles. Depending on the road conditions (all roads outside St Ives were unpaved), a horse and trap or a brougham generally travelled at 7–8 miles per hour.

The groom was responsible for the three or more horses stabled, as well as occasionally driving the doctor on his rounds. The preferred vehicle for doctors was a brougham (pronounced 'broom'),[142] because it had a canvas cover for wet or cold weather. A local carriage builder was Wood and Sons which moved from Hemingford Grey to new premises in Station Road, St Ives, after the railway came to the town. Dr Grove probably bought his carriages from them. As Dr Grove always visited patients dressed in a morning coat and top hat, the conventional dress for his profession, getting soaked to the skin in an open trap was to be avoided! Keeping the brougham and trap in working order added to the groom's workload. As Reginald grew older, during his school holidays, he went out on these house visits with his father, or sometimes with the medical assistant; Reginald often drove himself, but he probably drove only the trap rather than the larger brougham.

There was probably a young lad, who lived in the town, who helped the groom as the stable boy. William Brown was the groom listed in the 1871 National Census living with the Groves in the Bullock Market. Only the names of two other grooms, who worked for Reginald's father, over the years, are known. Sadly, one of them, a Mr Paine, died in mysterious circumstances some time after his employment ended, as described in Chapter 9.

The groom needed to have an excellent general knowledge of horses and had to make sure that they were regularly fed, groomed and cared for, as well as watching out for symptoms which need treatment. For minor problems, the groom was responsible for applying simple remedies. He usually had the job of buying the feed stuff, too, which included oats and hay.

Cleaning the horse's tack, clearing out the stables, putting out fresh hay in the feeder, giving a morning feed of oats, removing the dung, and laying new straw were all tasks for the early morning. Those horses not taken out by Dr Grove needed at least two hours' exercise each day carried by the groom. For 'saddle-horses' he would walk, trot or perhaps take them for

---

[142] The *brougham* was a light, four-wheeled, horse-drawn carriage named after Lord Brougham, who had this type of carriage built to his specification.

a canter up the Ramsey Road and beyond. Once back at the stables, the horses often needed to be washed down and given a drink. As the property in the Bullock Market led down to the river, the groom took them to the water's edge when the river was not in flood. The riverbank was not built up at this time and was a gentle incline into the water, like The Waits nearby. At Slepe House, Darwoods Pond at the end of the stables came in handy for the horses to be washed and have a drink after being out.

Ensuring the horses were well shod was another responsibility, with the blacksmith generally coming to the stables. Once reshod, it was good practice for the new shoes to be worn in by undertaking only short journeys. Henry Standen was the local farrier or 'shoeing smith', as he called himself, whose forge was in West Street a stone's throw away from the Bullock Market.[143] Standen's son, Samuel was running the family business before the First World War at the same address, and called himself a 'blacksmith'. Others who plied this trade were William Clack, whose forge was in Carlisle Terrace, and William Taylor in Globe Place.[144] New saddles and harnesses were bought from Marsh Reuben, the saddle maker, whose workshop was in Crown Street, a hundred yards away from the Groves' first home.

In the years before Reginald's father died, the groom was an old man called Baker. 'He loved the horses and would not give them up', Reginald remembered.

> He was never too tired to be out with or looking after them; he might have been up all night but everything woud be washed up and spick and span first thing in the morning and I never saw him out of temper.[145]

The cook's role

In 1871 the Groves did not employ a cook. As the daughter of a farmer, Reginald's mother knew how to cook, but as her family grew larger and entertaining the socially elite in St Ives became more important, employing a cook became essential. In homes which only employed a cook and general maid, Mrs Beeton said that 'the general custom is, that the cook should have the charge of the dining-room. The hall, the lamps and the doorstep are also committed to her care, and any other work there may be on the

---

[143] J. Harrod's *Directory of Huntingdon* (1877).

[144] *St Ives Business Directory 1885.*

[145] Ibid, footnote 12.

outside of the house.' By 1881 a cook was employed, but given her age and lack of experience it is more likely that Mrs Grove had oversight of the dining room and the cook kept to the kitchen.

Mrs Beeton recommended an early start for the cook as an hour lost in the morning,

> will keep her toiling, absolutely toiling, all day, to overtake that which might otherwise have been achieved with ease. Her first job was to make the dough rolls for breakfast at 8.00am and then, after having lighted the kitchen fire, carefully brushed the range, and cleaned the hearth, proceed to prepare for breakfast. She will thoroughly rinse the kettle, and, filling it with fresh water, will put it on the fire to boil. She will then go to the breakfast-room, or parlour, and there make all things ready for the breakfast of the family.

Then, Mrs Beeton continued,

> her attention will next be directed to the hall, which she will sweep and wipe; the kitchen stairs, if there be any, will now be swept; and the hall mats, which have been removed and shaken, will be again put in their places. The cleaning of the kitchen, pantry, passages, and kitchen stairs must always be over before breakfast, so that it may not interfere with the other business of the day. Everything should be ready, and the whole house should wear a comfortable aspect when the heads of the house and members of the family make their appearance.[146]

Breakfast for adults could be quite substantial in a middle-class home – cold game pie, devilled kidneys, ham, steaks, eggs, a variety of bread and rolls, but Reginald left no record of what was served. However, there is some evidence that in middle-class homes at this time breakfast was quite spartan for younger children. Gwen Raverat said that as a child she only ate porridge, toast and butter with jam spread thinly twice a week – a real treat! But with jam, out went the butter – 'Butter and jam on the same bit of bread would have been an unheard of indulgence, a disgraceful orgy'.[147] By the end of the century Kellogg's introduced cornflakes and breakfast habits began to change.[148]

---

[146] Beeton, ibid.

[147] Raverat, chapter 2.

[148] Calder, Jenni, *The Victorian Home* (B. T. Batsford, 1997), p. 40.

Dr and Mrs Grove with the older children, when home for the school holidays, would have breakfast together, summoning the cook to the parlour by using the bell system in common use by then to 'bring in' the breakfast. As Mrs Beeton said,

> it is the cook's department, generally, in the smaller establishments, to wait at breakfast, as the housemaid, by this time, has gone up-stairs into the bedrooms, and has there applied herself to her various duties. The cook usually answers the bells and single knocks at the door in the early part of the morning, as the tradesmen, with whom it is her more special business to speak, call at these hours.[149]

However, in the Grove household it is likely that the housemaid in her uniform of a white pinafore, white lace headpiece and long dark dress, answered the door, rather than the cook, to give a more professional impression to patients.

Preparation for dinner would then occupy the Cook's attention, whether it was fish, poultry, meat joints or vegetables. Unless guests were staying or being invited for dinner, the evening meal was not an elaborate one. Under Mrs Grove's direction, the cook would prepare pastry, soups, gravies, ragouts and so on. And when

> the dinner hour has arrived, it is the duty of the cook to dish up such dishes as may, without injury, stand, for some time, covered on the hot plate or in the hot closet; but such as are of a more important or recherché kind, must be delayed until the order 'to serve' is given from the drawing-room. Then comes haste; but there must be no hurry,–all must work with order. The cook takes charge of the fish, soups, and poultry; and the kitchen-maid of the vegetables, sauces, and gravies.
>
> Everything must be timed so as to prevent its getting cold, whilst great care should be taken, that, between the first and second courses, no more time is allowed to elapse than is necessary, for fear that the company in the dining-room lose all relish for what has yet to come of the dinner. When the dinner has been served, the most important feature in the daily life of the cook is at an end. She must, however, now begin to look to the contents of her larder, taking care to keep everything sweet and clean, so that no disagreeable smells may arise from the gravies, milk, or meat that may be there.[150]

---

[149] Beeton, ibid.

[150] Beeton, ibid.

The housemaid's role

24-year-old Maria Prior was the Groves' housemaid in 1881, having replaced Catherine Wilkinson who had been listed in the Census ten years before. Like the cook, the maid lived in and got up early at 6.00 in the summer and by 7.00 at the latest in the winter to start work. She had a variety of cleaning and other jobs in the house like making fires, carrying coal to fireplaces, washing, cleaning grates, lavatories, silver and brass, and bed-making. The work was hard, involved carrying heavy loads (like coal to fireplaces or hot water for baths) or mangling wet cloths. The hours were long, perhaps 12 hours a day, with Sunday as a day off. Heavy horsehair mattresses had to be turned before beds were made. Washday each Monday might well be a longer day as it required getting up earlier to make the fire and heat the water.

Her first job was to open the shutters of all the rooms on the ground floor, take up the rugs and sweep the breakfast room. The fireplace had to be cleaned out, the ashes removed and put into a cinder pail and taken outside for use in the outdoor privy. The grate then had to be black-leaded and then the fire was relaid. It was a dirty job, carried out on the maid's knees.[151] Once this had been done, and in winter, the fire lit, the maid every morning cleaned the stone steps at the entrance of the house, the halls, the passages, and the stairs which led to the kitchen. Her general duties, besides these, were to wash and scour all these places twice a week, with the tables, shelves and cupboards

Dusting was the next duty, and polishing the furniture in the downstairs rooms. In winter she would go upstairs, and bring hot water for the jugs in Dr and Mrs Grove's bedroom. In summer she would open the windows of those bedrooms not in use to let in fresh air. After the couple had got up, she would go in later to make the bed. This was a full bed remake, with the bedclothes placed over a horse or the backs of chairs, and the mattress aired. The bed was then remade carefully. The bedrooms were also swept and dusted. Mrs Beeton stressed that it

> is not enough, however, in cleaning furniture, just to pass lightly over the surface; the rims and legs of tables, and the backs and legs of chairs and sofas, should be rubbed vigorously daily; if there is a book-case, every

[151] The term 'housemaid's knee used by the medical profession to describe the painful inflammation of the knee (prepatellar bursitis) which often occurred was aptly chosen.

> corner of every pane and ledge requires to be carefully wiped, so that not a speck of dust can be found in the room.[152]

And so, the day carried on, with more cleaning throughout the house, including Dr Grove's consulting room when he was out on his patient rounds. In the evening the housemaid was expected to help in the kitchen by 'washing up the dinner-things, the plates, plated articles, and glasses, restoring everything to its place; cleaning up her pantry, and putting away everything for use when next required'.

Each year, the whole house was cleaned top to bottom after the end of winter. During his last Easter school holiday in 1887, Reginald described a spring clean at Slepe House which caused quite a disruption. Arriving back from a shopping day in Cambridge accompanying his mother, they found 'the house was crammed full of painters, sweeps etc, spring cleaning'. The next day he complained that 'the house was turned quite upside down with painters'. He left for school the following day so it is not clear how long the spring clean took. Generally, in April or early May all the domestic staff would throw open every window on a fine, warm spring day, air each room, take the rugs outside to be beaten, dust everywhere, clean down the walls and paint the woodwork. As coal fires threw out a massive amount of dust, this activity was needed each year until the advent of central heating. Smut and flakes of soot which floated in the air of most homes (called 'blacks') were a continual nuisance, requiring furniture and fabrics to be cleaned.[153]

The increasing use of gas, and later electricity[154] as the century came to a close, reduced the amount of dirt, but the annual spring clean continued. Cleaning was all done by hand until the 1900s when some mechanical aids began to be used – carpet sweepers, for instance. Reginald did not say when these began to be used at Slepe House.

The nursemaid's role

In well-off households these maids usually came from a slightly 'better' background than the rest of the servants. With the Grove family, the

---

152 Beeton, ibid.

153 Ralph Waldo Emerson, the American writer, was told when he visited England that no one wore white because it was impossible to keep it clean. (Flanders, Judith, *The Victorian House*, p. xl.)

154 The first electric lights used in domestic premises were at Cragside, Northumberland, the majestic home of the industrialist William Armstrong in 1880.

nursemaid was a reliable, local, young girl, perhaps from a farming background like Maria's. The only one that we know about is Jane Bedford, aged 20 at the 1871 Census. She came from the village of Warboys which was seven miles away to the north of St Ives. Besides looking after the children and keeping them clean, she was also responsible for mending the children's clothes, ironing and keeping the nursery clean.

A nursemaid had charge of the children as soon as they had been weaned until they were four or five years old. Boys stopped being dressed as girls at this point and were 'breeched' or put into young adult clothes. Due to the high child mortality of the period, this was an important event. From then on, the children would spend time in the mornings with a governess or start at a local school.

The under-governess's role

The need for a nursemaid ended as Maria Grove's child grew older and the Groves employed a young girl called Lucy Mayhew, aged 21, in 1881 as an under-governess instead. The distinction between a servant, such as a maid and a governess, or even an under-governess, like Lucy, was great. Gwen Raverat recalled that 'the gulf between a servant and a governess was then unbridgeable; it was as if a shrimp had tried to turn into a tiger'.[155]

Reginald's parents wanted all their children, including their daughter Mabel, to be educated privately. From Reginald's diary it is clear that two of his brothers went to boarding school when they were seven or eight, and his sister Mabel when she was 16.

Before boarding school, the boys received basic education from the under-governess, and when time permitted, their mother. Lucy's role in 1881 in looking after the boys probably came to an end after a couple of years as they would have gone to a local day school in the town before being sent to boarding school. There were a number of private schools to choose from in St Ives. For instance, Harrold Winter ran a 'school for gentlemen' at Burleigh House[156] across the road from the Groves in the Bullock Market.[157] A Mr Honeybourne, already mentioned, ran a 'grammar' school in Cromwell Place which later moved to Manchester House. Although

[155] Raverat, chapter 4.

[156] Burleigh House is now a Grade II listed building; formerly it was called Blue Gate House and was built in the early 18th century.

[157] J. Harrod's *Directory of Huntingdon* (1877).

it was called a grammar school, it was not an endowed one, founded as Uppingham had been in the 16th century, but was a private, fee-paying school. Before this, a Mr J. S. Bruce was the Principal of the Commercial & Collegiate School at Manchester House which, as its name suggests, catered for older pupils. By 1881 Honeybourne had moved to Manchester House, and Bruce's school had either moved or closed down.

It is possible that Lucy might have been kept on to teach Mabel who was 10 in 1881 until she went to boarding school six years later in Kensington. Or she, too, might have gone to a local private school before that; besides the ladies' school at Slepe Hall mentioned in the last chapter, there was a School for Young Ladies in Church Street, run by Mrs Hannah Patrick, and another ladies' school at Lime Tree House, whose headmistress was Mrs Mary Sparks.[158]

Such was the household, upstairs and downstairs, in which Reginald grew up.

[158] 1885 *St Ives Business Directory.*

CHAPTER 4

Society and Leisure

'In such a place as St Ives any man should use to the uttermost every opportunity he may have to strengthen the social life and spirit...'[159]

Revd Luke Paget, Vicar of All Saints Parish Church, St Ives, 1886–87

A QUESTION OF CLASS

The 19th century saw the rise of a new middle class; a number of factors caused this growth, but the twin causes were industrialisation and the advantages, for those who profited, of the means to pay for a good education for their sons and daughters. The demand was met by the small private and larger public schools which proliferated. Industrialisation gave employment and wealth, and spawned a growing consumerism. As the social historian Lawrence James puts it, 'the middle class expended as much time, energy and ingenuity on spending money as they did earning it'. The consequence was to show off wealth in the style of living, the house lived in, leisure activities, and so on. The spread of department stores, some of which became household names and – like Harrods – still trade today, offered the well-off middle classes the opportunity to indulge their new tastes.[160] The Groves were no exception after Reginald's father became established in his country practice.

Of course, identifying the traits of a particular class is generally difficult, although education, occupation and wealth were factors then, as they are now. Reginald's paternal grandfather was a draper from Staffordshire and was considered lower-middle-class, as he was 'in trade'. His sons, through their grammar school education, both entered professions whose stature was raised in the mid-19th century largely because of the new requirement for exam-based qualifications – in medicine in the case of Reginald's father, and in law with his Uncle Francis (Frank). The term 'gentleman' might well be applied to them, but not to their father. And as Reginald was educated at one of the new public schools, as well as gaining professional

[159] Henry Luke Paget, *Elma K. Paget* (Longmans Green, 1939).

[160] James, Lawrence, *The Middle Class: A History* (Abacus, 2010).

qualifications, in medicine, that term could be applied to him as he grew up.

And as today, fluidity between classes, as well as within a class, was commonplace. Individuals moved upwards or sometimes downwards on the social ladder, as Charles Dickens showed in his novels. A professional person like a lawyer or a doctor might describe themselves as being a 'gentleman', while a white-collared worker would not.

THE SOCIAL ROUND

Although Reginald was only at home in the school holidays, it is clear that his parents were hospitable, especially when they moved to their larger residence at Slepe House. Aunts, uncles, cousins and friends visited and stayed for weekends. A visit from a Dr Dyer who came for Christmas dinner in December 1883 when Reginald was 14 is an example of one visitor. Dyer worked at the Huntingdon County Hospital[161] and knew Reginald's father well.

And there was considerable entertaining between those middle-class St Ivians whom Dr and Mrs Grove knew – fellow professionals – solicitors, veterinarians, surgeons, town hall officers, teachers, businessmen and ministers of religion. In a small country town like St Ives, all those of any consequence knew each other.

This middle-class community grew larger from the mid-century onwards. They can be identified by the directories published by Kelly and other similar lists under the term 'Private Residents' or 'Gentry etc'. In the *Cassey Directory* of 1862, published just before Reginald's father moved to St Ives, 27 names were given.[162] They all identified, or were identified, as being those of some substance and standing. However, not all professional people were classified as gentry. Oliver St John Cooper, for instance, who was a surgeon, was not in this list, and nor was Mrs Mary Mumby who ran the ladies' school from 10 Cromwell Place; but four of the residents of Cromwell Place were on the list.

Fifteen years later, the *Harrod's Directory of 1877* listed 51 people under 'Private Residents', which was the designation then in use for the socially elite. Among them was Dr Grove who was still living in the Bullock Market.

[161] Diary 25.12.83.

[162] Cassey, Edward, *History, Topography, & Directory of Bedfordshire and Huntingdonshire* (1862).

He was also shown in the 'Professionals and General Trades' section. In the Private Residents list, eight lived in Cromwell Place which was now seen as a desirable location for the genteel. This list formed the core of middle-class society in St Ives; they knew each other and set the social scene. There were others from a similar background who were part of this circle who were not listed: Mrs Winter, who ran a ladies' seminary in the Bullock Market, and Cornelius Winter[163] who ran a 'school for gentlemen' from Burleigh House; and opposite where Reginald lived were two who would have been included as educated professionals. Not everyone who lived in Cromwell Place was classed as a 'private resident'. Henry Mitchell, who lived there was a 'dealer' – probably of livestock – and Abraham White was a 'beer retailer'.

The status and social standing of the head of a family were determined by a number of factors. There is no doubt thar Dr Grove's standing was enhanced by his public appointments; his public offices were listed in the *St Ives Business Directory of 1885* when he was 47 years old and indicated his standing in the St Ives community:

> Surgeon and medical officer workhouse and Somersham district, St Ives union and medical officer of health, St Ives urban sanitary district and certying [sic] factory surgeon, Slepe House.

Added to this was his role as a churchwarden; his rank of Surgeon Major in the Volunteer Reserves, and roles on a number of bodies like the Rowing Club and the National School Board show Dr Grove as a very public man. He was not the only doctor in St Ives, as there were perhaps two or three others with practices in the town, including his friend Dr Mence (who eventually signed his death certificate), but Dr Grove became a well-respected public figure.

The entry for George Game Day, a local solicitor from Wallingford and Day, and well known to the Groves, showed someone of similar standing:

> Solicitor and town clerk, clerk to the justices of the Hurstingstone division, to school board and sanitary authority, Bullock Market.

Day's partner, Edward Wallingford, had a similar profile:

> Solicitor and clerk to the guardians,[164] school assessment and attendance committees and to the rural sanitary authority and superintendent registrar and clerk to Warboys School Board, Bullock Market.

---

[163] It is unclear whether the Winters were related.

[164] The St Ives Union – the Workhouse.

Dr Grove and Messrs Day and Wallingford exercised considerable civic authority and were respected as men of local standing. Another man, William Wigston Warner, was one of the first Mayors of St Ives, serving on five occasions, the last being in 1897.[165] His father, John, was a butcher before moving into the leather business,[166] and in 1850 built the impressive Stanley House which stands in Market Hill. The exterior was built with early Victorian Italianate details, such as three first-floor balconies, and inside was an elaborate curved staircase which led to the drawing room when the house was used as a family home.

The *1885 Business Directory* lists a number of names of professional and business families which were to play a prominent part in the town's civic life well into the mid-20th century – Coote, Barton, Kiddle,[167] Turner, Ruston, Wadsworth and Warren, besides Day and Grove.[168] Frederic Warren, for instance, was Mayor in 1881, 1885 and 1890. His son, Frederic Maurice, was Mayor in 1912 and 1926.

A trend developed for those like Dr Grove and George Game Day to move out of the centre of the town to larger houses away from the bustle of the market. In the second half of the 19th century there was a piecemeal development as the town expanded and new houses and villas were built in Needingworth Road, London Road and Parkside. Day built a large house called Rheola in Broad Leys[169] while keeping the offices of his law practice in the Bullock Market. Other substantial houses in St Ives (which were not used as schools like Manchester House or Slepe Hall) were The Priory, occupied by the Warren family, Stanley House,[170] the grand residence of William Wigston Warner, and The Vicarage, Burleigh Hall and The How occupied by a succession of different families. The number of live-in servants was also an indicator of standing, being associated with the size of

165 On his death in 1905 he gave a larger piece of open land to the town now called 'Warner's Park' for recreational purposes. The old ridge-and-furrow system used in medieval farming is still visible today.

166 John Warner died in 1879 but William took over the business from his father and diversified into farming. He died a rich man, with the content of his will being detailed in the London *Evening Standard.* He left £47,302.

167 Edward Kiddle was Mayor in 1927, 1938, 1939, 1940 and 1941, and Geoffrey Kiddle in 1952.

168 Reginald's daughter, Mary Grove, was Mayor in 1962.

169 This led into the less genteelly named 'Pig Lane'.

170 Stanley House was bought by the Town Council in 1924 and used as the town hall to this day.

the house and, by implication, the wealth of the occupiers. In this respect, the Groves early in their marriage had three live-in servants compared to the three servants at the Ansleys who lived in a large house in Ramsey Road called The How, and the Revd Goldie's five servants at The Vicarage.[171] The Warren family, living at The Priory, employed four servants, including a nurse.[172] In contrast, Henry Barton, living with his wife in Bridge Street, had a shop assistant boarding and one domestic servant.[173]

These families all formed the core of St Ivian society.

Henry Barton, who ran a pharmacy store, lived above his shop, as did W. M. Turner, who ran a similar store in Market Hill. Interestingly, Barton sold wines and spirits in addition to medicines. His ledgers were passed to the Norris Museum when the family business finally closed in 1987. They give a fascinating insight into his customers' medical complaints, drinking habits and creditworthiness. One of the Groves' neighbours in Slepe House, for instance, was a Mr Clemison in Cromwell Place, who ordered cognac every month, and bottles of sherry and port from time to time, in addition to some of Barton's pills as a general tonic.[174]

Men who dealt with the sensitive affairs of their neighbours, whether Day with legal matters, Dr Grove with medical complaints, or Barton with the alcohol orders of his customers, had to be completely confidential in their social dealings, too.

In other towns, social and business links were formed through friendly societies, temperance movements and Freemasonry. Some friendly societies were organised into lodges like the Odd Fellows, as were some temperance societies. The St Ivo Lodge of Good Templars was formed in 1879 when this group bought a building for meetings which had been previously used by The Salvation Army.[175] The Templars were a temperance movement that began in the United States in 1851, and within a few years their lodges spread across to Europe. The St Ivo Lodge was affiliated to the Grand

---

[171] The Vicarage was a substantial house in large grounds near the church. It was demolished in 1964 and besides a new, smaller, modern vicarage being built, the site was large enough for a block of two-storey flats, Clare Court, to be built, too. Mary Grove, one of Reginald's daughters, lived out her elder years in one of them.

[172] National Census 1881.

[173] National Census 1871.

[174] Hudson, Noel, *St Ives: Slepe by the Ouse* (1989) p. 90.

[175] Before The Salvation Army used the building, it was used by a sect called the Swedenborgians and their church was called the New Jerusalem Church (see Chapter 19).

Lodge of England. Their building in St Ives was called the Temperance and Mission Hall.[176]

A Freemasons' lodge was formed in St Ives in 1897 also called, confusingly, the St Ivo Lodge.[177] The masons' meetings were held in a house in Wellington Street near the Quay.[178] Reginald was by then running his late father's practice, and as a local person of standing would have been asked to become a mason, but there is no record that he did, despite his Uncle Frank being one, and his youngest brother Tom becoming one later.

Those whose social standing was enhanced were those who served as local magistrates. One of Mrs Grove's brothers, Reginald's Uncle George, who farmed at Carleton Grange in Cambridgeshire, was one, and her personal standing was enhanced as a result.[179] The fact also that her brothers were tenant farmers employing large numbers of farm workers gave the Long family standing across Cambridgeshire. Reginald's grandfather, Hanslip Long employed 48 men and 13 boys, and farmed 1,200 acres in 1871.[180]

There were easily recognisable outward differences within the St Ives society which was replicated in other rural towns of the period. Some were professionals in law, medicine or the Church; with the latter, the social standing of the Vicar of the parish church, Revd Goldie, who had private means, was higher than Revd Lloyd from the Free church, for instance, or the minister of the Baptist or Methodist church. There were those in trade, like Kiddle and Rushton with their furniture and ironmongery shops, Coote[181] in the coal and coke distribution business,[182] and Turner and Barton with their pharmacy shops. There were those who worshipped in the parish church, and Nonconformists in a variety of chapels. Politically there were those who were Conservative like Dr Grove, and those who

---

176 Norris, Herbert, *History of St Ives* (1899), p. 61.

177 St Ivo Lodge No 2684.

178 There was a 'fine lodge room, with a raised dais and a dining room seating about 60 and used also as a billiard room'. *Kelly's Directory for Huntingdon 1914,* p. 59.

179 Kelly's *Directory of Cambridgeshire* 1885, p. 15.

180 National Census 1871.

181 Two of the Coote brothers who lived in Fenstanton, Howard and Thomas, were magistrates on the Cambridgeshire Bench, and this would have enhanced the family's standing. (*Kelly's Directory for Cambridgeshire 1883.*)

182 Coote and Warren's coal business had offices in St Ives and Cambridge. (*Kelly's Directory for Cambridgeshire 1883.*)

were Liberal like Revd Lloyd. There were disagreements and fallouts, but these were more about matters of principle, rather than social snobbery. For instance, as related in later chapters, Lloyd led the opposition to Goldie in 1875 as the latter tried to get elected to the Board of the British School, which had a Nonconformist leaning. The middle class in St Ives generally got on well together and disagreements did not get in the way of their social life. If there were difficulties, it was much more a matter of personality; while Reginald never made any mention of it, Goldie seemed to rub many people, Nonconformist and Anglican, up the wrong way!

Invitations for social events were given and received within this social circle. Confusingly, Reginald used 'dinner' to describe both the midday meal and the one in the evening. The midday meal was generally called 'luncheon', and during the working week, with the husband of the house at work, was a light meal for his wife, taken with the children or eaten alone. It might be soup or a sandwich.

The evening meal, dinner, was often held late in the evening at 8 or 9 o'clock, as the time had been gradually pushed back due to the length of the commercial day, prolonged in the cities by suburban commuting. This was less the case in a rural town like St Ives, but the timing of meals changed, too, influenced by the introduction of tea in the late afternoon. Afternoon tea was established by the mid-century as a light meal of bread and butter, cake and fruit, and tea. This was very much a middle- and upper-class meal. The best china crockery was used with specially designed tableware for the occasion for crumpet and muffin dishes, holding hot water in the base to keep the contents warm. High tea was a meal at the end of a working day for the lower-middle and working classes, and was a substantial meal with cooked fish and meat, and bread – and of course tea. The tea that Reginald had at both boarding schools was like this.

If guests were invited, particularly at the weekend, then formal dress was worn. Dinner was planned by the mistress of the house with great care and executed to perfection.

Eastlake emphasised the importance of good design for dining:

> a well-appointed dinner-table is one of the triumphs of an English housewife's domestic care. That the cloth should be of fine and snow white damask, that the decanters and wine glasses shall be delicate in form and of purest quality; that the silver shall look as bright and spotless as when it first came wrapped in tissue paper from the silversmiths; that the

> epergne[183] shall be filled with choicest flowers – these are points which she will consider of as much importance as the dainty skill of the cook's art itself.

Some invitations seemed to be quite informal; early in January 1883 just before Reginald's birthday, he noted: 'Mr and Mrs Laycock to dinner'.[184] But a meal that he and his parents were invited to in 1886 was held at one of the grander houses in St Ives, The How, off the Ramsey Road. Sir James Paget, the famous surgeon to Queen Victoria, and his wife Lady Lydia were on holiday in St Ives visiting their son, the new young vicar,[185] and staying at The How. They invited the Groves for dinner, specifically for Paget to chat to Reginald about medicine as a career, as well as talk about a young relative who was going to Uppingham in Reginald's house. Reginald said that he had a 'jolly evening', the conversation went on late, and he got home about midnight.

At some time after the family moved to Slepe House, the Groves adopted a family crest which was stamped on their cutlery. While there were a few silver pieces, their main cutlery set was silver plate.[186] The crest was put on the bowl of the dessert, salad and tablespoons, and on the top of the handle of the knives and forks.[187] There is no evidence that the Groves from Staffordshire, who had quite humble origins, had any heraldic coat of arms. But, like many aspiring Victorian families, they chose one as a statement of their new social standing. The Grove crest was that of a dog, possibly a mastiff.[188] It is a heraldic pose – 'talbot passant sa collared'.[189] It is a rather fine-looking beast and no doubt the crest impressed the dining guests at the Groves'.

Mrs Beeton gave sample menus based on the availability of meat, fish, vegetables and fruit during different seasons for her readers. The suggestion

---

[183] This was an ornamental centrepiece for a dining table to hold fruit or flowers.

[184] Diary 05.01.83.

[185] Paget and his wife spent some time in St Ives on holiday, and the rest of the summer was spent in the Pyrenees. (Paget, Stephen, *Memoirs and Letters of Sir James Paget* (Longmans, 1901), p. 360.)

[186] Electro plated nickel silver (EPNS) is an alloy of nickel, copper and zinc that's covered with a layer of pure silver in an electrochemical process. It is also known as silver plate.

[187] On the death of Reginald's wife Hilda in 1954, the cutlery set was divided up amongst their children. I have a number of spoons which were passed to me by my mother, Frances.

[188] Other heraldic designs used greyhounds.

[189] *The Book of Crests Volume 1 Heraldry Today* (Bookcraft, Bath, 1984), p. 245.

shown below for a dinner in August for six people was one that, even in a provincial town like St Ives, the hostess who wanted to impress her guests would have provided. Grouse was in season, trout easily available, as were strawberries, pears, plums and French beans.[190]

> **First Course:** *Macaroni Soup, Crimped Salmon and Sauce Hollandaise. Fried Fillets of Trout.*
> **Entrées:** *Tendrons de Veau and Stewed Peas. Salmi of Grouse.*
> **Second Course:** *Roast Loin of Veal. Boiled Bacon, garnished with French Beans. Stewed Beef à la Jardinière. Vegetables.*
> **Third Course:** *Turkey Poult. Plum Tart. Custard Pudding. Vol-au-Vent of Pears. Strawberry Cream. Ratafia Soufflé*

Another example of a menu for a grand dinner given in October 1885 by George and Maud Darwin[191] in their Cambridge home for Sir William and Lady Thompson was:

> **First Course:** Clear Soup, Brill and Lobster Sauce, Chicken Cutlets and Rice Balls and Oyster Patties
> **Second Course:** Mutton, Potatoes, Artichokes, Beets. Partridges and Salad.
> **Third Course:** Caramel Pudding. Pears and Whipped Cream. Cheese Ramequins. Cheese Straws. Ice. Grapes, Walnuts, Chocolates and Pears.[192]

The style of dining for formal dinner parties when the Groves set up home was 'à la Française'. Besides describing dishes in French ('boiled mackerel à la Maître d'hôtel' or 'peas à la Française'), this meant that the food was placed on the table in front of guests, roasts carved by the host, and then everything was passed around by the servants, guests and hosts. Elaborate floral decorations were placed between dishes. This style changed as late Victorian dinners at home were organised in a new style called 'à la Russe'. The interpretation of this varied but in essence meant that dishes were placed on a sideboard with the roasts carved there; the food was then served to the guests who ate from a dining table that was clear of tureens, decorations, and so on. At the end of the meal decorative desserts, jellies and ices were placed on the table in display, rather than

---

[190] Beeton, section 2041.

[191] George Darwin was Charles Darwin's second son, a Fellow of Trinity College, and a Professor of Astronomy.

[192] Raverat, chapter 5.

being served from the side.[193] The dining table merely had cutlery laid, wine glasses,[194] linen napkins – perhaps folded with a bread roll hidden in the centre, a simple table decoration, candelabra and bowls of fruit. It was a simpler style.

Besides the immediate social circle in the town itself, it extended to smaller outlying villages, too. In September 1882, when Reginald was 13, he visited the Herbert family to see his friend Dennis who was the same age, with his ten-year-old younger brother Ted. The Revd Henry Herbert was the Rector of St Margaret's, Hemingford Abbots.[195] Reginald and his brother joined the Herberts at their Harvest Festival tea and the service afterwards.[196]

Reginald missed Christmas at home during his years as a chorister. Singing in King's College Chapel on Christmas Day itself meant that the boys did not travel home until a few days afterwards (see Volume 2). But at Uppingham he was always home well before Christmas Day itself. The meal served on Christmas Day in the Grove household was one easily recognisable today. Mrs Beeton said that

> A Christmas dinner, with the middle-classes of this empire, would scarcely be a Christmas dinner without its turkey; and we can hardly imagine an object of greater envy than is presented by a respected portly paterfamilias carving at the season devoted to good cheer and genial charity; his own fat turkey and carving well.[197]

Plum (Christmas) pudding was a standard dessert made with perhaps a pint of brandy, according to Beeton!

This was the traditional meal served at Christmas in the evening. Reginald's entry for 1885 was: 'did not have dinner till 4.00pm. Mr and Mrs Iago, Mr Kwell Daison and his little girl were the whole company,

---

[193] A variety of ices became more widely available in London such as pine, lemon, orange, ginger, strawberry and cherry, according to A. V. Kirwan, in his *Host and Guest: A Book about Dinners, Wines, and Desserts*, written in 1864. Whether they were sold in St Ives is not known.

[194] Three glasses – one for sherry drunk after soup; one for hock drunk with oysters or with fish after the soup; and one for claret drunk with the dessert.

[195] Dennis went on to have a distinguished career, being elected as an MP for Watford in the 1918 general election. He served as an MP until 1943. He was made Baron Hemingford that year and died a year before Reginald.

[196] Diary 26.09.82.

[197] Beeton, section 1005.

besides ourselves. After dinner, played games of all sorts.' The Groves clearly were in the habit of inviting those who might otherwise be on their own, as next year for Christmas dinner 1886 he noted:

> Dinner at 5.00pm. Mr (Revd) Paget, Mr Whitins, and Mr Pollock came, making 13 but 2 ate at another table; Mr Paget, Mr Whitins and Mr Pollock had to go when dinner was over to the Hunt,[198] but got back at 9.00pm. Had very good games until 12.00pm.

FOOD AND DIET

Besides Mrs Beeton's guide for middle-class living, there were a huge range of magazine articles and other books providing advice about living styles, manners, the management of servants, and what meals to cook and how to entertain guests. Meat played a prominent part in the eating habits of the middle and upper classes – beef, mutton, pork, veal and ham. And these were washed down, certainly for formal dining, with ales, wines and spirits. At both ends of the social scale drinking was in earnest, although excess was not mentioned by Reginald at all in his diaries.

Another popular guide for the hostess was *Modern Cookery for Private Families* by Eliza Acton,[199] which was first published in 1845, revised in 1855, and remained in print throughout the 19th century. Acton dedicated it to 'The Young Housekeepers of England', such as the young Maria Grove, and it became an invaluable guide with well-written and easy-to-follow recipes. In her Preface she wrote:

> It cannot be denied that an improved system of practical domestic cookery and a better knowledge of its first principles, after still much needed in this country, where from ignorance, or from mismanagement in their preparation, the daily waste of excellent provisions almost exceeds belief.

She was concerned for proper diet and home-cooked food needed to be wholesome to promote good health.

> The amount of positive diseases which is caused amongst us by improper food, or by food rendered unwholesome by a bad mode of cooking it, seems a great evil still. The influence of diet upon health is indeed a subject of far deeper importance than it would usually appear to be considered,

[198] What this was is unclear, but at that time of night it cannot have been a hunt with hounds.

[199] Acton, Eliza, *Modern Cooking* (Longman, Brown, Green and Longmans, London, 1845, 2nd edition).

> if we may judge by the profound indifference with which it is commonly treated.[200]

Dr Grove would have agreed.

Acton lived in Suffolk for much of her life running a ladies' school in Ipswich, and then in other nearby locations before writing poetry and then her bestselling cookery book. Although she died in 1859 when Maria was 15 years old, it is not too fanciful to think that Acton may have known the Long family, farming on the Cambridge/Suffolk border given the extent that middle-class families knew of each other in a county. Acton's guidance gave instruction on preparation, the essential ingredients for each dish and cooking times, despite the heating unreliability of coal-fired kitchen ranges.

There were a number of 'firsts' – the first recipe for Brussels sprouts, the first recipe for what Acton called 'Christmas pudding', which was normally called plum pudding – which is what Reginald called it. The word *spaghetti* – which she spelt *sparghetti* – was used for the first time in an English cookery book. While the book gave mainly English recipes, there was a chapter on curries, and recipes for Eastern 'chatneys' (chutney), reflecting the growing influence of British interest in the Indian subcontinent.

Mrs Beeton's suggestions for *Plain Family Dinners*, month by month to include seasonal ingredients, give an idea of what could have been served up in the Grove household. For a Sunday dinner in January the suggestion was boiled turbot, with oyster sauce and potatoes; a roast leg or loin of pork with apple sauce, broccoli and potatoes, followed by cabinet pudding (a steamed pudding with dried fruits) and damson tart made with preserved (i.e. bottled) damsons. For a Thursday in September she suggested brill and shrimp sauce, followed by roast hare, which would have been plentiful around St Ives, gravy, redcurrant jelly; mutton cutlets and mashed potatoes; or scalloped oysters, instead of a pudding.[201]

There were seven butchers in St Ives that sold fresh meat;[202] frozen

---

200 Acton, ibid.

201 Spours, Judy, *Cakes and Ale* (2006), National Archives, p. 35.

202 There was wide choice for the St Ivian housewife to use: William Sparrow, in Crown Street; George Robinson (and farmer) in Bridge Street; and William Sharon in the Bullock Market. Because much pork was eaten, there were four butchers who specialised in this meat – George Hewson, Merryland; Pork Butcher & Green Grocer Thomas Watts, Crown Street; Edward Anderson, The Waits; and Thomas Anderson in Bridge Street. (*St Ives Business Register* 1885.)

lamb from New Zealand became available during Reginald's childhood[203] and was reasonably priced, but, given St Ives' rural location, and the ready availability of fresh meat, it was not a product in demand in the town. Fish,[204] cheese, milk, vegetables and fruit were bought locally in the town, a stone's throw away in the Bullock Market and within easy walking distance from Slepe House. In any event, delivery boys also took customer orders to their homes. There were nine greengrocers selling vegetables and fruit which were grown locally by market gardeners.[205] More exotic fruit became increasingly available as the century drew to a close. Bananas and pineapples could be bought cheaply due to refrigeration in ships transporting these from the colonies; before, they had been available only for the rich when hothouses cultivated these specially. On two occasions Reginald mentioned being given oranges by his mother and aunt when he was laid up sick in bed at King's.

In the second half of the 19th century preserved, processed and packaged foods became readily available. Condensed milk, imported from Switzerland and the United States from the 1850s onwards, besides satisfying the Victorian sweet tooth, was deemed safer than fresh milk, which before pasteurisation was a potential health risk. It was used in desserts, sweetmeats and baking recipes.

Processed foods saved time in the kitchen and enabled more ingredients to be available. Interestingly, unlike today's awareness of the dangers of harmful ingredients in processed foods, in Reginald's time they were seen to be healthier and better than man-made products. Everyday menus, especially for desserts, changed. Packaged baking powder made cakes and puddings much easier at home. Before powdered gelatine became available, 'isinglass' was needed; made from stock from calves' feet or heels, boiled and sieved, it took much time. Powdered gelatine meant that elaborate jellies could be made. Custard powder sold in tins meant that heating milk

---

[203] The first cargo of frozen meat was brought Australia to England in 1877, and three months later another cargo of frozen meat was brought from South America to France, with lamb from New Zealand to England a short time afterwards. (Paterson, Michael, *Life in Victorian Britain* (2008), p. 57.)

[204] There was only one fishmonger in St Ives – Edward Collinson, in the Bullock Market. However, locally caught river eels were eaten by the townsfolk.

[205] Fresh vegetables and fruit were sold by Miss Sarah Adams in Market Place; John Johnson in Crown Street; Mrs Charlotte Hammond and then Mrs Charlotte Horner, both in West Street; Mrs Susannah Grant in Wellington Street; David Smith in The Waits; George Burdett in East Street; and finally George Burgess in Bullock Market. (*St Ives Business Register* 1885.)

and eggs, which easily curdled, became unnecessary for the many steam puddings that were enjoyed.[206] The invention of bottling and tinning changed the Victorian menu. Tinned meat was introduced from Australia in 1874 and nicknamed 'Sweet Fanny Adams'.[207]

Other processed foods became available such as factory-made biscuits (from 1869)[208] and margarine (also invented in 1869) used for cooking. There were also dried vegetables, tinned soups, bottled pickles, tinned meats like beef and tongue, tinned fish (like salmon), jam and tinned fruit (such as peaches, apricots and pineapples). Two grocery stores in the town sold dry and tinned goods: John Stevens in Merryland, and George Burdett in East Street. For the discerning social hostess wanting a greater range there were many more grocer's shops in Cambridge which was only a 30-minute ride away on the train; Charles Cole & Co in Fitzroy Street was one example.

By the end of the 1890s many of the world's brands or processed products recognised today had been established: Campbell Soups were manufactured from 1869 onwards, as were Heinz products, in the year of Reginald's birth. Tomato ketchup was first sold in 1876 and marketing the number '57' brand on large wall posters then began.[209] Philadelphia Cream Cheese was on sale in 1880, Maxwell House coffee and Del Monte canned fruit in 1892; Cadbury's milk chocolate in 1897; Nabisco cereals in 1898; and Quaker Oats in 1902.

While Reginald mentioned that he was given a vegetarian meal when he was 13 at King's Choir School, he never mentioned other meat-free meals again.[210] The first group of people to abandon meat-eating in England was

---

[206] Alfred Bird was a chemist in Birmingham who invented Bird's Custard in 1837, made out of cornflower, because his wife liked custard but was intolerant to eggs. (Spours, Judy, *Cakes and Ale*, p. 43.)

[207] Fanny Adams was a child who was brutally murdered in Alton in 1867 and her dismembered body discovered. Her name sadly became associated with regulation tinned mutton produced for use by the Royal Navy in 1869. This replaced salted beef used as standard rations. Canning was still a new technology and the process did not always work well; also poor-quality offal was slipped in. Without being airtight the meat turned very quickly, and the sailors at the dockyards in Southampton and Portsmouth (30 miles from Alton) joked about the putrefying meat being bits of Fanny Adams. The grisly story became Navy slang for disgusting mutton or stew and so, by extension, anything worthless. Sweet Fanny Adams meant 'nothing at all'.

[208] Peek Frean's factory began production in East London and 'Fine Navy Biscuits' were produced for the troops in the Franco-Prussian War of 1870. In 1899 they manufactured the first chocolate biscuit.

[209] Sweet, Matthew, *Inventing the Victorians* (2001), p. 48.

[210] Diary 24.05.82.

the Bible Christian Church, led by The Revd William Cowherd in Salford, near Manchester. He gave his first sermon advocating a vegetarian diet in 1809. Vegetarianism grew in popularity, with a Vegetarian Society formed in 1847 to promote its benefits.[211] Reginald's father would have been interested in the health benefits of this diet and notable advocates were later to be Isaac Pitman (who invented the shorthand system), Dr Thomas Allinson (who founded the wholemeal bread company still trading today), Dr Anna Kingsford (the women's suffrage and antivivisection campaigner), George Bernard Shaw (the playwright) and Bramwell Booth (William Booth's son of The Salvation Army). The first vegetarian restaurant opened in London in 1849, and by the time Reginald was at Guy's Hospital Britain had 52 vegetarian restaurants.[212]

LEISURE LIFE

The last 30 years of the 19th century saw a massive growth in leisure activities throughout England. The rhythm of working life changed for society as statutory holidays under the 1847 Factory Act began to make a distinction between work and leisure time for the working classes. While the act applied only to industrial businesses, the shift towards defined working patterns began and over time impacted across society. In addition, improved working conditions, ease of travel on the growing network of trains, and a rising standard of living gave many, especially the growing middle class, more time and money to spend enjoying themselves.

There were a vast range of clubs and societies, outside church, chapel and civic activities, available for the middle-class townsfolk of St Ives and something to suit every interest and taste; below is a list. Those marked with * were those his father was involved in, which, when he was older

---

[211] The initiative to launch the Vegetarian Society came from those associated with the Alcott House Academy on Ham Common, near Richmond, Surrey. This was founded by a businessman called James Pierrepont Greaves. He set up the school in 1838, following the example of Bronson Alcott and naming it in his honour. Alcott had run a similar school in Boston, USA, based on the ideas of the educational reformer Pestalozzi. In 1842 the Ham Common school was renamed The Concordium, still in Alcott House, and they began publishing journals, first *The Healthian* and then *The New Age*. The April 1842 issue of The Healthian contained the earliest known printed use of the word 'vegetarian', and for the next five years all known uses of the word were from people closely connected with Alcott House. Though health was part of their approach, the basis of their vegetarianism was asceticism – living as simple and morally accountable a life as possible.

[212] Sweet, Matthew, *Inventing the Victorians* (2001), p. 107.

during the holidays, Reginald would visit, too. The date, where known, of the foundation of each group or society is shown in brackets, taken from Norris's *History of St Ives*.[213]

Angling Society* (1881)
Athletics Society
Brass Band
Choral Society
Cricket Club
Cycling Club (1877)
Football Club
Fox Terrier Coursing Club
Friendly Institute (1837)
Friendly Society (1841)[214]
Good Templars (1879)
Horticultural Society* (1879)
Hunts Agricultural Society (1838)[215]
Literary Institute (1866) – previously called the Young Men's Christian Association
Mutual Improvement Society (1852)[216]
Ornithological Society
Pleasant Sunday Afternoon (PSA)
Quadrille Party (dances)
Reading Club
Recreation Club
Rowing Club* (1865) – sometimes referred to as the 'Boat Club'
Saturday Evening concerts
Temperance Society (1848)
Whist Club*

---

213 Norris, pp. 60–61.

214 This was a branch of the Manchester Unity Friendly Society called 'The Stranger's Refuge'. Norris reported in 1899 that it had 350 local members. Friendly societies provided mutual benefits such as paying medical costs in an era where state support was non-existent or minimal.

215 This society was organised at St Ives and held shows at Huntingdon, St Neots, Ramsey and St Ives alternately.

216 This was one of the earliest societies in St Ives and a debating society which met in the hall of the Public Institution with the purpose of broadening the minds of those who came. Topics debated were slavery, Catholic emancipation and the repeal of the Corn Laws. A contentious topic debated in 1866 was about geology and the Christian faith.

At his death, patients, friends and family recalled Dr Grove's enthusiasm in supporting a wide range of clubs and activities. Reginald followed in his footsteps.

ST IVES ROWING CLUB

Rowing had become increasingly more popular after the publicity of the first University Boat Race in 1829; ten years later, the establishment of the Henley Regatta started to make rowing fashionable. Boat clubs began to be set up in towns and cities across England; Maidenhead, like Henley on the Thames, became well known after the Guards Boat Club was founded. The iconic painting by Edward John Gregory called 'Boulter's Lock, Sunday Afternoon', which depicts a myriad of skiffs by the lock on the Thames on the day after the Ascot Races in the 1880s, is a testament to the popularity of this sport.

And St Ives was no exception, as the St Ives Boat Club[217] was formed in April 1865,[218] just after young Dr Grove first came to St Ives. No records survive of the start of the club except a newspaper article[219] some years later that the club rules dated from 1864–65. A plaque in the Boat House states that the founding committee was Revd John Linton[220] as President, Mr Westby as Captain, Mr C. P. Tebbutt as Treasurer, with Dr Grove being on the committee. It cost 10/6d (£66.37) per season to be a member but 'any lady or gentleman paying an annual subscription of not less than 5/- (£31) shall be an honorary member of the Club but not entitled to vote'. This was definitely a sport for a gentleman.

No record survives as to why Dr Grove became interested in rowing, but his enthusiasm was certainly passed on to his son. Perhaps it stemmed from the applause that Reginald received as a boy aged 13 when he sang at an event at the Boat Club after Christmas in 1882: 'sang two sacred songs in a concert and was "encoured" [sic] in one'! After his medical training, he rowed for the Club and then became its President, as described in Volume 3.

One distinguished member of the Club during was John H. D. Goldie, the son of the Vicar in the '70s and '80s. Goldie grew up in St Ives, was

---

[217] The date was 1865 from club rules cited by Herbert Norris in his *History of St Ives* written in 1889.

[218] Carter, Mary, *19th Century St Ives*, p. 92, gives the founding date as 1860 but this year is not confirmed by the newspaper reports cited.

[219] Norris Museum press cuttings 1796–1914.

[220] It is not known to which church Revd Linton belonged.

educated at Eton and St John's College, Cambridge, and went on to a career as a barrister. He captained the St Ives Rowing Club in 1869 when he was 20 at Cambridge. In addition to being the President of the Cambridge University Boat Club, he was the stroke[221] and captain of the crew that won the University Boat Race in the three years of 1870, 1871 and 1872. As the Oxford crew had defeated Cambridge for the previous nine years, the victorious Cambridge crew exulted in their results. A public dinner was held in honour of Goldie at St Ives in 1872 which Dr Grove would have attended. He spent his holidays in St Ives, rowed for the local club, and was very popular. His younger brother was a cox. His rowing career developed on leaving Cambridge as he captained Leander[222] from 1873 to 1876, was their Treasurer from 1882 to 1895, and umpired at Henley Royal Regatta. The local newspaper reported Goldie's death on 1 April 1896 aged 47. Today, the club's administrative centre on the banks of the Cam is called the Goldie Boathouse. The second Cambridge boat in the Annual Boat Race which has competed since 1965 against Isis, the Oxford second boat, is called 'Goldie' after this son of St Ives.

Dr Grove was an enthusiastic supporter of the St Ives Boat Club. As already mentioned, the river gradually declined as a commercial thoroughfare, and by the mid-1870s was being used more for leisure. In June 1874 the Boat Club organised a regatta[223] which soon became an annual activity. 11 years later, on 25 April 1885 at the club's annual meeting at the Corn Exchange on Market Hill, Dr Grove was elected one of two Vice-Presidents with Mr W. W. Warner, who was an Alderman and had been Mayor in 1877.[224] The newspaper report[225] said that there was a 'good attendance'. Another annual meeting took place (date not known) at the 'Priory Rooms' with the permission of F. Warren, and Dr Grove presided. He proposed that the Mayor (Mr C. Coote) be President for the next year – it was usual to elect the Mayor to this position, but he also took a keen personal interest in the club.

Reginald's younger brothers, Ernest and Ted, rowed at King's School, Ely, in competitive rowing events – in April 1887 Ted coxed a four against

---

221 A 'stroke' is the rower who sits nearest the stern of the boat.

222 The prestigious Leander Club in Henley-on-Thames is one of the oldest rowing clubs in England.

223 Little, Bryan, and Werba, Herbert, *St Ives in Huntingdonshire* (1974), p. 40.

224 He went on to be Mayor in 1883, 1887, 1892 and 1897.

225 Norris Museum press cuttings 1796–1914.

Ely Theological College with Ernest as one of the crew. In March 1888, the year after he left school and had begun rowing for his college, Sidney Sussex, Reginald became a member of the St Ives Club.[226] A few months later there were some 'Scratch Races' held[227] when Reginald was a crew member; his brother Ted was the cox and his father was a judge.[228]

Another newspaper article on 6 July 1889 reported that the annual 'four-oared boat race' held between St Ives and Huntingdon crews 'would take place the following week on a Thursday evening at 7.15pm'. The St Ives crew was made up of H. Lines (bow), his good friend A. R. Ulph (2nd), E. Kiddle (3rd), and Reginald as stoke, with W. Ward as cox. Reginald was 20 at the time and came down from Cambridge to participate. The course for the race was 'the usual one' at Houghton Whale,[229] and the St Ives crew planned to row upstream to the race position beforehand. By his second year at Cambridge, he had become a keen member of the Sidney Sussex rowing club.

By 1894, after his return to St Ives from his medical training, Reginald was chosen as captain of the St Ives Club.

THE ANGLING SOCIETY

Reginald enjoyed fishing but was never a member of the local angling club. The St Ives and District Angling Society was founded 1881 when he was 12. The Great Ouse teemed with a wide variety of fish, from the humble gudgeon, bleak and dace, carp, roach, chub, perch, rudd, tench, bream to much larger fish. The Society held the fishing rights for the Great Ouse from Houghton Mill, upstream of St Ives, down to Overcote Ferry – a distance of about seven miles.[230] Overcote Ferry was located at the Pike and Eel public house near Needingworth, and Reginald and his father used to cross the river using the ferry on their medical rounds to Over (see Volume 3).

The public house was aptly named, as both pike and eels were found in abundance in the Great Ouse. Pike could grow extremely large and one,

---

[226] Norris Museum press cuttings 1796–1914, *Hunts County Guardian,* 24.03.88.

[227] The newspaper report said that the club was 24 years old, which meant that it was founded in 1864.

[228] Norris Museum press cuttings 1796–1914, *Hunts County Guardian,* 14.03.88.

[229] A location somewhere between St Ives and the Hemingfords which has not been identified.

[230] Norris, Herbert, *History of St Ives* (1889). Also confirmed by Colin Leach, Chairman of the St Ives Angling Society, in an interview with the author on 23.06.2018.

weighing 19½ lb, was recorded as being taken in 1881 in 'Nix's Hole'.[231] Another, weighing 15½ lb, was caught at Portobella.[232] An eel caught in 1869 at St Ives Staunch, downstream of the railway bridge, weighed 7lb. But neither was the largest fish caught; sturgeon occasionally swam up the river in winter when the Ouse was in flood. As Norris said:

> Being a monstrous fish, and a stranger, it is much sought after by gentlemen both for the sport it affords and for its rarity ... a specimen caught on 12 June 1859 was netted in the sixgate[233] pit and was six foot long and weighed over 60lbs'.

It's tempting to say this was a 'fisherman's tale', but as others were recorded as being caught of a 'large size', one being preserved in a glass case by a Mr Brown, it may well be true.[234] There were some instances recorded of salmon trout being caught, an 18lb one being netted in the Hemingford Mill pits in February 1868.

The Angling Club flourished under the enthusiastic leadership of the secretary, Mr Collinson, who publicised angling events in the local newspapers, as well as specialist national ones like *The Fishing Gazette*, and *The Times*. This attracted visitors to events and competitions who were supplied with regular information about fishing conditions and catches. What tackle the anglers used is unclear. Chub were caught with a fly as they fed on insects, but generally for coarse fishing a rod, reel, float and hooks were the standard equipment used. However, some fish, like roach, tench and bream, were caught by the locals using dragnets, and bream[235] were certainly sold, like eels, in St Ives to eat.[236] They required a soaking in salt water to get rid of the strong muddy taste of the river before cooking.

Anglers came down from London by train and stayed at the White Horse Hotel (which was the club's headquarters) in St Ives. Besides the

---

[231] The location of this spot is unknown.

[232] See footnote 593 in Chapter 11.

[233] This was a large, deep pool between Hemingford Grey and Hemingford Abbots, just beyond the Manor House, along the backwater. Further up was another large pool called the Four Gate Pit which was known as '*The Frying Pan*', because of its shape, by Reginald's son, David Grove and his family. (National Ordnance Survey May 1888–1913.)

[234] Norris, p. 92.

[235] A bream caught in the Ballast Hole was recorded by Norris as weighing 4½ lb. This was a large, deep pool between St Ives and Holywell on the south side of railway line to Cambridge just before it crosses the river. (National Ordnance Survey, May 1888–1913.)

[236] Norris, p. 93.

White Horse, visitors also stayed downstream at Holywell where Mrs Metcalfe had lodgings for anglers, as did Mrs Hemmington at Overcote, a little further down towards the Bedford Level.[237]

Dr Grove became the first President of the Angling Society.[238] In April 1888 at the Annual General Meeting he said that he wanted to step down as 'he had spent a lot of time carrying out the role'. He was persuaded to be re-elected and 'expressed the hope that he would be well supported during the coming year. He would again do his best to promote the interests of the Society – (applause).'[239]

In June 1889, a special meeting was held at the Unicorn Hotel, in the old Bullock Market, to revise the Club rules followed by the Annual General Meeting. Dr Grove said at the meeting that he had been involved for the previous eight years but was again persuaded to stand again. But ill health dogged him and by 1892 a Mr Dendy Sadler had replaced him and Dr Grove was elected as one of the Vice Presidents.

After his father's death, and his return to St Ives, Reginald was also elected as one of 13 vice presidents, with the MP for Huntingdonshire, the Hon A. E. Fellowes being another.[240]

The mantle had now been passed from father to son.

ST IVES TOWN FOOTBALL CLUB

It was in December 1886, when Reginald was nearly 18, that during the holidays he went to a meeting at Copley's, the solicitor, who was trying to start a football club. It certainly looked possible and Reginald's enthusiasm for forming scratch teams for informal games was well known.

The next year the St Ives Town Football Club was formed, and Dr Grove was elected Vice-President in the autumn of 1888.[241] At this stage Reginald was at Cambridge and there is no record of his further involvement.

HORTICULTURAL SOCIETY

There was a flourishing horticultural society in St Ives and an annual show took place in the 1870s and 1880s on a Thursday each July. The first

---

237 Flanagan, Bridget, *Artists along the Ouse.*

238 Handwritten notes of an address given to the Angling Society after 46 years' service by the

239 Norris Museum Newspaper Cuttings book 22.06.89.

240 *Hunts County Guardian* 30.04.98

241 Norris Museum press cuttings 1796–1914.

show started in 1876 when Reginald was seven but was limited to St Ives residents and offered cash prizes, the top award being 10s (£63). Most of the prizes were two or three shillings (£12–19) which was a handsome prize for a working man. Next year the show was opened up to nearby villages. The shows took place either on a public space like the tennis ground, or on land supplied by a patron such as Henry Goodman in 1883, who was Mayor that year and allowed a field that he owned in Needingworth Road to be used. James Hankin, who was the Secretary of the St Ives Branch of the National Skating Association, was the show's Treasurer for some years.

By the time of the fifth show in 1880 the open classes for roses section had achieved national recognition, and entrants from around England competed for a massive prize of £5 (£634) for 24 distinct varieties of roses. As there was no similar show at Huntingdon, the St Ives show was effectively recognised as the county show. There were stalls in large tents displaying a vast range of flower, fruit and vegetable exhibits, including grapes, melons and peaches grown under glass. The 1883 show had over 500 exhibits including singing birds – canaries, goldfinches, bullfinches, linnets, blackbirds and thrushes. At the 1879 show the band of the Volunteers played, no doubt arranged through Reginald's father (see Chapter 10).

The show dominated the town with bunting hung, and businesses closed for the afternoon. Special trains were laid on to bring visitors to the attraction, as well as take them home after the evening ended at 11.00pm. Dr Grove was one of the members of the General Committee which ran the show with 22 others – men from the town but also from surrounding villages like Earith, Bluntisham, Holywell, Houghton, the Hemingfords and Fenstanton. In total there were 46 officials who took part. The judges were ordinary men for the 1888 show appointed as they knew about the products being exhibited; 'Messrs Ingram of Huntingdon; Thomas Tilbrooke, gardener to Mr Bateman Brown; Hopkins, gardener to Lord de Ramsey; Meyers, gardener to the Earl of Sandwich; T. Smith, gardener to Miss Cheere from Papworth Hall and R. Hobday'.[242]

For the 1888 show there was a brass band (the Rushden Temperance Silver Prize Band) that played 'a capital selection of music with their performances being greatly appreciated'.[243] On this occasion there was also entertainment provided by the 'Celebrated Yokohana Troupe' with a flying

242 *Hunts Guardian* 21.07.88.

243 *Hunts Guardian* 21.07.88.

trapeze, juggling and balancing feats on a high wire and trick cycling feats. 'The addition to the usual bill of fare occasioned much congratulatory comment', the local newspaper said. Dancing in the evening, admission 6d (£3), lit by Chinese lanterns, and a fireworks display finished off the evening.

These flower shows were quintessential English occasions bringing townsfolk and villagers together.[244]

[244] http://allotmentheaven.blogspot.com/2012/07/st-ives-flower-show-from-1876.html (18.11.19)

CHAPTER 5

Family and Friends

'your affectionate Grandmother M. G. Grove'

Georgiana Grove, née Barnes, in a letter to Reginald, 1886

Reginald's family on both his mother's and his father's side were close and they kept in contact with frequent letters, birthday presents and visits. His mother's parents had both died before he could really know them – Grandfather Long in 1873, and Grandmother Long three years later when Reginald was seven years old. But his mother's Long brothers and sisters and their children were numerous, and Reginald's visits to them are described in a later chapter. They all lived on the Cambridge/Suffolk border and were farmers.

On his father's side it was a very different story. His father only had a younger brother, Francis (or 'Uncle Frank' to Reginald), and he was unmarried until late in life and had no children. Reginald had no Grove first cousins. His father's mother, Mary Georgiana (née Barnes), was widowed when her two sons were very young, so Reginald never knew his Grove grandfather, a draper from Staffordshire. His grandmother's family were pawnbrokers from the same county.

So Reginald's father's family were from the Midlands, and were in 'trade', and his mother's family were tenant farmers from East Anglia.

MAMA AND PAPA (MATER AND PATER)

In his early diaries Reginald called his parents 'Mama and Papa' which was the term used by all middle-class children; in the fifth form at school, when he was 15, they became 'Mater and Pater',[245] a term used by young adults.[246]

His mother spoke with a Suffolk accent; his father with a Midland one. His mother was six years younger than his father.[247] Both parents were

245 This means 'Mother' and 'Father' in Latin and was a term commonly used by young adults.

246 Diary 04.07.84.

247 William Richard Grove was born in 1838, and Maria Elizabeth Long in 1844.

quite short – his father was about five feet tall, and his mother a couple of inches taller.[248] The only portraits that have survived show them in middle age, with both having put on some weight. Reginald's father wears a full beard which was fashionable until the end of the century. When the young doctor courted the farmer's daughter who became his wife he could well have sported long, combed sideburns which were nicknamed 'Piccadilly Weepers' or 'Dundrearies'.[249]

Gwen Raverat was a child in the 1880s and grew up in Cambridge in a middle-class family like the Groves'. Her father was a don, who also had a full beard and smoked, as did Dr Grove. In her early childhood she remembered she was 'much confused' because his beard and the tobacco he smoked seemed to be exactly the same colour and texture. She thought that perhaps he smoked his own moustache, but that because his hair was darker this made for darker kind of tobacco. Did Reginald ever think the same?[250]

His parents made great financial sacrifices to educate Reginald and his brothers and sister privately; after schooling, they funded Reginald's university and medical training as well as Edward's training as a civil engineer and Richard's as an architect.

Birthdays in the Grove family were always remembered with cards and gifts; as Reginald's birthday in January was always before he went back to Uppingham after the Christmas holidays, a family celebration was held. Their birthday present to him on his 13th birthday was a book of Shakespeare's poems, and on his 14th two more books – a Greek New Testament and Defoe's *Robinson Crusoe.* On his 15th birthday he was given a gold set of collar studs (and a set of shelves for his study at school), and the next year a pair of rather stylish pince-nez glasses. He was away with his uncle and aunt at their farm in Shippea Hill on his 17th birthday,

---

[248] From a family photo taken in 1893/94 (Grove Family Archive).

[249] In the 1830s and 40s the fashion was for the clean-shaven look as seen in early photos of Dickens, Disraeli and Ruskin. By 1860s the fashion had changed to facial hair with beards being the norm, starting with sideburns in the '40s broadening to fully fledged side-whiskers, which were sometimes called 'mutton chops'. Long, combed sideburns were also called 'Piccadilly weepers' or 'Dundrearies' (after a dim-witted character in a play by Tom Taylor). Dr Grove may well have had this style when he went to St Ives as a young doctor. Gradually the fashion changed and beards eventually met under the chin by the early 1850s. This style became the 'Newgate frill' or 'chinstrap', so that the neck and jaw were hairy while the rest of the face was clean-shaven. But the stampede for a full beard was sparked off by the Crimean War in the 1850s when British officers were allowed to wear beards. Beards then became the mark of a manly hero.

[250] Raverat, chapter 1.

but his mother gave him a copy of Tennyson's work, and his father a silver pencil case. In 1887 on his 18th birthday he went with them both to a tea at the workhouse where the children put on a singing entertainment in his honour, and some of the old ladies pulled his leg. His present from his parents was a dressing case with a pair of razors. He was becoming a man.

He always sent them a present for their birthdays as these occurred during term-time at school. For her birthday in 1886[251] he bought his mother a copy of Longfellow's poems, from Hawthorn's, the bookshop in Uppingham, for example.

From his diaries it is clear that his relationship with his parents was an affectionate but respectful one. Letter writing at school to his mother was at least weekly, and with her letters to him, she often sent copies of the local newspapers which he liked to read. When he was at King's Choir School she frequently visited him, sometimes with his father, to take him out for a meal or listen to him sing in the choir. When he caught German measles at Easter 1883, she came bearing gifts of jelly, sponge cake and oranges to cheer him up. Both parents attended the choir festivals held twice a year at King's in which he sang and encouraged him in his choral music. Hampers sent by her to him at King's and Uppingham were always well received!

She was keen to make sure he learnt to dance as he approached adulthood. As described in a later chapter, he went through acute embarrassment in the Christmas holidays when he was nearly 17. He and others had been invited for tea and supper by the Copley family, and afterwards there was an impromptu dance, but Reginald refused to take part. He felt hugely embarrassed.

His mother took matters in hand and arranged dancing lessons for him during the Christmas holidays of 1886 with a Mrs Barley who held lessons for 24 young people. After initial difficulties, it was a great success for Reginald and he was glad of her pushing him, as 'instead of disliking dancing I now enjoy it very much'.

As explained in Volume 2, discipline during his childhood at home and at school was firm; in his early years his mother had this responsibility which passed to his schoolmasters during term-time, and then to his father during holidays as he grew older. At home he was never caned. At the fore seemed to be the advice given by Revd T. V. Moore in his piece in *The British Mothers' Journal* on 'The Family as Government', that 'the great

[251] 13 October. It was his mother's 42nd birthday.

agent in executing family law is love'.[252] The recollection of Mary Denison, of her father, a vicar, when she was brought up in the 1900s may well have been Reginald's and his siblings' experience:

> All he did was to talk to me in a quiet voice, but it was far worse than any punishment. In two minutes or less you were in tears – unless you tried to keep them back. You wished so much not to be naughty, not to give trouble to mother.[253]

Occasionally his father was a little tetchy but that might have been as a result of lack of sleep from a patient emergency call out the night before. Before he left school, his father's health was affected by the onset of illness which lasted until his death in 1895.

In his 17th and 18th years, when in the Sixth Form at Uppingham, he received a number of 'jaws' from his father, which was the expression used then for a serious parental talk – mainly about school work, his examinations and his career in medicine. His mother also spoke to him at the end of the 1886 Christmas holidays to tell him he was spending too much time with his sweetheart, Mary Long, to the detriment of his schoolwork. To be fair, their meeting was clouded by the fact that his mother was not feeling well, as she had a bad cold and headache, and remained in bed all day when she asked to have a private word with him in her bedroom. Being told that he was spending a lot of time with Mary and 'always went everywhere where she did' mortified him. But he took the admonishment on the chin.

From the reports in the local newspapers at his death in 1895, Dr Grove was a kind and compassionate man seeking to serve his community and be a good husband and father.

> He was very highly esteemed amongst all circles in the town, and he took a deep and practical interest in everything concerning the welfare of the borough; indeed, he will be sadly missed and especially will his loss be felt by the poorer classes.[254]

Reginald was to follow in his footsteps.

---

252 Moore, T. V., *British Mothers' Journal* May 1856, p. 99, cited by Flanders, Judith, p. 34.

253 Burnett, John, *Destiny Obscure: Autobiographies of Childhood, Education and Family from the 1820s to the 1920s*, p. 36, citing Mary Denison's *Church Bells and Tram Cars: A Vicarage Childhood.*

254 *Hunts County News* December 1895.

GRANDMOTHER GROVE

Georgiana Grove

Reginald never knew his paternal grandfather, William Grove,[255] who died in 1841. At the time of his death when he was only 31 he lived in Lane End, Uttoxeter,[256] Staffordshire, and had a draper's shop. He had married the beautiful Mary Georgiana Barnes in 1837 by licence[257] in the parish church of Uttoxeter. Their witnesses were Thomas Griffin, Louisa Williams Barnes and Joseph Barnes. Louisa was her sister and Joseph was her grandfather, as her father had died just before the marriage. Her father had been a pawnbroker and on his death, his wife, Susannah, Georgiana's mother, took over running it. The Barnes family were well known in Uttoxeter and various members of the family lay buried in the churchyard.[258]

Early in 1841, William's young 24-year-old wife, Georgiana, as she liked to be called, was left with two young sons, three-year-old William Richard, and two-year-old Joseph Francis. It was a huge tragedy, but not uncommon in this period, as life expectancy was low and disease prevalent (see Volume 3). She had been married just three years. Her portrait, painted before her marriage, shows a graceful young woman, with hair parted in the middle and looped coils of long hair on each side of her head, in the style of the 1840s. She never remarried and struggled to bring up her children on her own, not able to run her husband's shop.

Her mother Susannah had continued to run the pawnbroking business and moved in to live with her daughter; they then ran the pawnbroking business together and Georgiana managed to support her two sons at the local grammar school. For the next 30 years after he died she lived at Carter Street, Uttoxeter, running the business and supporting herself and her family. Her eldest son, Richard, Reginald's father, left home to train for a medical career, and Frank stayed at home to become a solicitor through

255 William Grove (1810–41).

256 Lane End and Loughton was a market town and part of the Potteries on the outskirts of Stoke-on-Trent. In 1851 it had a population of 15,000.

257 Some couples preferred not to have their 'banns' (or intention to marry) announced in public at their parish church. They could obtain a special licence, instead. One of the reasons for privacy was because of a difference in social standing. This may have been the reason – pawnbroking may have been looked down upon by the Grove family, although they were drapers and hosiers.

258 Notes made by Sylvia and Beryl Grove (cousins) from parish records on visits to Uttoxeter in 1976. Grove Family Archive.

being articled as a clerk to a local lawyer.[259]

By the mid-1860s Frank had qualified, was single, and worked in a law firm in chambers in the centre of Birmingham. In the late-1870s he moved to Kingston upon Thames, Surrey, and his mother, who was now in her sixties, left the business and went to live with him there until 1881. It may have been while they were living there that Frank met his future wife, Anna Putt, who ran a girls' school only ten miles away in Ealing, West London.

Frank moved in 1881/82 to Brixham, Devon, to a warmer clime on the south coast due to his poor health as he had some form of tuberculosis. His accommodation at 16 Fore Street was very modest, and he lived as a bachelor lodger above a shop run by a pharmacist. It does not appear that his mother moved with him, as Reginald noted in his 1882 diary that her address was c/o of a Mrs Mahone, at Claremont House in Hunstanton St Edmunds (as the seaside town was then known). This was probably a guest house where she went to reflect on where she wanted to live now that she and Frank had parted. Why she did not move with him is not known, but it was either because he could not afford to rent a suitable house for them both, or possibly because they fell out, as she did not approve of Anna Putt. It is noticeable that Frank married within a year of his mother's death which indicates it was only then that he felt free to do so.

At some point Georgiana moved to the south coast to live in Southsea, near Portsmouth. She had some relatives of her mother's family there[260],

[259] 1841 National Census: Georgiana was living in Carter Street, Uttoxeter, with her two children and Susannah H. Barnes (aged 55, her mother). In the 1851 Census she was living at the same address, with Frank (Francis) and a servant, her mother having died. In the 1861 Census the situation was the same although by now Frank was a solicitor's general clerk. A Susanna Clotilda Hinds, aged 23, was a boarder living there whose rent supplemented the family income. Interestingly, she was born in Barbados, West Indies, in 1837. From baptismal records from St Andrews Church, Barbados, 20 August 1838, her father was Cudjoe Hinds, an 'appointed labourer', and her mother Elizabeth. Virtually all the other fathers listed were also shown as appointed labourers, a term used for ex-slaves who worked on the sugar plantations. Susanna married Revd Arthur Vaughan in 1861 at St Mary the Virgin, Uttoxeter. She and her husband and six children lived in Lambley on the Cumberland/Northumberland border where he was the vicar. She was still at the same address in 1871; Frank had moved out and Georgiana had a lodger and servant living with her. At the time of the 1881 Census she had moved to be with Frank in Kingston upon Thames, Surrey.

[260] Her nephew, J. J. Staynes lived there with his wife at St Davids, Kingston Crescent, Landport. This is the only information found about them from Georgiana Groves' death certificate and that of Uncle Frank who died 18 months later. It would seem that Georgiana had a sister who married a 'Staynes' but no Census or other records have been found to throw further light on this.

and by now in her mid-sixties her health may well have been poor. A further attraction to Southsea was that one of her son's previous Medical Assistants, Dr B. J. Guillemard, was in practice there. He was the son of a well-known doctor in Cambridge whom Reginald's father knew. Guillemard also became a mentor to Reginald, writing to him frequently at school. This was when he was at St Ives, as well as after he left, giving advice about a career in medicine. By the time he finished his practical training at a general practice, he had become a family friend. Guillemard established his own practice in Southsea, at 22 South Parade, in the 1880s. Georgiana knew him from her visits to St Ives and trusted him both professionally and as a family friend. Her move to Southsea may well have been because of the medical care he could provide as she became infirm. If she was living with her nephew and niece in Landport, Portsea, then his surgery was only just over 3 miles way.

She was still able to visit Frank in Brixham, but stayed at a guest house when she did. During Reginald's boyhood she frequently wrote to him and generally remembered his birthday, although her finances did not stretch to presents, apart from a copy of *Tom Brown's School Days* on his 13th birthday. After her death she left him a diamond pin that belonged to Reginald's grandfather, which he was given by his father at Christmas 1886.

The correspondence from her that survived is three letters written from Brixham in February and March 1885 and July 1886 to Reginald. Signed 'your affectionate Grandmother M. G. Grove', they are in the Grove Family Archive. Her swirling copperplate handwriting is difficult to read, but the letters clearly express her affection for him. In one she complained that Ernest and his brothers never wrote to her or Uncle Frank and said rather dryly that 'she hoped they were better employed'.[261] Reginald noted receiving two of them in his diary but did not comment further. In one of March 1886 she mentioned reading in *The Daily Telegraph* about some Uppingham boys finding the body of a vagrant in a derelict house in the nearby village of Glaston. She hoped her grandson wasn't one of them. He wasn't but it didn't stop him and two friends taking a morbid look at the spot, as described in Volume 2!

In the same letter she mentioned Uncle Frank's involvement with the Conservatives in the Torquay constituency. That year the Conservative

[261] Letter to Reginald 25.02.85.

candidate, Richard Mallock, was defeated by the Liberal, Sir Lewis McIver. Uncle Frank supported the Tory, and was involved in the election the following year when Mallock overturned the 348 majority, winning by 80 votes. Uncle Frank went to Torquay for the declaration of the result and stayed overnight. Grandma signed off her letter by saying: 'I must say goodnight for the rest of the household is gone to bed, with kindest love which Uncle Frank would join if he had been here'.[262]

Her last letter to Reginald was written in July 1886; two months later she died in Landport aged 70 at the home of her nephew and niece, the Staynes. Tragically, she died a painful death over a two-week period from blocked intestines. Thankfully, her niece was at her bedside when she died. A Dr Way issued her death certificate; whether he was an associate of Guillemard is not known.

But Bernard Guillemard, with Uncle Frank, Reginald, and Dr Grove attended her funeral. There is no record of her will so it is likely that she died with little to leave her sons, apart perhaps from her portrait which passed to her eldest son, Dr Grove, and then to Reginald, then to his son David, and then to his son John, Reginald's grandson.

After Christmas that year, Uncle Frank sent Reginald a photograph of her which has not survived.

UNCLE FRANK

Reginald's Uncle Frank was a couple of year's younger than his father and was single for most of his life. Trained as a solicitor, he moved jobs and towns at least four times during his life from Uttoxeter where he was articled, to where he practised at the Atlas Chambers, in Paradise Road, Birmingham.[263] The city was adynamic thriving commercial and industrial centre, which grew in prosperity through the 19th century and was known as 'the city of a thousand trades'.[264] During this period, Joseph Chamberlain was Mayor from 1873–1876 and under his leadership, Birmingham was transformed, as the council introduced one of the most ambitious

---

[262] Letter to Reginald 13.07.86.

[263] Kelly's *Birmingham Commercial Directory* 1876

[264] For most of the 19th century, industry in Birmingham was dominated by small workshops rather than large factories or mills. These made a wide variety of goods such as buttons, cutlery, nails and screws, guns, tools, jewellery, toys, locks, and ornaments.

improvement schemes outside London. [265] It was an obvious choice for an ambitious young lawyer as commercial legal work grew as the city itself grew. In the centre, where he had chambers a new thoroughfare was constructed in Corporation Street which became a fashionable shopping street. Chamberlain also was behind the building of the Council House and the Victoria Law Courts in Corporation Street where Frank represented clients. While practicing in Birmingham he lived at two addresses[266] until he moved south to Kingston on Thames, in Surrey in the late 1870's.[267]. It was at this stage that his mother joined him.[268] A further move later took place to Brixham in Devon and after his marriage to Southsea[269]. As already mentioned his last move may have been due to ill health due to tuberculous or consumption as it was known to the Victorians.

Shortly before he got married in the summer of 1887 a fire burnt his office down in Brixham. He was living at 16 Fore Street, which was a row of Victorian shops which led down to the harbour. It was a modest address for a solicitor. At No 14 was a paperhanger, at No 18 a draper and at No 22 a butcher.[270] Vittory Green, who was a chemist and druggist, lived at No 16,[271] and Frank lodged with him before he got married. No details exist

[265] Birmingham City Council bought the city's gas and water works, and worked to improve the lighting and provide clean drinking water to the city, income from these utilities also provided a healthy income for the council, which was re-invested into the city to provide new amenities. Under Chamberlain, some of Birmingham's worst slums were cleared

[266] In 1873 he lived at 88, Bennett's Hill, Birmingham which was an apartment in an impressive four storied terrace in the centre of the city and then by 1876 he was staying at The Oaks, St Paul's Road, in Balsall Heath, Birmingham. This house has since been demolished.

[267] Kelly's *Directory for Birmingham* 1873, p. 398, and 1876.

[268] He and his mother lived at Rose Cottage, Adelaide Road, Kingston-on Thames, Surrey (although in the Kingston Electoral Register of 1881, it is listed as 'Ross' Cottage). The road is now in Surbiton and within 5 minutes' walk of Surbiton Station built in 1838 which Frank would have used to travel in to London. The road was a mix of housing- there were large Victorian villas with names like 'Moray House', 'Adelaide Lodge', 'Woodlands', and 'Landsdowne House'. There were three cottages: 'Rose', 'Harescomb', and 'Nightingale'. These cottages have ow been demolished but some of the large Victorian villas remain. The fact that Frank lived in a small cottage, with his mother and one domestic servant, while surrounded by the prosperity of others in large detached residences, point towards his modest financial state.

[269] Kelly's *Birmingham Directory* 1876, *The London Gazette*, Kingston 1880 *London City Directory*, Brixham 1881 (The Lodge of True Love and Unity Brixham Lodge), Brixham 1887 (marriage) and Southsea 1889 (Probate Record).

[270] *Kelly's Directory* (Devon) 1889, p. 82.

[271] The ground floor of No 16 is now a Co-operative store and Fore Street is a pedestrianised street.

of where his office was or the damage by the fire, but it must have hit his business badly and been a huge blow to his marriage plans.

He was a bachelor most of his life, living with his mother, and met Anna Putt late in life. She ran a small, private school for girls in Ealing, West London. When they married in June 1888 he was 48 and she was 41, and he died two years later when they were living in Southsea. They had no children and Anna lived for another 50 years. She probably went back to running a school but she remained in contact with the Grove family for some years with Reginald staying with her as a lodger for a short while when he was carrying his medical training in London as described in Volume 3.[272]

Frank only left £90 (£11,412) to his wife. Six years after he died, his elder brother, having educated all his children privately, left £3,943 4s 10d (£500,026). Both were men in the respected and well-paid professions of law and medicine.

What had happened to Frank's legal career? Perhaps he was not very accomplished as a solicitor; or he made investment mistakes. Or perhaps his business never recovered from the fire. But the most likely reason is that increasing ill health hampered him. Writing to Reginald in 1886, his mother said that Frank was 'never strong'.[273] After he and his new wife moved to Southsea, their doctor became Bernard Guillemard. Frank died when he was only 49. For four days before he died he suffered from pleurisy and congestion of his liver, but the reality was that he died of congestion of the lungs.[274] A cousin on his mother's side, W. J. Haynes, was at his bedside when he died, as was his wife, Anna.

Sadly, ill health plagued him throughout his life and led to an early death.

Reginald's diaries for 1888 and 1889 have not survived so there is no evidence that he was at Uncle Frank's funeral, but in view of their friendship, it is inconceivable that he wasn't there to pay his respects.

Uncle Frank was one of Reginald's godparents and first saw his nephew at the christening held at All Saints, St Ives, in February 1869 when Reginald was a few weeks old. Seventeen years later he brought Reginald a christening

---

[272] In 1891, the National Census recorded that she was visiting a couple called Fletcher who lived at 21, Lamps Road, Southsea. Nothing further is know about her after this.

[273] Letter to Reginald 11.03.86.

[274] Death certificate dated 09.01.89 signed by B. Guillemard M.D.

mug engraved with the newly acquired monogrammed family crest on it!

Frank was a regular guest at Slepe House; on one occasion Frank travelled with his brother to Birmingham for a couple of days. Was this something to do with Frank's previous work in Birmingham? The brothers returned and Uncle Frank stayed on, went for a Sunday afternoon walk with Reginald, and then spent time fishing. They caught two perch. Nephew and uncle clearly got on well.

Frank kept a keen interest in Reginald throughout his boyhood, writing to him, and sending him money[275] or an unexpected gift like a 'jolly card case' when he came to stay with the family in the summer holidays.

Only two letters have survived from Uncle Frank to Reginald, the first written in January 1885 when he sent Reginald some autographs, some of which he thought were 'quite interesting'.[276] Reginald was collecting autographs as a hobby at the time. The other letter was written a year later 'in haste' just before his 18th birthday as 'an expression of my [unclear writing] joy at your success', having just heard about him gaining a scholarship to Sidney Sussex, Cambridge, in January 1887. He asked Reginald to congratulate Ernest for making a model ship, and recommended he got hold of some 'fine cord' used for fishing roach, for the rigging. Reginald received the letter the day after it was written, which is a good example of the efficiency of the Victorian postal service. He'd also written a couple of days before, sending him a photograph of Grandma Grove, some tools for Ernest and 'other things for other members of the family'. That letter did not survive but the tools must have been to help Ernest in his model boat making.

Uncle Frank, Reginald noted from his letters, 'was smit' with Anna Putt. As the wedding was held down in Devon during the last few days of term, Reginald could not be there. Uncle Frank wanted him to visit the couple in the summer holidays to compensate. His father and mother went down by train to Paignton where the marriage took place at the ancient parish church one Saturday in early June 1887. He drank the couple's toast in tea at teatime when the wedding breakfast was taking place. He nearly forgot to do this, as he was very busy entertaining a group of important visitors to Uppingham, as described in Volume 2.

---

[275] Uncle Frank sent 5/- (£31.00) out of the blue in October 1882 when he was 13, and Reginald went out and bought a book with the money.

[276] Letter from Uncle Frank 22.01.85.

Hot from the press, the next day, Sunday, he had a letter from another guest at the wedding, Miss Mayhew, who had travelled down with his parents, to tell him about the festivities. Two days later a photograph of the newly married Mr and Mrs Grove arrived. Sadly, this photograph has not survived and there is no record of what Frank or Anna looked like.

But what has survived is the little white card, with a silver border, sent to Reginald to announce that the wedding had taken place.[277] It was customary with Victorian weddings for the bridesmaids to go to the bride's father's house the day after the wedding to arrange for the new couple's wedding cards to be sent out. The groom supplied these before the ceremony and were folded cards with his name on the left-hand fold, on the right-hand one the words 'with Mr & Mrs J. F. Grove's compliments', and her name on a separate card insert. As the couple were older than most in getting married, it is not known whether Anna had bridesmaids; if not, someone else would have been designated for this responsibility. Both groom and bride would have left a list of those to receive these cards, one of whom was his nephew and godson. Whether Reginald visited them that summer is not known.

The couple moved to Southsea and when Frank died 18 months after their marriage they were living at 2 Victoria Gardens, 24 Victoria Road.[278]

As mentioned earlier, his cousin was at his bedside, just as his wife had been at Frank's mother's death nearby, 18 months' previously.

Very little about Anna Grove's life after her husband's death is known. She kept in contact with Reginald as he mentioned getting letters from her when he was at Sidney Sussex, Cambridge. At some stage she moved back to live in London, perhaps earning a living by teaching again. While he was training to become a doctor at Guy's Hospital in London in the early 1890s she was living in Newington, near the Oval Cricket Ground and he lodged with her for a short time on the second floor at 27, St Agnes Place in 1894 in a single, furnished room where he had the use of the sitting room[279]. There were no other lodgers. This was a house in a three storied terrace which was a typical development of the period in what were then

[277] Grove Family Archive.

[278] This was a three-storeyed, substantial, semi-detached house which still stands today. Given the amount left in his will, it is likely they rented part of this house, rather than the whole house.

[279] Electoral Register, Southwark, Newington West 1894.

the suburbs of south London.[280] All his lodgings when he was in London were in the same vicinity in south London, which was an easy journey of less than two miles to Guy's. His fiancée, Hilda Stevenson also lived nearby in Brixton until they married three years later.

What happened to Anna after this is not known.

REGINALD'S SIBLINGS

Brothers Ernie, Ted and Tom, and his sister Mabel

Reginald was the eldest in the family and was closest to his brother Ernest, who was a year younger. Ernest was a self-assured and adventurous boy who was allowed by his parents, when he was only 11, to travel by train to Cambridge to meet Reginald at school at the start of his Christmas holiday, and travel back with him. His second brother was Edward ('Ted'), three years younger, and then Richard (or 'Tom', as the family called him, after his middle name). The gap with Tom was five years. All the siblings seem to get on well and as they grew older, take part in the same holiday activities like messing about in boats in the summer and skating in the winter.

Regular letter-writing wasn't a chore but an enjoyable way of keeping in touch with one another; equally, letters were exchanged with the Long cousins who were their age and whom they met up with during the holidays, either going to stay on the farms where they lived, or the cousins coming to stay with the Groves.

The two younger boys went off to boarding school, initially small, private schools to prepare them for entry to public school. Across the country there were numerous such schools which proliferated throughout the second half of the 19th century, catering for the educational needs of the children of the growing middle class. Uncle Frank's wife ran such a school for young ladies in Ealing, West London, as an example. As already seen, St Ives had several schools and this was replicated in towns and cities throughout England. No academic or professional qualifications were

[280] An interesting footnote to the later history of this property, which Anna Grove rented, was that St Agnes Place became a 'squatted' street in the latter part of the 20th century which resisted eviction orders for more than 30 years. When a number of derelict houses were scheduled for demolition to extend Kennington Park in 1969, squatters occupied the properties and a High Court injunction prevented the demolition. The street was run by a housing cooperative until 2005, when Lambeth London Borough Council obtained an eviction order. The street was demolished in 2007. (https://en.wikipedia.org/wiki/St_Agnes_Place 15.1020)

needed to open a school, although many were run by clergymen and no teaching qualifications for the staff were needed. Aged 23, Vincent van Gogh, after being sacked from his sales job in an art dealer's in 1876, promptly got a job teaching at a boys' school in Margate. The Headmaster moved the school to Isleworth, a village by the Thames, near Richmond, Surrey. Van Gogh moved with him.[281] In his letters to his brother, Van Gogh described his life at this type of school.

Reginald never mentioned if he had been at a boarding school before he went to King's Choir School, but as he was ten when he went it is unlikely. Before his brothers got into the King's School, Ely, they did as Reginald made a note of their addresses in his diary so he could write to them. In 1881 Ernest was at a school in West London run by a Revd T. Wood, but won a scholarship that autumn to King's, Ely, when he was 12, having tried unsuccessfully to become a chorister at King's Choir School, Cambridge. He was put in Hereward Hall[282] which had been opened earlier that year. That term, he joined the Literary Society,[283] a debating society, perhaps encouraging Reginald to join a similar society when he went to Uppingham.

Ted was at a school in Paddington, West London when his older brother went to King's Ely. Reginald wrote in his diary that their mother took him for his first term in September 1881. But in September 1884, aged 10 he also joined King's School, Ely as a King's Scholar like his brother.

Reginald visited his brother's school when he was home and his holiday did not clash with theirs. He went to their Sports Days and Christmas Entertainments with his parents to see them when he was at home. For instance, in December 1886 he went to see his cousin Dick Long, who was also at King's, perform in the 'Sorcerer; which was the school Christmas drama production. His brothers were also in the cast. His brother Ted

---

[281] Van Gogh's first school was in Ramsgate run by a Mr Stokes. Stokes later moved his school to the village of Isleworth, and van Gogh moved with him in late-June to Linkfield House at 183 Twickenham Road. Unfortunately, Mr Stokes did not keep his promise to pay van Gogh a salary after a month's trial, so he left and joined another school down the road at Holme Court, 158 Twickenham Road, run by a 47-year-old Congregational Minister, Revd Thomas Slade-Jones. He was paid a salary of £15 p.a. (£1,900) plus board and lodging.

[282] Hereward Hall was the first purpose boarding house of the School and the first outside the College, the Cathedral precinct. It was built with government grant assistance when the school separated as an entity from the Cathedral and provided much needed additional accommodation. (email from Elizabeth Stazicker, School Archivist 04.10.20.)

[283] The Elean School Magazine, December 1881.

played the prima donna ('looked an awful good girl'!) and Ernest was in the chorus. Their mother, father and sister Mabel were there too, having stayed overnight at the old coaching inn, 'The Lamb' in Ely. Reginald was very pleased to sit next to Mary, his sweetheart, throughout the evening. She went to see her brother.

In Dr Grove's view, the school was an excellent one. At the Speech Day held in July 1883, he seconded a vote of thanks by Revd Canon Luckock's to the masters by speaking of 'the kindly feeling which existed between the boys and the assistant masters'.[284] Six years later, when Ernest had moved on to train for the army at Woolwich College, and Ted was still at King's, at the Speech Day in seconding a vote of thanks for the donors of prizes he said that

> he listened with pleasure to the report by the Headmaster, and expressed the hope that the teaching of Classics, which had gained such distinction in that School, would always maintain its excellence. He was glad to see that the laboratory was an established fact. He hoped the boys would not forget that it was not merely by their own exertion that they had won prizes but that it was greatly owing to the excellent teaching they had received (applause). He hoped there would be a special prize for chemistry next year.[285]

Ted trained as a civil engineer after leaving, sharing lodgings with Reginald when both were living in London in 1891, as described in Volume 3.

Mabel, the only girl among four brothers, remained at home while they went off to school until she went to a small boarding school herself at 'St Leonards' when she was 15. It is not clear whether this was St Leonards-on-Sea in Sussex or near her Uncle James and Aunt Louise at St Leonard's, in Bow and Bromley, Middlesex. Small boarding schools for ladies were common in most towns, as the number in St Ives demonstrated.

She regularly wrote to Reginald, and when she was at that school sent Reginald a small box of flowers for his study at school. In April the following year she was taken by her father to another boarding school in Kensington, the address of which Reginald never noted in his diary. On completing her education, she remained at home helping out.

However, it seems that she may have developed a rebellious spirit in her

---

[284] Ibid December 1883.

[285] Ibid December 1889.

late teens as a letter written by Ernest in 1890 when he was out in India to Reginald expressed his concerns.

> Has Mabel given up the idea of hospital nursing? I hope she will, I don't think it is all her run of life. It might do her good and it might do her harm but I fancy it would be difficult to find anyone to hold her in check. Then she might get the sack which would do all the harm in the world. Does she give much dick [sic] at home. It seems to me she thinks herself too big a swell for the whole lot of us.[286]

Mabel was 19 at the time and did not take up nursing. She continued living at home, taught in Sunday School at church until she married Revd Bernard Wilder in 1894. He was the Rector of a country church in Suffolk and no doubt they met through her Long relatives nearby. She was 23 years old; he was 27 the same age as Reginald. Her father was able to walk her up the aisle but sadly he died the following year.

There is no record of where Tom went to school but it was neither Uppingham nor King's Ely. He went on to train as an architect, as described in Volume 3.

BEST OF FRIENDS: ARNIE ULPH

Reginald and Arnie ('Arnold')[287] Ulph, who was 18 months older, were good friends and met up at every holiday to play when they were younger and then to row, fish, bike, play football and skate together when they were older.

The Ulph family were prominent shopkeepers in St Ives, and the family business was an ironmongery in Bridge Street. Arnie's grandfather was John Birt Ulph, who was one of newly elected Improvement Commissioners of St Ives in 1847 and acted as Treasurer besides his other civic roles.[288] His son, also John Birt Ulph by name, married to Charlotte, 13 years his junior, lived in Crown Street initially, but by 1871 there were seven children and they had moved to 6 Cromwell Terrace some years before

---

[286] Letter from Ernest to Reginald 30.11.90 (Grove Family Archive).

[287] Arnie joined the family business, lived at home until he married a local girl, Jessie Johnson, in 1892.

[288] Ulph had also been a Trustee of Turnpike Trust which built the arched New Bridges causeway south of the medieval bridge in 1822. He was also a shareholder in a group of Nonconformists who bought land to use as a cemetery to avoid burials being taken by the Vicar in the churchyard of the parish church.

the Groves moved to Slepe House, part of Cromwell Terrace, themselves. The ironmongery business did well. In the 1881 Census Ulph stated that he employed '5 men and 3 youths'.[289] In 1885, when Arnie was too young to help run the business, he took on Mr F. T. Rushton as a junior partner, and the shop became known as Ulph and Rushton,[290] based in Crown Street. Arnie did join the business later as his father's assistant and became a metal valuer. Rushton was to develop the business under his own name eventually. By the time of the First World War, Arnie was still living in Cromwell Terrace, but was 'a collector of district rates and hardware valuer'.[291]

The two families got together in the school holidays for meals and games; in September 1882 when Reginald was 13, for example, he went to tea at the Ulphs and played charades, took part in a play, sang and played music.

They both enjoyed cycling. Arnie had his own cycle which might have because his father was stocking them in his shop; he was happy for Reginald to ride it.

SCHOOL FRIENDS – THE WARREN BOYS

The Warren family were coal merchants and respected and prominent residents of St Ives, and friends of the Groves'. In fact, besides the coal business, Warren also farmed, and in the National Census of 1881 was shown as farming 100 acres and employing 6 men and 21 boys.[292]

Besides Frederic and his wife Anna, there were six children of which two brothers, Frederic and Harold, were friends of Reginald's. Frederic was a year younger than Reginald, and his brother two years younger. They joined Uppingham in January 1884, but were in a different house to Reginald. Frederic left the year after Reginald and went to King's College Cambridge, so was at university with him. They sometimes travelled back from school together with Reginald getting a lift in their pony and trap from Huntingdon to St Ives.

Their father, Frederic Warren, was the business partner of Charles Coote who came from London to take over running the coal business

289 National Census 1881.

290 *St Ives Business Directory* 1885.

291 Kelly's *Directory of Huntingdonshire* (1914), p. 64.

292 National Census 1881.

of the coal and corn[293] in 1873 after Coote died at the early age of 33. Coote had built an imposing house in the grounds of the old monastery, a quarter of a mile from Slepe House, called The Priory,[294] which his partner, Frederic Warren, took on from his widow. He took an active role in local politics, being Mayor in 1881, 1885 and 1890.

Dr and Mrs Grove went to Uppingham for prizegiving in July 1885 and brought with them 16-year-old Kitty (Katherine) Warren, the sister of the Warren brothers. Although she was the same age as Reginald, he never mentioned any attraction between them. Once at Uppingham, Kitty went home with her brothers, and Reginald and his parents made their own way back, spending time looking over Peterborough Cathedral, as described in Volume 2. On another occasion, the boy's father visited Uppingham to see his son Frederic who was ill. He sent Reginald a note while he was staying at the Falcon Inn and invited Reginald to have breakfast with him the next day. Forty-two-year-old Miss Sarah Vardy, the ex-governess of their younger children,[295] was there with Warren and so the three sat down together for a hearty cooked breakfast. She must have been invited to see how two of her charges had turned out.

GEORGE LLOYD AND THE LLOYD FAMILY

George was a good friend of Reginald's, but seven years older. Like the Ulphs and Warrens, the Lloyd family were prominent residents of St Ives.

George wrote frequently to Reginald, and vice versa, throughout his time at Uppingham, often to give him advice about medicine as a career. In February 1887 he wrote a 'very long letter on what work I was to do at Cambridge'. Reginald took it to discuss with Howson, his chemistry teacher, who 'almost before I had read it' was much taken by its contents. As described in Volume 2, Howson's response was that he should have some extra private tuition in physics which he would give him. Reginald had his first tutorial with 'about 8 other fellows' when tea was provided before the session began![296] Lloyd's letter proved insightful as Howson took notes from it so he could help others going to Cambridge as medical students.

---

[293] The firm of Coote and Warren continued in St Ives as a family business until 1944 when it was taken over by Charringtons. (Burn-Murdoch, Bob, *Victorian St Ives* (2007), p. 37.)

[294] The house was bought by St Ives Rural District Council in 1950 and has been used as offices since then.

[295] National Census 1881.

[296] Diary 08.02.87.

Reginald referred to his friend as 'George Lloyd', rather than George, and unfortunately none of the correspondence has survived, but it's clear from Reginald's diary notes that George was a trusted confidant.

George's father (Thomas) was the minister of the Independent Free (Congregational) Church in Market Hill St Ives. The church had been built in 1863–64 under the leadership of Lloyd with the support of leading nonconformist citizens such as Thomas Coote, George Newton Day and Potto Brown. The spire was deliberately constructed to be a few feet higher than the parish church. Lloyd, who was Welsh, was 14 years older than his wife Annie, whom he married when she was 20. They lived on the Quay initially, only a short distance from the Groves in the Bullock Market. They were sufficiently well off to employ a governess for their children, as well as two maids, who all lived in.[297] As one of the local clergy, Lloyd and his family were well known in the town and were firm friends with the Groves.

In 1874, the private school for girls called Slepe Hall in the Ramsey Road went up for sale. The school had its origins in one run on the site of Reginald's second home at Slepe House, Cromwell Terrace. As described in an earlier chapter, the old house had been sold and demolished in 1848 and the Rugeley family, who ran the school, built New Slepe Hall to replace the old one.[298] It stood in three acres of grounds.

In the 1870s the school belonged to a Mrs Marshall, whose daughter Grace ran it before she, in turn, married and moved away in 1874. When Mrs Marshall put the building up for sale in 1877 great interest was apparently shown by the Roman Catholic Church. This led several prominent members of the Independent Free Church to buy Slepe Hall, and they installed Lloyd and his wife to run the school as a private, nonconformist school for girls. Lloyd continued as the Minister of the church, and was described as 'the kindest and best of men', although apparently many who listened to his sermons 'hoped against hope that they would soon come to an end!'[299]

Lloyd had a great interest in missionary work at home and abroad (especially Madagascar), as well as the anti-slavery movement, the temperance movement (which met in the newly built public institution[300]

[297] National Census 1871.

[298] The house still stands and is now a hotel.

[299] Carter, Mary, *19th Century St Ives,* p. 76.

[300] The Public Institution was built by a local, wealthy, non-conformist businessman, Potto Brown and was used for a variety of meetings, including debates.

in Crown Place), the study of science, church history and travel. He also gave practical help to the poor of the town.[301] He had a great concern for the impoverished in St Ives and the surrounding areas, and he persuaded his wealthier friends to buy medical supplies which he could take to the poor whom he visited on his pastoral visits, especially to outlying districts.[302] He kept the medicines in his saddlebags.[303] Did Dr Grove see this as competition to his medical practice? Given Dr Grove's own compassion for the poor and needy, he would have been delighted that they received help at the hands of a Good Samaritan whom he respected. Such was George's father.

For all his long-winded preaching, Lloyd believed in women's education. Innovations were made by him at the school when he began, such as three terms per year instead of two, and they stopped the practice of two girls having to share the same bed.[304] By 1881 there were 19 pupils aged 11–17 who boarded. Lloyd was still the minister of the Free Church, but his wife, Annie effectively ran the school as the head, with their daughters acting as teachers together with a couple of their friends.

With the Lloyd children, three maids completed the household.[305] A number of the pupils were from villages nearby like Swavesey, Willingham, Oakington and Warboys, but others were from further afield – London, Swansea and Hemel Hempstead. But 16-year-old George was away at boarding school himself at Amersham Hall School under the headmastership of Mr West in Caversham.[306] Interestingly, two of his fellow schoolboys were born abroad – one in Natal, South Africa, and the other in Tobago in the

---

[301] Robb, Betty, http://saintives.org.uk/slepe.htm (pupil at Slepe Hall School from 1930 to 1940).

[302] During his ministry Free Church congregations were formed into a union of chapels in Houghton, Hemingford Grey, Woodhurst, Hartford and Godmanchester.

[303] Carter, Mary, *A Remarkable Journey* (2005), p. 35.

[304] Civic Society of St Ives Annual Report 2015.

[305] National Census 1881.

[306] Amersham Hall was a 'school for the sons of dignified gentlemen' in England founded in 1829. By the time George Lloyd was a pupil it was located in Caversham in Oxfordshire (now Berkshire). It now houses the Queen Anne's School, Caversham. The Grey Coat Hospital Foundation took over the buildings in 1894 and Queen Anne's Caversham School was founded. Reginald's daughters went to this school in the period 1910–1925. One of his nieces, Beryl Grove, the daughter of his brother Tom, was a housemistress at the school in during the 1940s to 1960s. (Talbot, Daniel, *The Scarlet Runners,* Third Millennium Publishing Ltd, 2008.)

West Indies.[307] It's possible that his schooldays with these two sons of the Empire may have contributed to George making a career by emigrating to Australia after qualifying as a doctor. Reginald's sister, Mabel, was friendly with Mrs Lloyd, and it was possible that she might have been a day pupil at the school when she was younger. Reginald noted in his diary in the Easter holidays in 1886 that two of Mabel's school friends came to tea at Slepe House as they had been staying at Mrs Lloyd's school.

The school was empty over the holidays, so putting up guests was another way of increasing their income. At the end of that year, Mabel came home from school, arriving on the same train from London with George. After Christmas, Reginald and Mabel went for tea at the Lloyds' and spent an agreeable time playing chess. Their brother, 16-year-old Ernest, went on the same day to one of the daughters ('Miss Lloyd') for the first time to learn French. Which one is not known but it is probable that it was Martha, the eldest, who was later co-principal with her mother. She was a remarkable woman who had studied in France and Germany and taught Anglo-Saxon, as well as being known as a mountaineer.[308] When her mother died on 17 November 1912 Martha ran the school until she retired in 1928.[309] She died in 1943.

Annie and her daughter supported the London Missionary Society and Martha was a director for many years.[310] Lloyd's health deteriorated and he retired from being the Minister of the Free Church in 1883. Some friends took him on holiday to Germany but he died suddenly. He was replaced by Revd Arthur Turberville who was the minister from 1886 to 1890.[311] Annie carried on as the school principal with Martha and five other teachers for the 24 pupils. George no longer was at home but went to study at Cambridge in October 1881, at St John's College. After graduating he went to St Barts Hospital, London. Initially, he did not enjoy living in London as much as Cambridge, and told Reginald how he felt. But he persevered and gained his MB in 1884 and his BChir in 1889.

---

307 National Census 1881

308 Martha was an early member of the Ladies' Alpine Club which was based in London. She was the first woman to climb the Sudlenspitze. https://en.wikipedia.org/wiki/Martha_Lloyd_(principal) 14.05.19.

309 Civic Society of St Ives Annual Report 2015.

310 Her father was the Secretary of the Baptist Missionary Society.

311 Apparently, 20 years later he joined the Church of England. (Mary Carter, *A Remarkable Journey*.)

He went out to Mackay in Queensland[312] on the east coast of Australia in 1890, and was appointed the Medical Officer of Health. Sadly, he died in 1909 aged 45.

HENRY BERRY

Aged 18, and in his last year at school, Reginald and his great friend Henry Berry walked much of the way to their respective homes, rather than take the train at the end of the Easter Term 1887. Reginald always referred to Henry by his surname, as was customary amongst boys at boarding school. When he was 13, Berry had joined the school in January 1882, a year earlier than Reginald. Both were in the same house. He was nine months older[313] than Reginald and was the son of Revd T. M. Berry, the rector whose parish was St Swithun's, Sandy, in Bedfordshire. Berry was the captain of the house, and Reginald was a fellow praepostor in that last year at school. In that year they both sat scholarships at Cambridge – Reginald at Corpus Christi, and Berry at Pembroke College. Berry was successful but Reginald was not.

[312] Eleven years after his death a major public health incident affected the town when a major cyclone and hurricane-force winds caused huge damage and loss of life. Bubonic plague broke out, causing more deaths.

[313] Henry Berry died in 1935, aged 66, having lived in Egypt.

CHAPTER 6

Bob Bensly, Reginald's Best Friend

'Perhaps you will take pity on me and let me have a letter or two these holidays. I find it fearfully dull being in bed all day long.'

Bob Bensly, December 1886

FRIENDS AT KING'S

His best friend from King's College Choir School was Robert (Bob) Bensly,[314] who died aged 17 from a respiratory condition. Their friendship was a close one and his death deeply touched him. Bensly was nine months younger than Reginald, but despite their age difference their friendship grew.

Reginald first mentioned him in June 1882 when two new boys, Radcliffe and Bensly, were 'put up' (i.e. joined) the choir. A few days later Reginald and he sang a duet together. Their friendship began to grow, and during the short school holiday at the end of the month, Bensly sent Reginald a postcard.

Bensly's family lived in Cambridge on Parker's Piece. It was a requirement that all choristers had to board at the school, so, despite living in town, their son was a boarder like Reginald. This may have suited them as a family as they seemed to move quite frequently. They had previously lived in Hastings,[315] and Bensly had been born in Grantchester, near Cambridge, as had a younger brother, William.[316] His elder sister, Louisa, was born in Cambridge. He had an elder brother, too, whom he mentioned in his letters, but nothing more is known about him apart from the fact that he studied in Germany.[317]

His father, Robert Lubbock Bensly, was a skilled Middle East linguist who became Professor of Arabic at the University of Cambridge by the time

[314] His name was spelt 'Bensley' in the National Census records and also by Reginald in his diaries. However, the blackboarded announcement of his death issued by his parents in February 1887 spelt his name 'Bensly'. This spelling has been used in this book.

[315] National Census 1881.

[316] William Bensly went on to become an Assistant Master at King's Choir School from 1898 to 1899. (*A History of King's College Choir School*, R. J. Henderson, p. 127.)

[317] Letter from Robert Bensly 26.08.86.

his son had joined the choir.[318] When the family was living in Hastings, Bensly's father's occupation was listed as 'Hebrew Lecturer'. His mother, Agnes Dorothea, was German (née Von Blomberg) but born in Russia. She became a naturalised British subject later. Robert and Agnes (who was three years younger than her husband) had married in Sachsen, Germany, in 1860. Bensly's middle names were Von Reibnitz[319] to reflect his mother's heritage.

Reginald and Bensly continued to sing in the college choir together; Reginald sang second treble with him in an anthem in August and again in October 1882. Bensly gave Reginald a special birthday present for his 14th birthday the following January – 'a hand painted china jar painted by himself'. Back at school, they went into Cambridge one afternoon and bought a fife, although its use was unclear. Both boys caught measles in March, and while Bensly was sent home Reginald stayed on at school; Reginald received a letter and book from him a few days later, and then Reginald himself was sent home to convalesce.

Their friendship continued during the last two terms at King's in the spring and summer of 1883. Both tried for a scholarship to Marlborough College[320] in Wiltshire in June, and travelled together to take the examinations. Reginald mentioned that the day before he went to see Mrs Bensly in town to talk about travel arrangements. They stayed there for three days sitting various examinations and taking a break in between by exploring nearby Savernake Forest on two of the evenings. This is a 4,500-acre forest near the town of Marlborough. Neither was successful in gaining a scholarship.

Reginald, of course, went to Uppingham, and Bensly gained a place at Haileybury College[321] in Hertfordshire.[322] After they went to different schools they kept in touch through letters.

After his first term at Uppingham, Reginald stayed with his Long family relatives at Carleton Grange, and on the way back home by train after the

---

318 Bensly's father died in 1893, and his mother in 1900.

319 Given in a memorial card printed at his death in the Grove Family Archive.

320 Marlborough College was founded in 1843 by a group of Church of England clergymen with the main aim of educating the sons of clergy. By 1870 the College's reputation both for scholarship and as a forward-looking, Christian boarding school was established. http://www.marlboroughcollege.org/ 12.11.18.

321 Letter from Robert Bensly 19.12.86.

322 Haileybury College was founded in 1862 after the closure of the East India College. By the 1870s it had become well established and had c.500 pupils. (https://www.haileybury.com/24.12.18.) Reginald was to send his eldest son, William Stevenson Grove, there. It may well have been because his best friend had gone there.

New Year he stayed a short time in Cambridge and saw two of his friends – Bob Hudson and Bensly. A couple of days later, after his 15th birthday, he then stayed with the Benslys in Cambridge for a few days, meeting his sister and brothers.

On the invitation of the Vice Provost of King's, Reginald visited the college and school during the summer holidays of 1885, and Bensly joined them for a tricycle ride through the villages of Shelford and Hauxton; in the evening they went to see their old Headmaster, Revd Reynell, and played whist. This was the last time they saw each other.

BENSLY'S ILLNESS

Bensly wrote to him in October 1885[323] from Great Yarmouth to tell him what his plans were for the winter. He apologised for not writing for a year or so, and, although not saying it, this was probably due to his unfolding illness. He mentioned that he hadn't been able to study much over the preceding six months, and said: 'I have had an attack of inflammation of the lungs in [the] spring while at Bournemouth from which I am only now recovering'.

This is the first and only reference made to his illness. With the length of his illness and the fact that he spent many months in warmer climes, he would have died from either tuberculosis or a chronic obstructive pulmonary disease such as chronic bronchitis. With the latter, after the initial infection, the disease lies dormant. It can then be reactivated by a weakened immune system due to other illnesses[324]. This may have been the case with Bensly, as he caught a serious bout of gastric fever lasting three months a year after his illness was first diagnosed. Consumption, as TB was then known, was a virulent and often fatal disease in the 19th and early 20th centuries. Sadly, for such a young man, whatever the nature of his illness, it proved terminal.

In his 1885 diary Reginald gave Bensly's address as being Bournemouth,[325] as well as at Stanton House in Lowestoft, Suffolk. It appears that Bensly's illness may well have become evident earlier in the year and he was moved from Haileybury to a smaller school in Suffolk, perhaps to be near the sea

323 Letter from Robert Bensly 22.10.85.

324 Notes taken by the author from discussions with Dr Jenny Eades MBBS, BSc, DRCOG, MRCGP on pulmonary diseases.

325 The Benslys continued to live in Cambridge but the address at 'Wynchbury', West Cliff, Bournemouth (address shown in Reginald's 1885 diary) could have been a relative's one in which he stayed temporarily; the weather on the south coast was more clement.

so he could benefit from the salt air.

In his letter Bensly said that he had rather wanted to go on a round-the-world voyage, but instead he was going with his mother to Algiers, staying probably until May. He promised that he would write once he got there. Given this exotic North African location,[326] it seems strange that Reginald recorded this news in such a matter-of-fact way. True to his word, Bensly wrote three weeks later[327] from the Hotel Kirsch in the Mustafa district of Algiers. Set on a hill, it overlooked the large bay. Bensly's eight-page graphic letter gave a full account of his travel out to Algeria with his mother. The four-day sea journey from the Port of London to Bordeaux was very rough as they sailed through the Bay of Biscay on the French Atlantic Coast; 16-year-old Bensly thought it great fun, but the seaman called it 'a regular snorter' and it was extremely rough, delaying the trip by an extra day. The SS *Albatross*[328] was a large vessel and had been used as a troopship in the spring to take soldiers out to the Sudan where Britain was involved in the Mahdist War, one of numerous colonial wars of the late-19th century. The ship rode higher in the water than it should have and consequently rolled frequently in the waves.

There were only 12 passengers, mainly ladies, he told Reginald, who 'retired to their cabins rather quickly and uttered most dismal groans from time to time with some Irish ladies even went further and shrieked out for priests to come and attend them'. But he wryly commented that 'as we did not happen to have shipped any their desire could not be gratified'. Bensly said that his mother wasn't among the groaners and, while not well, she spent most of the time on the deck house during the day. What was hardest, he said, was 'dressing, washing and eating as everything not battened down' in their cabin flew all over the place. During mealtimes, the crew tried to make sure the passengers could eat 'but our knife and fork and food were at liberty to dance about as much as they liked which they took advantage of much more often than was pleasant!'

In Bordeaux they spent a couple of days seeing the sights and took the 'Rapide' train[329] to Marseille on the Mediterranean coast. The journey

---

[326] Algeria had been a French colony since 1830.

[327] Letter from Robert Bensly 23.11.85.

[328] The ship's name was given in the letter above.

[329] Run by the railway company, Compagnie des chemins de fer du Midi. Today the train journey takes just under seven hours.

lasted 14 hours. As a sleeper it was rather uncomfortable. They arrived early in the morning to embark on their next vessel to Algeria; Marseille was the second-largest city in France and main port of departure for the French colonies of Algeria, Tunisia and Morocco. The sea journey to Algiers took 36 hours and the bad weather continued in the Gulf of Lion as they sailed across to North Africa. The exotic smells of the 'unadulterated oriental', as Bensly described it, were overpowering. After a couple of days, they moved to a large house in the suburbs up in the hills above the city called the Hotel Kirsch run by a German, as the hotel name suggested. No French guests stayed there probably because the memories of the 1870–71 Franco-Prussian War were still fresh. Other guests were English, so French was not spoken. Bensly had thought that French would be spoken all the time and he would return speaking it fluently. It was not to be.

WINTER IN ALGIERS

There were stunning views over the Bay of Algiers and a horse-drawn bus took guests down to the city every half-hour. Bensly was fascinated by the seething mass of Arabs and Jews dressed in colourful clothes in the market there; many of the former arrived by camel caravan from the interior.

On Boxing Day Bensly wrote to describe his Christmas at the Hotel Kirsch. He'd been grateful for Reginald's two letters since his arrival; the second had been delivered on Christmas Day which was a blessing, as his Christmas 'wasn't a very happy one',[330] as everyone was away from home. He and his mother had been to the English church which was decorated with bright flowers, very different from home, and with sunny, warm weather he missed being able to skate! At the evening meal (soup, fish, roast beef, crawfish, turkey, plum pudding,[331] ices, cheeses, cakes – ten courses in all!) a toast was raised for absent friends. He expected his father, sister and younger brother to come out in the spring. They'd need to take a house rather than stay in the hotel, due to the expense. Reginald received this letter and a New Year's card three days later, so the postal system by boat and rail was fast. Reginald wrote again from Uppingham to his friend in the New Year 1886.

---

330 Letter from Robert Bensly 26.12.85.

331 He said that the 'plum pudding was an awful failure as it came out quite black and spoiled, some people gave up in their attempt to eat it others swallowed it in silence for the honor [sic] of Old England'. A wonderful example of the English stiff upper lip of the English abroad!

Three months later in March 1886 he received another letter[332] from Algiers. Bensly had been severely ill with gastric fever, which had been very debilitating and he had not fully recovered. But his father, sister and brother had by now come out and the family had moved into a rented house, Villa Robert, 100 yards from the hotel. They now employed a French servant to housekeep and cook for them. A remarkable character, Bensly described her as

> rather an earthshaking monster to wait on us, her voice is something terrible in its shrillness and capability of piercing through floors and walls and doors and her weight, well I should just like to know what it is; for all that she cooks very well, beats down Arab vendors of eggs, fish etc as if she had been used to it all her life whereas she has only been in Algiers a little over a year and above she does not eat too much and is quite satisfied with four bottles of wine a week and as the vin ordinaire only costs 4d a bottle that is not likely to ruin us.

With his family together, they met the English expatriate community; many wintered there rather than the South of France to enjoy the warm weather. One mentioned by Bensly was Sir Peter Coats who owned Coats Sewing Cotton.[333]

The Bensly house in Cambridge was now rented out,[334] but the family visit was quite a short one as there was a family wedding to attend. Bensly thought he 'would stay on for a couple of months'. He said that he 'hadn't the least idea of what is going to happen to me next summer. I think one thing is fairly certain and that is that I shan't pass very much of my time at Cambridge but I shall try if possible to be there part of the long vacation.'

RECUPERATION ON THE SOUTH COAST

Reginald wrote back but some time elapsed before Bensly wrote[335] again, this time from a hotel in Penzance, Cornwall. He had sailed in June from Algiers to Marseilles, and then by a luxury[336] P&O[337] steamer en route from

---

332 Letter from Robert Bensly 13.03.86.

333 The company still manufactures sewing thread.

334 Letter from Robert Bensly 01.07.86.

335 Ibid.

336 'Equal to a first-class hotel, we had fresh meat, poultry, bread milk etc every morning.'

337 The Peninsular and Oriental Steam Navigation Company was formed in 1843. It operated mail, passenger and cargo services between the England, Spain and Portugal, Egypt, India, the Far East and Australia. The opening of the Suez Canal in 1869 speeded the voyage considerably to the Far East.

the Far East via Gibraltar to Plymouth. He was well enough to go on an excursion to the Scilly Isles with his mother which he enjoyed and described in some detail, staying overnight on St Mary's, the largest of the islands. He was again uncertain about what would happen to him, but supposed they would stay in Penzance for a few weeks longer. Evidently, he and his mother moved to a hotel in St Ives, Cornwall – the Treginaldenna Castle[338] and the move seemed to have benefited him, as he said that his health had improved considerably – 'the air of St Ives has set me up a bit'. Their house in Cambridge was shut up and his father was living in Caius College. Bensly's illness and how to treat it was causing the family to live separate lives.

A visit to a consultant in London was planned to assess his condition, and he thought he might winter in somewhere like Davos in the Swiss Alps or again in Algiers. In Algiers he had learnt to use a camera and with his letter he sent Reginald a couple of plates showing his handiwork. In fact, the consultant, Dr Bristow, was down in the West Country and saw him at his hotel. He advised staying in a warm climate over the winter in either the South of France or Algiers, and then in the summer, next year, to stay in the Alps.[339]

On 12 September Bensly turned 17.

BACK TO ALGIERS

He sailed with his mother from Falmouth up the Channel and arrived in London before going for some weeks to stay in Harwich on the east coast. They stayed briefly at the Great Eastern Hotel[340] and then moved into lodgings[341] temporarily.[342] Sadly, his health took a turn for the worse, and he was confined to bed while staying in Harwich, but recovered enough to be able to travel by train to Liverpool and from there by ship to Algiers.[343]

Thankfully, this voyage through the Bay of Biscay was without

[338] This large hotel is still operating today. It was built as a private residence in the 18th century, with grounds covering 72 acres, and became a hotel in 1871 leased by the Great Western Railway Company (GWRC) five years before Bob and his mother stayed there.

[339] Letter from Robert Bensly 07.09.86.

[340] This huge hotel was built in 1864 by the Great Eastern Railway Company, dominated the harbour and served as a stepping stone for passengers travelling from London to steamships sailing for the Continent.

[341] 29 Esplanade, Harwich, Essex.

[342] Postcard from Robert Bensly 02.10.86.

[343] Letter from Robert Bensly 19.12.86.

the storms that they experienced the year before. However, his health deteriorated on the voyage 'from want of fresh milk',[344] and writing to Reginald in December he said that

> for the last month I have hardly left my bed although I am a little better it will take a very long time to pick up again all the strength I have lost. Perhaps you will take pity on me and let me have a letter or two these holidays. I find it fearfully dull being in bed all day long.

Weakened by his illness, he could only write with a pencil from his bed. This time, they stayed in a villa about two miles from the city centre with eight other English people. With separate sitting rooms there was one large common room where they ate together. His father and sister came out to join them for what was to be their last Christmas together.

From other contemporary accounts of nursing someone with the disease, it was exhausting. Laura Forster, the daughter of a clergyman, had a brother and sister with consumptive illnesses, and she described in her diary of 1864 a typical routine: 'At 12 [midnight] I gave [her sister] her pill; at three her draughts, at four thirty I made her breakfast; she coughed again at six, but only a little, and soon after I got up and put on her some embrocation'. After her brother's death, some five months after writing this, she said: 'I do not fear death but the valley of the shadow is a weary place to place to live in', referring to the well-known verse in Psalm 23.[345] The physical and emotional burden on Bensly's mother must have been considerable.

On Boxing Day Reginald received this letter written in pencil. He realised that Bensly was 'terribly bad' and that his illness had worsened. Taking up his friend's plea, Reginald wrote back, enclosing a photograph, and Bensly wrote back quickly. His friend's letters cheered him. Bensly's next letter, again written in pencil, gave news of life in the expatriate community and tales of the Arab merchants visiting the house trying to sell their wares; he was given a large, curved dagger in a carved sheath over a foot long to display on his bedroom wall.[346] Bensly's letter took just four days to reach Reginald at St

---

[344] One cause of the spread of TB is now known to be unpasteurised milk. However, today a person with TB is advised to have a healthy balanced diet through eating cereals, millets and pulses; also vegetables and fruits plus milk and meat, eggs & fish, oils, fats and nuts and oil seeds. Drinking fresh milk would have helped Bensly.

[345] Flanders, Judith, *The Victorian House* (2003), p. 304, citing *The Journal of Laura Foster*, May/June 1864.

[346] Letter from Robert Bensly 11.01.87.

Ives. Despite Reginald's involvement with his sweetheart Mary, and getting ready to return to school, he began a reply the same evening and finished it off a couple of days later, giving news about trying to get into Sidney Sussex Cambridge; Bensly received this three days later and sent him a postcard thanking him.[347] The speed of the postal service was extraordinary.

He was up to writing but it was his last letter to his friend.

Reginald wrote back and sent a copy of the latest Uppingham School Magazine with his 'Our Concert' article, of which he was very proud (see Appendix 4). Two days later, Reginald received some French and Arabic newspapers from his friend. Reginald thought that perhaps he'd sent them 'as a curiosity' and to show him he was still alive. Included with these was a piece of paper in Arabic script. Written in large and then smaller writing were the words 'Abd Al Aziz'. This spelt out a name; it was of the 32nd Sultan of the Ottoman Empire who died in 1876.[348] Why Bensly wrote this name down and sent it is not clear. Perhaps, as Reginald inferred, it was his way of emphasising the exoticness of his life in North Africa. The paper is now in the Grove Family Archive.

HIS DEATH

Sadly, Bensly never received his copy of the magazine, as he died on 10 February. Reginald found out about his death by chance as he was glancing through the *Standard Newspaper* on 18 February and saw a notice of his friend's death printed in the 'Deaths' column: 'The first name I came to was poor Bob Bensly, he died on the 10th'. As he read this he thought that his friend perhaps had received the magazine on the day he died. He found out later this was not the case:

> I am awfully sorry for his people[349] and I very much feel his loss myself for though we had not seen each other for some years we had nevertheless corresponded very regularly.

Bensly was buried the day after according to the custom of this Muslim country. While he faded fast and was bedridden since arriving in Algiers, his death at such a young age and the fact that burial was in Algiers were a

347 Postcard from Robert Bensly 23.01.87.

348 He was the first Sultan to travel to Western Europe when in 1857 he visited Paris, London and Vienna.

349 This expression was used commonly at this time to refer to someone's parents or family.

deep shock to his parents and family.

'In the midst of life, we are in death.'

Mrs Bensly wrote shortly to Reginald afterwards with a card about her son's death. Her letter carried the customary black border for mourning.

> Villa Lacourt
> Mustafa Superior
> Algiers
> 15th February 1887
>
> Dear Mr Grove,
>
> I know you will mourn with me the loss of our beloved son – he died fully prepared and resigned after much suffering on the 10th and according to the law has been buried as soon as the 11th in the beautiful English Cemetery here. He had been suffering so much the last 10 days that at first we felt almost thankful to have him at Peace but from day to day we realised more and more how much we have lost in him. Your knew him well and you will not think it only a fond mother fancy when I tell you that we can remember no one cross word or unkind thought of his. His character was singularly pure and noble – full of love and utterly unselfish. Perhaps it was this great unselfishness that made him bear many a pain or weakness without complaining and led us to neglect little things, which, taken in time might have been improved and healed.
>
> Though aware of his danger, we could not help at times hoping for [writing unclear] health and one of his favourite plans was joining you at Cambridge in working once more with you as he did at King's School. Your last letter was his last pleasure – he was too weak to read it alas but he kept it under his pillow and made me read him a few lines at a time. Allow me to thank you for your kindness to him in writing so often. I shall never forget it and shall be glad if any future time, when you are in Cambridge we can do you some little service to show how we appreciated your friendship.
>
> Believe me,[350] sincerely yours,
>
> Agnes Bensly.

The School Magazine arrived there after his funeral.

Her words brought out Reginald's grief. As he recorded in his diary,

> It was just a mother's letter and yet every word was true and yet hardly good enough for him. I'm afraid I altogether gave way and had a good cry. I am sure it could not have been unmanly.

[350] Her son also ended his letters to Reginald using these same words.

Reginald felt the tension of keeping a stiff upper lip with expressing how distraught he really felt. His Headmaster Edward Thring's credo was directed towards making a boy 'manly, earnest and true', as explored in Volume 2.[351] And manliness embraced the vulnerability of experiencing the raw emotions felt at the death of a friend.

Thring was good friends with Mrs Juliana (known as Julia) Ewing, the author,[352] who died prematurely at Easter 1885, 20 years after they had starting writing to each other. He only met her twice as she lay dying. The first occasion he sat with her, comforted her and prayed with her with, 'her wasted hands in mine'. On the second, a few days later, according to her sister, Horatia Gatty, he

> gave great consolation by his unravelling of the mystery of suffering, and its sanctifying power; as also by his interpretation that the life which we are meant to lead under the dispensation of the Spirit who has been given for our guidance into Truth, is one which does not take us out of the world, but keeps us from its evil, enabling us to lead a heavenly existence on earth, and so to span over the chasm which divides us from heaven.[353]

Faith was at the heart of his ministry.

On her death, Thring was asked to conduct the funeral service by her husband Major Ewing, which he did despite the desolation he felt at her passing. Thring took comfort himself in one of her books, *Laetus Sorte Mea* (Happy with my lot), and wrote that 'my lower heart is heavy, whilst my higher heart is full of a new faith and peace'. The following day he read her book again and 'at first could scarcely get through the mist of tears but I was strangely comforted as I read'.[354] He knew the pain of grief and was not ashamed to share this with his pupils. Like his Saviour, he was 'a man of sorrows and familiar with suffering',[355] and stood as a role model for boys like Reginald in their grief.

Reginald was aware that the Benslys were going back to Cambridge immediately. He knew he should write to them, but didn't know how to put down his thoughts without 'appearing a hypocrite'. He concluded that

---

351 Thring, Edward, *Education and School* (1864), p. 269.

352 She wrote *Jackanapes*, the story of an orphaned son of a cavalry officer who on joining the Army himself as an adult, died in battle, saving the life of his childhood friend (see chapter 14).

353 Gatty, Horatia, *Juliana Horatia Ewing and Her Books* (SPCK, 1885), p. 80.

354 Thring, Edward, Diary 24.05.84 cited by Parkin p. 473.

355 Isaiah 53:3.

if he ever went abroad 'as my own master and am able to go to Algiers I will go and pay a pilgrimage to his grave'.

Sadly, he never made that journey.

In the Easter holidays, after his walk home from Uppingham with his friend Berry, Reginald visited Bensly's parents in Cambridge. He said that Mrs Bensly was 'very nice' but seemed, not unnaturally 'very cut up indeed'. Reginald talked about his plans for the future once he left school and his accomplishment on walking home. Seeing her son's friend and hearing about his hopes brought back painful memories for her. She wanted to give Reginald some of Bensly's things but they were still being sent by sea and had not arrived yet. She wrote in September from their address in Cambridge to say that their luggage had taken several months to arrive and then she had been ill. It was only then she was able to contact Reginald and send him some keepsakes which

> our dear boy wished you to have. In a little notebook kept by his bedside in the brass bowl sent you I found these words: In case of my early death my brass bowl and my Ottoman dagger[356] to W.R. Grove in remembrance of his many kind letters he sent me during my illness. He had chosen these things when he first came to Algiers and had them instantly by his side. I know you will value them as having belonged to Bensly.

Reginald's reaction to her letter is not known as he stopped writing his diary on 29 July 1887, the day after leaving school.

But it is a measure of his friendship that he kept every letter to his dying day that Bensly sent him after he became ill.

[356] This was the dagger mentioned in his letter to Reginald 11.01.87.

CHAPTER 7

Country Cousins

'Catching hares again all day long till about 4.00pm, caught 52, but one escaped and one had its back broken.'
Reginald Grove diary, 6 January 1885

Growing up in a Huntingdonshire market town, and then attending Uppingham School in another market town in Rutland, the countryside was only a stone's throw away during his boyhood years.

There were numerous occasions when Reginald travelled with his father around the local villages on his rounds in a pony and trap, or went for walks, or cycled along country roads. The same applied when he was at school at Uppingham, as Thring encouraged all the pupils in countrywide pursuits to learn directly about natural sciences, as described in Volume 2.

He had numerous relatives who were farmers, and he spent many holidays on their farms when he was back from school. It was his maternal uncles and aunts who introduced him to country life on their farms and nurtured his love of the English countryside. While he lived in a small market town and the countryside was little more than five or ten minutes' walk away, staying with his relatives on their farms was an exciting and to some extent a toughening experience. Living on remote farms there was no piped water or gas lighting, and heating was by a large fire in the main living room and the kitchen range. There were outbuildings to explore, hayricks to climb, mice and rats to catch, and, as he grew older, walks in the fields to shoot birds or game.

Reginald's mother, Maria Long, came from a large family of farmers from the Cambridgeshire/Suffolk area. The Long family had farmed in the North Cambridgeshire area since the late-18th century. Maria was born in 1844, one of ten siblings, and she outlived them all, having been a widow for 35 years. She died at the age of 86 in 1930 when Reginald himself was 61. The Long relatives – uncles, aunts and cousins – were to loom large in Reginald's childhood. The Long family was large and, as sometimes the same first name was handed down to another generation, keeping track of who was who is difficult 150 years later. For instance, at the funeral of Alderman William Warner, five times Mayor of St Ives, which was held at the Free Church in December 1905,[357] five Longs were listed as mourners, in addition to Reginald's mother, Reginald and his wife, one of whom can be placed.[358]

Reginald had seven maternal uncles, the eldest being Richard Kent Long[359] (1830–64) who died before Reginald was born. Then there was Uncle Hanslip[360] (1836–1916), Uncle George[361] (1839–1902), Uncle Daniel[362] (1842–1920) and Uncle Lawsell[363] (1852–1935). Reginald never knew two of his uncles who died when they were both four years old – William (1840–44) and then John (1846–50). Of his three aunts on his mother's side, there were Aunt Martha[364] (1832–1912), Aunt Louise[365] (1834–1919) and Emily[366] (1849–95).

Family ties were strong, especially as most of his Long relatives lived within a reasonable train journey's distance from St Ives as well as near each other in various villages in Cambridgeshire. He had numerous cousins on his mother's side of the family, many of whom were his own age, whom he saw quite often when he visited them or they and their parents stayed at St Ives during the school holidays. Those of his own age, especially Hansie (Hanslip) and Dick Long (Richard), whose sister, Mary, Reginald fell in love with, regularly wrote to each other. An especially enjoyable and memorable holiday took place in the summer of 1886 when the cousins

---

357 Cambridge Independent Press 22.12.05.

358 Mrs G. Long was Warner's sister in law. Mr D. Long, Mr and Mrs D. K. Long and Mr R. Long have not been identified.

359 Richard Kent Long married Emma Sharp in 1857.

360 Hanslip Long married Elizabeth Slater in 1864. He was the third Hanslip to bear this name in the Long family. The first Hanslip Long was born in 1769.

361 George Long married Elizabeth Warner in 1864. She had been born in St Ives, Huntingdonshire.

362 Daniel Long married Sarah Ellis Ann Bowring Ellis. The date is not known.

363 Lawsell Long married Emma Horsley in 1878 and his marriage certificate states that he was a 'gentleman'.

364 Martha Long married James Mardall in 1860. He was shown as a 'landowner' in the 1871 National Census when they were visiting her brother, Hanslip, and his wife.

365 Louise Long married James Gosling in 1858.

366 Emily Long married Arthur Kent in 1871 and they lived in Chippenham, Cambs. He died in 1881 and she in 1895. After his death she lived in Cambridge and Reginald used to visit her when he was at Sidney Sussex College.

rowed down the River Lark to Ely and back. This is described in some detail later in this chapter.

There were four uncles whom Reginald visited during his holidays from school – Uncle George, Uncle Dan, Uncle Hanslip and Uncle James. He visited a fifth, Uncle Lawsell, but never stayed at his farm in Carleton which was near Uncle George's.

FARMER LONG OF CARLETON GRANGE FARM

Uncle George and Aunt Elizabeth Long

On a raw January morning in 1881 Reginald, whose twelfth birthday was in a matter of days, travelled to Carleton Grange Farm, Carleton, Cambridgeshire by train with Uncle George. His uncle had probably come to St Ives, especially to collect him and take him back for his first holiday on a farm. The trip was one of the first entries in his first diary during his Christmas holiday from King's Choir School, Cambridge.

The Long family had farmed in the North Cambridgeshire area since the late-18th century and Uncle George was a tenant farmer. Crops grown were wheat, barley, oats and beans. Carleton Grange was a substantial estate and the farm building itself was large.[367] Uncle George's wife's name was Elizabeth. Because there was another aunt called Elizabeth, who was married to Uncle Hanslip, the Grove family called her 'Aunt George'. Uncle George and wife were tenant farmers in the hamlet of Carleton, and did not have any children of their own. The Long household numbered ten in 1881: besides his uncle and aunt, there were two of their two nephews[368] living there, a lodger, a governess and four servants.[369] George Long was a magistrate serving on the Cambridgeshire Bench.

At Church Farm nearby lived Uncle Lawsell and Aunt Emma. In 1851 there were five large tenant farms in and around the small hamlet of Carleton[370] on the North Cambridgeshire and Suffolk border. It was seven miles from Newmarket and five miles from the Six Mile Bottom

---

[367] Kelly's *Directory of Cambridgeshire, Norfolk and Suffolk* 1883, p. 71.

[368] Ellis Long, aged eight, and Algernon Kent, aged six.

[369] National Census 1881.

[370] The name was often spelt Carleton but its full name was Carlton-cum-Willingham (*Kelly's Directory 1883*). Lawsell Long was listed as a farmer at Church Farm, and George Long was also shown as a farmer at Carleton Grange. Both were his mother's brothers and so uncles of Reginald.

railway station,[371] and while well farmed it had numerous wooded areas, the remains of the ancient woodlands that used to cover the whole area.

With a population of just over 300 in 1883, the three main landowners were a Miss Soames 'lady of the manor'[372] of Lopham's Hall,[373] Lord Dacre of Carlton Parva, and a Mr Hall. Lopham's Hall dates back to the Tudor period and is now a listed building. Wheat, barley, oats and beans were the main crops farmed in the Victorian period. With a small church, one alehouse called the Axe and Saw, and a village school with around 50 children, it was a sleepy farming community.

That said, over the years, the local press[374] reported a number of crimes – turkey rustling, poaching, sheep worrying, and a case of bigamy. However, 30 years before Reginald was a regular visitor to his relatives, there was a case heard before the Cambridge Assizes in February 1852, and a Benjamin Revell aged 23 was convicted of what was called 'an unnatural' or an 'abominable' offence. Such was the offence that the evidence was 'of course unfit for publication'. As the death sentence was passed, his crime was either sodomy with a young lad or possibly bestiality. Both offences had been capital ones since the 16th century, and no distinction was made between the two acts. However, Revell's sentence was commuted to penal servitude to Western Australia.[375] In 1861 these offences were made liable to penal servitude rather than hanging; the Penal Servitude Act of 1857 actually abolished this punishment, but transportation went on until 1868, the year before Reginald's birth.[376] In the same year public executions were outlawed.

A year before Reginald's first visit to stay with his uncle and aunt, the public house in the village was the scene of a tragic suicide when the publican hanged himself on the premises, leaving a widowed wife and

---

[371] *Kelly's Directory of Cambridgeshire, Norfolk and Suffolk* 1883.

[372] Ibid.

[373] In the National Census of 1871, Hester Olley aged 81 lived at the Hall together with his two unmarried daughters, Ursula and Lucretia both in their forties. Hester is noted as farming 308 acres and employing eight labourers and three boys. On his death the Hall passed to Miss Soames.

[374] http://www.carlton cambridgeshire.org.uk/index.php?title=Historic_Newspapers (05.03.2019).

[375] *Cambridge Chronicle and Journal* 24.07.52.

[376] http://notchesblog.com/2016/09/06/prison-sex-in-the-mid-victorian-english-convict-system 14.04.19.

young family.[377] The story was fresh in everyone's minds when he visited in January 1881, and passing the Axe and Saw on the way to and from the farm was a reminder of the terrible tragedy that had happened there.

The Carleton Grange Farm itself was occupied from 1817 until around 1875 by the Nash family; nearby Church Farm,[378] covering 1,040 acres in 1851, was leased to William Long (1797–1883), brother to Hanslip who had taken it on by 1851.[379] The National Census of 1851 listed Hanslip Long as a farmer employing 25 men and 35 boys. This was Reginald's grandfather who died in 1873 when he was four years old. One of his sons, also called Hanslip, farmed at Shippea Hill Farm further north on the county border (see below).

Grandfather Hanslip[380] Long was a tenant farmer who was married to Martha (née Kent) from Little Wilbraham in Cambridgeshire, just six miles east of Cambridge itself. In the 1871 Census, 20 years later, 69-year-old Hanslip employed 48 men and 13 boys, and farmed 1,200 acres.[381] The couple also farmed at Swavesey, a village not far from St Ives. Grandmother Long died three years after her husband, when Reginald was seven. The farm then passed to another son, Reginald's Uncle George.

The farmhouse, barns and outbuildings nestled below a chalk

[377] The newspaper report stated that 'considerable excitement was occasioned in this village on Sunday Morning by a determined act of self-destruction committed by George Woods, landlord of the Axe and Saw beer shop. At about half-past six o'clock the report of a gun was heard by several persons sitting in the house and it was soon ascertained that the landlord had gone down into the cellar and there shot himself with a gun, which he placed close to his right side, inflicting a serious wound. He was picked up and endeavours were made to staunch the blood. Dr. Tandy happened to reach the village soon after, and attended to deceased, but found it to be a hopeless case. Dr. Head, hearing of it, also went, but the poor fellow died about eight o'clock the same evening. Deceased who was 35 years of age, leaves a widow. He was noticed during the day to be moping and gloomy, but otherwise these seems to be no reason for the dreadful act.'

[378] It is not known who owned the land in the 19th century but in 1910 the Land Tax records show that the farm was leased from Viscount Hampden. The house and premises were taxed at two acres and eight rods. The land was taxed at 496 acres and two rods. In addition, there was Carlton Wood which was nine acres and one rod.

[379] *A History of the County of Cambridge and the Isle of Ely:* Volume 6. Originally published by Victoria County History, London, 1978

[380] Hanslip was a family name handed down over three generations: Hanslip Long, born 1769; Hanslip Long, Reginald's grandfather born 1801; and then Hanslip, born 1836, his uncle. This uncle's eldest son, Hanslip was one of Reginald's cousins and a good friend, mentioned often in his diaries.

[381] National Census 1871.

escarpment; a photograph taken in 1912 shows a large house with outbuildings. It has since been pulled down and nothing remains to show where it stood.

On that first visit in January 1881, Uncle George and young Reginald changed trains at Cambridge and took the Newmarket line, getting off at Six Mile Bottom station where a pony and trap awaited them. The hamlet of Six Mile Bottom got its name from the distance to the start of the Newmarket Racecourse and the fact that it also lay in a valley bottom. The station served the village from the 1860s until 1967, when it was closed.

Once they arrived at the farmhouse they had something to eat and drink before driving in the trap 12 miles over to the small village of Chippenham, on the road to Mildenhall to see another family member. This was his Aunt Emily, one of his mother's sisters, who was married to Arthur Kent. The village itself had only 800 inhabitants.[382] Uncle Arthur and Aunt Emily lived at La Hogue Hall Farm, which was a large holding of 1,700 acres. His father, Lewis Kent, had been the tenant farmer who employed 44 men and 25 boys.[383] There were six cottages on the farm which housed some of the farm labourers. Arthur took over the farm probably in 1876 when his father died and after his marriage in 1871 to Emily. By the time of his father's death the young couple had two children, with a third born later that year.

The next morning Reginald was given a shotgun to go out into the surrounding fields with his uncle to shoot; he did not record their success or their quarry, but it is probable that they were hunting hare. On Sunday morning he went with his uncle and aunt half a mile down the road to the little 16th-century church at Brinkley, where they worshipped each week.

Next day he took great delight in more hunting – this time his quarry was the mice in the large haystack near the farm.[384] This kept him occupied the whole day. What his success was, Reginald did not say. Before he left in the afternoon the next day he went riding on a pony kept on the farm. It must have been a cold spell as a couple of days after getting back to St Ives he went skating along the flooded meadows downstream to Holywell. In winter the Ouse often overflowed its banks, and the surrounding fields were flooded and iced over.

---

[382] https://www.british-history.ac.uk/vch/cambs/vol10/pp370-374 (14.03.19).

[383] National Census 1861.

[384] Diary 08.01.81.

He went back to school at King's the next day, but not before he had another spell skating on Hemingford Meadow. Sadly, Uncle Arthur died aged 33 a few weeks after he got back to school. Perhaps his uncle had been ill and this was the reason for the trip to Chippenham to see him. Aunt Emily was left a widow with five young children to bring up. Reginald again spent part of his summer holidays in 1883 on the farm when he was 14½ years old. It was just after he had recovered from a bout of measles. His father was travelling to a summer camp with a contingent of military reservists from St Ives, and Reginald accompanied them for part of the journey. Boarding the train at the station at St Ives at about 9 in the morning on Saturday 14 July, they travelled via Cambridge on the Newmarket and Chesterford Railway line. Reginald arrived at Six Mile Bottom station just before midday. Having been met by his uncle in his trap, his father and the other reservists travelled on to their camp.[385] Six Mile Bottom was a small hamlet perhaps two miles from the farm. The station served the village from the 1860s until 1967, when it was closed.

The next day, Reginald went with his relatives to church at Brinkley, a small hamlet less than a mile away; then in the afternoon he returned to Brinkley to post letters but got caught in a thunderstorm. In the evening he went for a drive with his aunt and uncle to the actual village of Carleton which was a few miles from the farm. He attended church on each of the three Sundays that he stayed at the farm. Exploring the farm for a boy his age was an exhilarating experience.

During the next week he shot at rooks in the fields with his uncle's shotgun, although his success was limited. When not shooting, he spent time in the hayfields; it's not clear whether he was helping with the harvesting or just relaxing there, but there was one diary entry in which he said he 'got up all the clover', so his holiday seems to have been partly a working one. Walking around the farm on his own or with his uncle and aunt was also another activity, as was riding a pony about the farm and across the fields. He was left alone with the servants at the farm on a few occasions while his uncle and aunt were away in Newmarket and Bury St Edmunds. One of their visits was to the market at Bury, presumably for business. His uncle went to Bury St Edmunds the next day, leaving Reginald to shoot at rooks all day; he came in at 9 when it began to get dark.

Aunt Elizabeth went off to St Ives by train one day to see her sister,

[385] No information is given in the diary as to where the camp was held.

Reginald's mother, the next day and he spent the day with his uncle driving about the farm, shooting rooks again. Two other uncles on his mother's side, Lawsell[386] and Dan, visited for tea with a Mr Pratt. During the two weeks he stayed at the farm he learnt about a lawsuit that his uncle was involved in. His lawyer, a Mr Salman, visited the farm to discuss the case which was heard at Bury St Edmunds the day before William returned home. He gave no indication about the nature of the case, but it is likely it was a civil rather than any criminal matter. He went with another relative, Uncle Ellis,[387] by train to Bury to sit in on the court hearing. This was probably heard at the Shire House in the centre of Bury St Edmunds. Uncle George had travelled there the day before, no doubt to prepare for the hearing with Mr Salman.

The case was heard in the morning and Uncle George won. It must have been a fascinating insight into the drama of a legal hearing for Reginald sitting with the men in the court, and he said that he enjoyed the day very much. Travelling home by the midday train, he stopped off in Cambridge where he remained all day before attending chapel at King's College in the evening.

He arrived home at St Ives at 8 o'clock, and as the next day was a Sunday he attended church in the morning and evening. The next day, 5 August, was the August Bank Holiday. Other relatives had arrived the previous day – Uncle Gosling and Arthur – and they all paid a visit to the St Ives market that day. Both guests went off by train to London in the evening.

The Longs then farmed in Swavesey, renting in Hemingford while their new house was built.[388] His aunt had been born in St Ives so knew the area well.[389] The first mention of him visiting them in Hemingford Grey was in January 1885 when he walked over, stayed for tea and went to church. There, Reginald paid them frequent visits while on holiday at home, generally walking or rowing upstream to see them. They bought a steam launch with which Reginald was impressed; he went for a short jaunt in it for the first time just before he went back to school in January 1885. In the Easter holidays, he rode over on his bicycle to Hemingford

---

[386] Lawsell Long (1852–1935) and Daniel Kent Long (1842–1920).

[387] Uncle Ellis may have been a brother of his Aunt Sarah (née Ellis), wife of Daniel Kent Long.

[388] Reginald specifically mentioned their farm in a diary entry when he 'went for a drive with Uncle George to his farm' (17 December 1886).

[389] National Census 1881.

Grey and went out in it again with his uncle, this time travelling upstream to Godmanchester and arriving back home late at 7.30pm.

Back home from school in March 1886 due to his eyesight problems, Reginald went down to the staunch[390] one morning with his Uncle Gosling[391] who was staying at Slepe House to meet Uncle George 'passing on his way to Shippea Hill with his steam launch'. Uncle George must have been on a leisurely trip by river to visit his sister and brother-in-law at Shippea Hill Farm. Cruising down the Ouse to Earith, and then to Ely on the Old West River, he may have made arrangements to see Reginald's brother who was at King's School, Ely. From Ely it was not far to cruise down to Prickwillow on the River Lark, mooring perhaps at the Fish and Duck past Prickwillow Bridge.

As described in Volume 3, Uncle George and Aunt Elizabeth returned to Swavesey after renting 'The Old Rectory' which was on the river in Hemingford Grey and settled into their new home, called the Priory, in Carters Lane.[392]

FARMER LONG OF THE HALL, GREAT BRADLEY

Uncle Dan and Aunt Sarah Long

Uncle Dan[393] was another of Reginald's uncles who was a tenant farmer on the Cambridge and Suffolk border and lived at Great Bradley Hall, near Haverhill, Suffolk. This was and still is an impressive building. Pevsner's *Suffolk (Buildings of England)* lists it as being 17th-century, and in about 1877 the Hall had a drawing room, two bedrooms and a dressing room added, which again Pevsner described as 'good 19th century'. A wing was added built at right angles to the rest of the house. A dairy also existed at right angles to the main structure of the house.[394] This was where Reginald came to stay for a few days in the Easter holidays of 1887.

Uncle Dan had a mixed arable and livestock farm on 1,700 acres. Like other members of the Long family he employed a large number of farm

---

390 Another term for a pound lock on the river, located about half a mile downstream from the medieval bridge.

391 James Gosling was married to Louise Long, Reginald's aunt. They lived in Chalk Hill, Elveden, in Suffolk, and farmed until their family business collapsed in the early 1880s and they moved to London.

392 National Census 1891 and 1901.

393 Daniel Kent Long (1843–1920) married Sarah Ann Bowning Ellis.

394 https://greatbradley.weebly.com/about-the-hall.html 28.05.19.

workers – 47 men, 22 boys and 14 women in 1881.[395] In the 1911 Census he was described as a 'farmer and grazier', and employed a farm bailiff which indicated his prosperity. His tenancy continued until his death, aged 78, shortly after the 1914–18 war had ended. Wheat, barley and oats were the cereals that he grew, together with peas, beans and root crops. As the farm had a dairy building, some of his cattle were for milking; others no doubt were raised for meat consumption.

The village had only 359 inhabitants[396] and was six and a half miles from the market town of Haverhill, and eight from Newmarket. The Longs had three daughters, Reginald's cousins, Elizabeth, Ida and Louise, and a son, Richard Ellis. Ida Mary and her husband Frederic Webb later lived and worked on the farm. Elizabeth was to marry a member of the local gentry, John Thistleton-Smith, a gentleman farmer and Justice of the Peace who lived at Pudding Norton Hall in Norfolk.

Reginald was invited to stay at the Hall before starting his last term at school. He wanted to take more brass rubbings, and the churches in the area had many to tempt him. He took the train from St Ives to Cambridge and then travelled on to Linton and walked to Hildersham, where he planned to take some brass rubbings. Unfortunately, due to building work in the chancel, the brasses were covered up so his plans were thwarted. He took the road again to another village called Horseheath, where he was able to take two good copies, 'one of them a very good knight in armour'. The clergyman who spoke with him was very kind and invited him for a glass of beer and biscuits which Reginald was delighted to accept, and he went on his way 'rejoicing'! Back on the road he met up with another young man from Rugby School who was 'on the tramp round the place alone'. They walked and chatted until they parted company – Reginald back to Linton and the Rugby lad to Baldock. By lunchtime he had walked 12 miles, and because his boots were too tight, found that the skin off the top of one of his feet had been stripped bare. He kept walking until he arrived at Haverhill at about 2.30pm and was met by his relatives there: 'everyone seemed very pleased to see me'.

Staying with his uncle and aunt was a young man called Archie Gold who was a 'pupil' – the equivalent of a farming apprentice – and who was 'the life of the party at dinner'. In the evening they both went out with

[395] National Census 1881.

[396] *Kelly's Directory of Suffolk* 1881.

Uncle Dan and his dogs rabbit hunting. Five were killed, and when they came back over the fields they killed ten rats around the farm. During the evening out in the fields Reginald heard the cuckoo for the first time that year. The next day he and Archie went out for a walk around the farm and paid a visit to Harry Wilder,[397] the son of the local vicar, to invite him for a game of tennis. He was off to the races at Newmarket with his father so they played tennis on their own to amuse themselves. Gold was a bit of an amateur photographer and took some pictures – one of which was of Reginald and Lorrie[398] larking about – 'embracing in a most scandalous manner'! After lunch he and Gold took the trap to Newmarket themselves to 'do some business for Uncle'. He complained that the drive back was 'fearful cold', but got warmed up playing another game of tennis. The evening was a jolly one, singing comical songs in the drawing room as Gold's brother turned up with a cousin. They were a very noisy lot but 'awfully nice and jolly'. It was a late night.

The next day the 2,000 Guineas Race was being held and the household started off at 11 to Newmarket for a day's flat racing – Uncle Dan and Reginald in the horse and trap, and the Gold boys on horses. They met some others who were undergraduates at Cambridge and then sat down to lunch with some family friends, the Channells. They watched the afternoon's races on the Rowley Mile, Reginald and his uncle from the heath, which was free, and the others from the grandstand. They saw the Prince of Wales riding by. Reginald did not place any bets, whether from moral objection or because he had no money to spare is not clear. That evening after they got back there was a large dinner party at The Hall, including the Cambridge friends and party, another Uncle, Lawsell, and his wife and another cousin, Henry Mardall. The Cambridge men left at about 10.00pm, but not before they had sung a number of comical songs and played cards for money. Reginald wisely avoided this as 'some of the fellows lost a lot', and he had a quieter evening playing cribbage with his two aunts. Another late night – this time until 1.00am.

An early morning start at 8.00am saw the Golds leave and Reginald resumed his brass rubbing quest, walking to another village nearby, Cowlings, with two of his cousins, Bessie and 11-year-old Ida. The brass

---

397 Harry Wilder was a year younger than Reginald and the son of the Rector of Great Bradley, Revd John Wilder, who had married Reginald's father and mother.

398 Lorrie was his cousin Louise Long, then aged nine.

wasn't very good and they returned, but the eight-mile round trip did his foot, injured a few days before while walking, no good. A quick visit after lunch in the trap with Lorrie to Little Bradley Church enabled him to take one of the five brasses there before rushing back, getting changed and then going with his aunt and a friend of hers, Mrs Frank Smith (who lived in London but had a house in Great Bradley), to Carleton six miles away to visit other Long relatives for tennis before dinner. It was a large dinner party with, besides the hosts, seven guests, including Reginald. But in contrast to the evening before, it was a quiet evening talking, although they played one game which involved lighting a candle from the next person while kneeling on one knee. He was back by 11.00pm and in bed by midnight.

There was another excursion the following day, despite the rain, but this time his uncle lent him the horse and trap and he went to Balsham Church, seven miles away. He was given a 'splendid lunch' to take with him, and after getting two sets of rubbings, one of which was a 'small battered knight', he did not get back to The Hall until 6. He left for home the next morning after he had walked down to the village church with his aunt and took a 'curious brass on the wall of Day the Printer' His uncle drove him to Newmarket, having said his farewells and promising to stay again during his next holidays in the summer. Whether he did we do not know, as he kept no diary after leaving Uppingham.

FARMER LONG OF SHIPPEA HILL FARM

Uncle Hanslip and Elizabeth Long

Uncle Hanslip Long and his wife Elizabeth lived at Shippea Hill[399] Farm near the village of Prickwillow in the east of Cambridgeshire very near both the Suffolk and the Norfolk borders. Reginald spent a number of holidays with them on the farm. Prickwillow lies on the banks of the River Lark which flows from Mildenhall in Suffolk into the Great Ouse just north-east of Ely. It is an unattractive, bleak village, 20 miles north of Carleton, and four miles from Ely on the edge of the Fens. In 1887 it numbered 1,297 inhabitants.[400]

Travel to the farm by train on the Breckland line that linked Ely with Norwich further east was easy for the family to get to and from Cambridge

[399] In the Ordnance Survey Map of 1836, the farm is called Shippey (sic) Hill Farm.

[400] Bartholomew, John, *Gazetteer of the British Isles* 1887.

and St Ives. The little station[401] was opened in 1845 as a railhead for fruit and vegetables grown in the area, and was surrounded by farms of which Shippea Hill Farm was one. Much of the surrounding Fenlands is a metre below sea level, so the word 'hill' is somewhat of a misnomer, although the farm itself was perhaps five metres above sea level.

Shippea Hill Farm was where Uncle Hanslip and Elizabeth his wife lived with their large family. Their 12 children were Reginald's cousins, of course, and Reginald was very close to two of them, Mary[402] and Hanslip ('Hansie'), who was his own age. His friendship with Mary is described in Chapter 8.

Reginald's cousins Richard (Dick) and George (sons of Uncle Hanslip) both went to King's School, Ely, with his brothers Ernest and Ted; as did Ellis Long, son of his Uncle Daniel.

Uncle Hanslip's tenant farm had a large acreage. In 1861 he farmed 1,200 acres and employed 46 men and 24 boys.[403] The 1871 National Census of 1871, when Reginald was two, recorded that he employed 58 men, 20 boys and 10 girls.[404] Ten years later, just before Reginald began visiting his cousins, he farmed 1,600 acres and employed 56 farm workers.[405] Given that Reginald made no mention in his diary of a dairy, cattle being brought in for milking, sheep being shorn or any husbandry being carried out on any livestock, the farm must have been an arable one.

The first time he mentioned visiting them was a brief stay in January 1884 just before his 15th birthday. A year later, Uncle Hanslip had been staying at St Ives and they both caught an early morning train to travel to the farm. There they spent the rest of their day together catching hares. Although it rained in the afternoon, their tally was an incredible 45 hares. Reginald did not say how, but the hares must have been caught through

---

401 Originally, the station was called Mildenhall Road although the country town of Mildenhall is eight miles away. In 1885 when a separate railway line was opened from Cambridge to Mildenhall, it was named Burnt Fen. In 1905 the station's name was changed again to Shippea Hill which it bears to this day. Fresh agricultural products are still delivered to Covent Garden market in London by train. It is the least used passenger station in Great Britain, according to the Office of Rail and Road estimates. It is a request stop. There is one train per day to Norwich, Monday to Saturday, and on Saturdays one train to Cambridge. (https://en.wikipedia.org/wiki/Shippea_Hill_railway_station] 12.03.19.

402 Mary Long was born in 1868 and was a year older than Reginald.

403 National Census 1861.

404 National Census 1871.

405 National Census 1881.

coursing with greyhounds or lurchers.[406] They relaxed in the evening around the farmhouse fire with card tricks being shown and musical entertainment. The local vicar, Revd Kingdon,[407] and his brother were guests. The following day there was more hare coursing with 52 being caught, although 'one escaped and had its back broken'. There was a different quarry the next day as he took the opportunity of killing some rats and mice at a haystack that the farm workers were threshing.

Threshing was a typical winter activity for farm labourers using handheld flails to separate a pile of grain. Horse-powered machinery had yet to take over this work at Hanslip's farm. As the men threshed, the rodents, which had used the stack as their home since the summer when the stack had been made, fled. Reginald and his cousin Dick were ready and waiting for them with their sticks. For two young lads this was great fun. Reginald did not record how many were killed, but for a farmer keeping the rodent population down was a matter of life and death. A harvest could well be eaten away by these pests.

In the afternoon his cousin Dick left for St Ives to visit Uncle George on his new farm at Hemingford Grey. Reginald and his other cousin, Hansie, and his uncle spent an enjoyable evening in front of the fire playing cribbage[408] and a card game called 'nap'. In the morning, after a walk around the farm with Hansie and his uncle in the crisp winter sunshine, he was driven in the horse and trap to Ely by his uncle and then a train took him back to St Ives by 5.30pm.

A few days later his cousin Mary and another cousin, Willie Mardall, came to stay at St Ives. The visits between cousins were frequent events in the school holidays. Walks in the countryside during the day and games like whist in the evenings made for relaxing times. Mary and Willie stayed for just under a week, which included Reginald's 16th birthday celebration.

In the summer holidays of 1886 Reginald went to stay with his cousins at Shippea Hill Farm. The River Lark ran nearby. After breakfast on his first day there Reginald and his cousins Hansie, Mary, Tattie, Elsie and Ethel rowed down to the river in two boats to Ely. This was about five miles away. One boat belonged to a friend James Pratt, and the other to

[406] Hare coursing is now illegal in Great Britain.

[407] This was the Revd Claude Drewitt Kingdon, Vicar of Prickwillow, who had studied at the University of Oxford.

[408] Cribbage is a card game usually played by two contestants.

a Mr Mosely. 'Mary and Alice were in my boat, going and coming back', he was to note in his diary. 'Had some lunch at Ely then went over the cathedral, went up to the top of the big tower and had a splendid view over everywhere. Got back in fairly good time.'

Given the flatness of the Fenlands surrounding Ely, the view was stunning. The following day, having spent the morning studying in Cambridge, Reginald got back to Shippea Hill after 3.00pm and in the 'evening went on the river with Mary, Alice and Will – had a jolly boat sail. Mary and Alice had to go to choir practice so Will and I took the boat back, met Tattie and walked home with her.' It was an idyllic few days in the country with his cousins, and especially with his sweetheart, Mary.

Once again during the Christmas holidays in 1886 he went to stay again for a couple of days while seeing his brother's school play in Ely. It was very cold and he went skating on a couple of days with cousin Dick on a mile-long stretch of ice on flooded fields alongside the river, as well as shooting with cousin Hansie; he had one shot at a pheasant but missed before going back by train to St Ives for Christmas with his family.

FARMER MARDALL[409] OF WHEATHAMPSTEAD AND HARPENDEN *(Uncle James Mardall and Aunt Martha)*

One cousin who did not live on the Cambridge/Suffolk border was Francis ('Frank') Mardall,[410] who was one of the sons of his Aunt Martha's. She had married James Mardall in 1860 who took over his father's farm on the Hertfordshire/Cambridgeshire border in the small village of Wheathampstead. When he was a young man, the farm of 150 acres, on Wheat Hill, employed 16 men and two boys.[411] By the time he married when he was 37, he had left farming and moved into business as a corn and coal merchant, still at Wheathampstead, but in a house in Gustard Wood.[412] His business prospered, and in 1870 he bought the Peacock

[409] In some National Census returns the name is spelt 'Mardell'.

[410] Francis ('Frank') House, Kingston Mardall (1872–1955), was one of James and Martha's children; the others were Henry b. 1861, James Daniel b. 1864, William ('Willie') b. 1867, Hugh, b. 1870, Norman b. 1872, Alice b. 1875 and Beatrice b. 1878. Both William and Hugh were born in St Ives, presumably staying with her sister, Maria and her husband Dr Grove. Perhaps they wanted his medical experience at the births?

[411] National Census 1841.

[412] A year later, at the time of the 1861 Census, three relatives of Martha's were visiting. They were her sister, Louise and her husband James Gosling ('farmer of 300 acres employing 18 labourers') and her brother, Hanslip Long ('farmer of 12,000 acres 46 labourers and 24 boys').

Brewery[413] in Harpenden for the huge sum of £16,000 (£2,028,960). This was a massive investment, and yet the following year he demolished the old house and built new premises, called Brewery House. He and Martha lived in the new house which had a brewery building onsite. He died in 1881 when he was 59. He must have planned ahead to transfer his assets to Martha as he left less than £4,000 (£507,240), given the huge investment made into the brewery 11 years earlier. Martha continued to run the business with the help of her three sons, and only a few years later deemed herself a 'brewer' in *Kelly's Trade Directory*.[414] In 1893 she bought out the other brewery in town, owned by the Healy family. The combined business became the Mardall Brewery.

The first mention of his cousins, Henry and Willie, was in Reginald's diary of 1881 when the two came to stay with the Groves in the Christmas holiday. Henry was then 20, and Willie 14, so both were older than Reginald. When the brothers went home, Reginald's sister Mabel, then aged only ten, went with them. It was quite an adventure for her to travel with her older cousins, but it was very common for all the Long cousins to visit their relatives.

Frank was three years younger than Reginald but they got on well. In August 1885, when Reginald was 16 and Frank 13, Frank came to stay with the Groves and both enjoyed going on the river and taking bicycle rides. Reginald then travelled back with Frank to stay with him and Aunt Martha. Martha was then running the brewery. Henry Mardell, Frank's older brother who was 24, was helping his mother run the brewery, and another brother, James, aged 20, had just joined the family business. Tennis and cricket were games they all enjoyed playing or, in Reginald's case, umpiring at a local tennis championship which Henry won for the third year running. Reginald was taken round the brewery and Henry took them shooting ('sport very poor, he only shot three birds and one of these he lost'), but as an adult he was the only one who carried a shotgun.

There were tricycle rides, a trip to St Albans Abbey, more tennis and a game of billiards before Reginald retuned to St Ives. These were happy times.

The Mardall brewery business prospered and was eventually sold in

413 It was called this because of a peacock weathervane on top of the building.

414 *Kelly's Hertfordshire Trade Directory 1886*, p. 652.

1897.[415] Martha owned land, too, and sold a large plot in Harpenden to a Robert Henry Wix which became St George's School in 1906. This coeducational school is still there.

FARMER LONG OF CHURCH FARM, CARLETON

Uncle Lawsell and Aunt Emma Long

Lawsell Long was Reginald's mother's youngest brother and was born in 1852. Lawsell was another first name used in the Long family dating back to 1721 when Richard Long married Elizabeth Lawsell.[416] Married in 1878 when he was 26 to Emma Horsley aged 23 in Southorpe village church, he was described as a 'gentleman'[417] in their marriage certificate.[418] To Reginald they were Uncle Lawsell and Aunt Emma, and they lived at Church Farm in the village of Carlton-cum-Willingham, Cambridgeshire, near Lawsell's elder brother George Long and his wife at Carleton Grange Farm. Lawsell lived at home with his father and mother (Hanslip and Martha Long) at a house 'near the Church at Carlton [sic]'.[419] His father was listed in the 1871 Census as farming 1,200 acres and employing 48 men and 13 boys. Lawsell took over Church Farm from the Trustees of his father's estate[420] in 1875 when he was 23 years old. His marriage came three years later. By the time the 1881 National Census was taken,[421] he and Emma had three children: Charles, Gerald and Herbert.[422] Sadly, a

---

[415] In 1897, the Mardall Brewery was sold to Richard Glover, a London-based businessman. By then it 37 'tied public houses, 8 of them in Harpenden. A *tied* house is a *public house* that has to buy at least some of its beer from a particular brewery; commercially it extremely advantageous for a brewery as sales are guaranteed. Mardall's beer sales were over 5,000 barrels per year and a 'considerable spirit trade was carried out'. Martha carried on living at Brewery House until she died in 1912. (Harpenden History website.)

[416] Their youngest son, born 1739, was named Lawsell but the name then skipped three generations; it was again used for one of Uncle Hanslip and Aunt Elizabeth's sons, Lawsell W. S. Long, who was born in 1880.

[417] His father, Hanslip Long, was a witness, as was Emma's father, Charles Horsley, described as a merchant.

[418] Marriage certificate dated 3 July 1878. His father, Hanslip Long, was a witness as was Emma's father, Charles Horsley, who was described as a merchant.

[419] Interestingly, staying there that night, besides Lawsell (aged 19) and his sister Emily (aged 21), were James and Martha Mardall and their two sons William and Hugh, and another cousin Arthur Gosling. It was quite a family gathering!

[420] The landowner was Viscount Hampden (1910 Land Tax Records. Church Farm (no 340)).

[421] National Census 1881.

[422] Charles was born in 1880, Gerald, in 1883, and Herbert in 1885 (National Census 1891).

daughter, Ella Margaret, died aged eight months in August 1881. By the time of the Census in 1891 the boys had a governess to give them lessons, a Miss Harriet Rex.

While Reginald mentions Uncle Lawsell on a number of occasions in his diaries, it does not seem as if he ever stayed at Church Farm. Reginald met him on a summer holiday to stay with Uncle George and Aunt Elizabeth at Carleton Grange in July 1883. Like his brother George's, Lawsell's farm was mainly arable but he also had a small herd of cattle, some sheep and pigs. Sadly, he went bankrupt in 1903 after a succession of bad harvests,[423] as described in Chapter 23.

[423] *Cambridge Independent Press* 11.12.1903.

CHAPTER 8

Mary, Reginald's First Love

'A rosebud set with little wilful thorns, and sweet as English air could make her, she.' [424]

Alfred Tennyson, 'The Princess' (1847)[425]

Mary was Reginald's first love. Despite writing to each other for an 18-month period, none of their letters survive. However, from his diaries it is clear that they were both deeply attracted to each other. Theirs was a shy but blossoming love in a chaperoned family environment. Reginald's love letters written to his fiancée Hilda Stevenson, seven years later, do survive. These letters show a tender-hearted man willing to express how he felt in deeply intimate terms, and his earlier ones to Mary are sure to have been similar.

Throughout his diary entries he never mentions her surname or who she is. He clearly felt she needed no introduction. In fact, Mary was a first cousin, one of four daughters of his Uncle Hanslip Long[426] who farmed in North Cambridgeshire. Uncle Hanslip was one of his mother's many brothers. He had married Elizabeth Slater in 1864 and they had 12 children. The Longs had big families.

Besides her sisters Helena, Ethel and Kathleen, Mary's other siblings were Hanslip (Hansie), Richard (Dick), George, John, William, Christian, Lawsell and Bertram. The Groves and Long cousins knew each other well, as they stayed with each other and the Groves enjoyed staying on the Longs' farm during some of their holidays. Her brother Hansie was the same age as Reginald and they got on well.

Reginald first mentioned Mary staying at Slepe House in January 1885 together with another young Long cousin, Willie Mardell. He described a musical evening when Mary played the violin and his father and he were on the flute. A few days later, Reginald celebrated his 16th birthday. Besides presents from the rest of his family, he received an oil painting

[424] Reginald read this poem in March 1886.

[425] Stanza 9 line 153.

[426] Uncle Hanslip Long (1837–1916).

from Mary which she had done. Three days later she returned home with another guest, Edwin Hudson. Reginald had a bad cold at the time and was not allowed to go out to see her off at the station.

Mary's birthday was on 7 April and while she had given him a birthday present Reginald did not reciprocate when he was away at school. They did not write to each other during the year, but he was on her mind, as after Christmas she wrote to him asking him to act in a play being put on at her home in a few weeks' time in the New Year. The play was being performed on 13 January. He was initially reluctant to accept, as it would mean he was not at home for his birthday, but later in the day he received her letter and wrote back to agree, hoping that he would 'do his part all right'. Clearly the invitation had struck a chord in his heart.

Two days later she wrote back and enclosed the play she wanted him to act in. This was scenes from Charles Dickens' novel *Nicholas Nickleby.*[427] She called the play *Dotheboys Hall.* Whether she wrote it herself or it was one that had been published for home use is not clear. But what is clear is that she chose Reginald to play the hero of the story, young Nicholas Nickleby. The handsome, young Reginald was to have the starring role! His brother Ernest was to be Smike, the simple-minded servant, Mary was Miss Fanny Squeers, the Headmaster's daughter, and various Long cousins[428] were assigned to take other parts. The vicar of St Peter's Church Prickwillow, Revd Kingdon, was to play Mr Squeers, the odious Headmaster. Reginald did not have much time to learn his lines, but that Sunday evening he did not go to church as he usually would have, but stayed behind and wrote out his lines and started to learn them.

The next day, two days before his 17th birthday, on a rainy day when the snow melted, Reginald left St Ives by the 11.27 train with Ernest and a young friend, Will Langhorne. It was a Monday morning. Just before he left Reginald heard that the Vicar of St Ives, Revd Goldie, whom his mother and father knew well, had died. Reginald was to miss his funeral at the end of that week, as on the day itself Mary 'pressed him to stay'. Love was beginning to blossom.

At Ely Reginald, Ernest and Will were met at 12.46pm (as Reginald

---

[427] *Nicholas Nickleby* was Charles Dickens' third novel and published in serial form in 1838–39. It featured the one-eyed Wackford Squeers as Headmaster of the infamous Dotheboys Hall in Yorkshire, as well as his wife and daughter, Fanny. Nicholas was the assistant master to Squeers.

[428] Richard Long (Wackford Squeers junior) – Mary's brother; Miss A. C. Long (Mrs Squeers and Miss Tilda Price) and Miss Helena Long (servant) – a sister of Mary's.

meticulously noted) by Alice[429] and Mary Long. They all then travelled on to the Longs' farm at Shippea Hill, East Cambridgeshire, near the Suffolk border. Whether this was by trap or train to Shippea station is not recorded. That evening rehearsals for the play began with no one knowing their lines very well. Overnight there was a hard frost which meant that there could be skating on the nearby fens, but Reginald and the others were hard at work in the morning rehearsing again. The play was being put on in the schoolroom in the nearby village of Prickwillow, and in the afternoon the cast went to view the venue. Revd Kingdon drove them back to the farm in his trap. A dress rehearsal was held in the evening – there was little time before the curtains opened the following evening. That night it thawed again.

The next day, a Wednesday, was Reginald's birthday; although his brothers Ernest and Dick were there, celebrations were put to one side while preparations for the play continued – the programme was written out and more rehearsals in the morning. The play was actually being staged in the second part of the evening's performance, as the first part comprised songs and musical pieces. The programme[430] they wrote out was as shown below.

Prickwillow Schoolroom
January 13th 1886
Programme

Part I

Consisting of vocal and Instrumental music

Part II

Scenes from *Nicholas Nickleby* entitled *Dotheboys Hall*

Dramatis Personae:[431]

Mr Squeers	Revd C. D. Kingdon
John Browdie	Mr W. H. Langhorne
Nicholas Nickleby	Mr W. R. Grove
Smike	Mr E. W. Grove
Wackford Squeers jun	Mr R. S. Grove
Mrs S. Squeers	Miss A. C. Long
Miss Fanny Squeers	Miss M. Mary Long
Miss Tilda Price	Miss A. C. Ambrose
Servant	Miss H. H. Long

Boys

---

429 Alice Long was a second cousin, born in 1851 and daughter of William and Henrietta Long.

430 The performance details were written out in full by Reginald on a Memorandum page of his 1886 diary. On the previous page he listed all 29 books he read that year.

431 Latin (the masks of the drama) used for the main characters in a play.

The stage was put up by the cast in the afternoon just in time for the doors to open and the audience to be seated. Considering that the audience numbered 70 and were drawn from the surrounding villages, it was a good turnout for a cold January evening. The cast performed well and Reginald felt that Ernest and he did 'pretty well'. Afterwards they enjoyed a good 'stand-up supper', as he described the meal.

The cast and musicians discussed the performance the next morning; in the evening the performance was put on again, but this time Part 1 was abandoned and instead music was played between scenes. Perhaps the audience had been restless for the first part of the entertainment; or maybe the scene changing needed music to create continuity and hold the interest of the audience.

There was a third performance on the Thursday evening, this time before the villagers. Reginald felt that the performance went very well and the audience had enjoyed themselves. On the Friday, when Reginald had intended to return to St Ives for the vicar's funeral, Mary's entreaty to stay swayed his heart and he stayed on at the farm; in the morning he went round the farm with his Uncle Hanslip, helped to take the stage down and in the afternoon, as it was raining hard, the young ones stayed in reading and playing music. In the evening his uncle and others in the family played 'nap'[432] together. Mary and he had a 'good talk' together. The following day after playing hockey with some of the others, Ernest and he were driven to Ely in the trap by his Aunt Elizabeth and Alice and, having caught a train to St Ives via Cambridge, got back home that evening at 6.00. Reginald wrote in his diary: 'have had a very enjoyable time of it and hope that I shall be asked there again'. He would.

Just over a year later Reginald wrote a thinly disguised account of the stage performance in the Uppingham School Magazine (see Appendix 3). He first became involved in the Autumn Term of 1886 when he took responsibility for printing and correcting proofs, rather than any writing. The then editor, Eccles, had to resign due to work pressures, so Reginald's friend Berry took on the editorship. The pair worked well together and Reginald assisted Berry as a subeditor. There must have been a shortage of material for the spring edition of 1887 so Reginald wrote his first contribution; significantly, he dedicated the article to Mary; not by name

[432] A card game for four players – 'Napoleon' or 'nap' for short. It became popular in the 19th century.

but by using her initials of M.M. as the author. Disguising the authorship of the articles was customary in the magazine, but by using her initials he made a small declaration of his love for her.

Berry read through the draft and praised Reginald and it was sent off to print. Reginald confessed to himself that it was 'awful rot', but it's a charming piece of writing. When published, Reginald was told by a boy at school, who did not know that he had written the article, that he thought it was 'not at all bad'. Reginald could not resist telling him 'in the fullness of his heart and under a strict promise of secrecy that I had written it'. A few months later in March he and Berry received a copy of the School Magazine from King Edward's Grammar School in Birmingham. The editors praised the Uppingham Magazine as the 'best of their contemporaries' and went on to congratulate the author of 'Our Concert'. In their opinion it was 'the most amusing thing they had ever read in a school magazine'. Praise indeed for Reginald.

Interestingly, while he sent a copy of the magazine to his father, Bensly, his friend from King's School who was in Algiers due to his illness, and his father's friend Major Dunn, he did not say that Mary was sent one.

Reginald did not feel he had taken anything as a model for the article, but 'if I have at all it is the concert at Wyton'. But the similarities are clearly there: the village hall or the schoolroom at Prickwillow, the references to 'the pater', to the 'girls', the layout of the programme – all point to the Prickwillow performance influencing the story, especially with his dedication to Mary.

After his visit for the Prickwillow performance, 18 January 1886, he sent off to London to get a photo of himself copied. A couple of days later he sent two photos to Mary before he returned to school the next day. Their romance was starting to develop. Shyly at first, and then more boldly, they were drawn to each other and exchanged letters, photographs and presents.

The day before Valentine's Day 1886[433] Reginald sent Mary some more photographs – presumably of himself. He does not mention getting a card from Mary himself, but he did get a 'jolly' letter from her four days later thanking him for the photos he had sent. Letters continued to be exchanged between them during the course of this Spring Term. He was prolific at

---

[433] The custom of sending Valentine's Day cards became increasingly popular in the Victorian era after the 1d post was introduced in 1840. Victorian Valentine's cards were flat paper sheets, often printed with coloured illustrations and embossed borders. The sheets, when folded and sealed with wax, could be sent cheaply by post.

letter-writing and he continued to write home to Mother, Father, his sister Mabel and others to whom he wrote regularly.[434] In spite of problems with his eyes (which resulted in a trip to London to see an eye specialist, as well as a few days' rest at home) and a series of examinations, Reginald remembered Mary's birthday. On the day before her 17th birthday on 7 April, he sent her a silver glove button hook with a note. Elsewhere in his diary Reginald noted on the accounts page that her gift cost 3s 6d (£22.00). She replied the day after receiving it with a thankyou letter which Reginald again described as 'awfully jolly'.

The Easter holiday saw him meeting up with Mary at Ely when both visited the grammar school where Ernest was a pupil for the school sports day. His mother, sister Mabel and brother Tom went with Reginald by train, and Mary attended to see her brother Tom compete. Mary told him she was keen to arrange some more theatricals in the holidays and wanted him to act again: a good excuse for them to spend time together. He sent her an Easter card which cost 4d (£2.00). Some days later, Mary wrote to say that the theatricals wouldn't be taking place in the holidays; she gave no reason. He wrote back the next day. Reginald's eyes were still troubling him and he had another visit to the oculist in London. On his return he received an invitation for a concert at Shippea Hill, but his mother or father said that he could not go, owing to the fact that the holidays were drawing to a close. In fact, the smallpox vaccination that he and the other family members had had the week before had resulted in his arm becoming painful, so in any event this was another reason for him not to go.

The next term Reginald neither wrote nor received any letters. She was then at a boarding school for young ladies at St Leonard's. Did she feel hurt that he had not come to visit her at Shippea Hill, and felt some sense of rejection? Did he feel embarrassed after their correspondence the previous term? However, in early June 1886 he wrote to her saying that he hoped she'd be at home to get the letter, so maybe she had returned by then. Mary replied a few days later, so obviously she had received it at her home. He wrote in reply, but for the rest of the term there was no further correspondence. Reginald went home for the summer holidays at the end of July.

[434] Brother Ted, Ernest, Mr Ewart (his father's Medical Assistant) his friends George Lloyd and Arnie Ulph. He also wrote to his friend Bensly who was by now staying in Tangiers because of his ill health.

On 10 August, when it rained for most of the day, he travelled early by train to Ely, stopping off at Cambridge to help Mary's brother Dick find a tutor for mechanics. He spent some time at King's College, and climbed up to the roof of the chapel to see workmen carrying out some repairs. In Cambridge he bought a little book for Mary. He and Dick were met in the late afternoon at Ely station by Uncle Hanslip who drove them in his trap to Shippea Hill where they stayed for a few days.

The first day there he did some studying, met the vicar, Revd Kingdon, who had performed in the play with him in January, and then played tennis doubles with Mary against Dick and Hansie on the grass court at the farm. They were just beaten by the boys. That evening he and Mary and some others in the house went down to Prickwillow village to join in a school 'treat'; this involved managing races for the evening. It sounds as if this was some form of sports day for the children. Reginald said that he 'rather enjoyed himself'. The following day he was up early to study, then at 8.00am he and Dick drove to Ely and then by train to Cambridge so Dick could see his tutor; Mary stayed at home but he and Dick caught the midday train back to Shippea station and played more doubles tennis with Mary and the two boys. This time they won. The next day, Reginald rode to Prickwillow to post a letter home and some others he had written. Rain during the rest of the day mostly put paid to tennis with Mary, although they were able to play a little in the evening.

He went off to Cambridge again with Dick for more tutoring but got a letter from his mother asking that he come home early from his holiday on Monday afternoon, as he had an invitation from Sir James and Lady Paget for dinner. They were the parents of the new vicar of St Ives Parish Church. Sir James was an eminent surgeon,[435] and meeting him would be extremely helpful for pursuing his career in medicine. While realising how important this dinner invitation was, his heart was torn as he wanted to stay and be with Mary. He vowed that after the dinner he would try and return to the farm. There was more tennis that afternoon with Alice Long and their friend Will Langhorne.

The next day was a Sunday and Reginald attended church, both in the morning as well as the evening, with the Long family. He went for a bathe

[435] Sir James Paget was knighted for his services to English medicine as a surgeon and pathologist. He discovered the cause of a form of deformity in the bone which then became known as Paget's disease. See Volume 3.

in the River Lark nearby which he described as 'jolly'. He didn't say who was with him, but, given the conventions of the time, Mary would not have come. At the evening service at Prickwillow Church, Revd Kingdon preached what Reginald called a 'splendid sermon on 'our mission in life' based on the passage in Luke 13 about Jesus' parable of the barren fig tree.[436] Reginald did some more studying the next morning, and played some more tennis with Mary and the boys and left with his cousin Hansie at 1.00pm. In the evening he went to dinner with Sir James and Lady Paget who were staying at The How in St Ives. He did not get home until midnight and said the evening was 'jolly'.

'Jolly' was a word well used by Reginald!

Reginald's plans to meet up with his cousins from Shippea Hill for a seaside trip to the Norfolk coast were thwarted a few days later. It had been planned that the Grove and the Long families would go by train to Hunstanton together; he was very disappointed that the Longs decided not to come, as they thought the weather was going to be too wet. An exclamation mark in his diary records Reginald's reaction. Reginald went on 18 August with his mother, the younger children and Miss Schiralm, their governess, his father having left the day before. His father stayed at Hunstanton until the end of the month because of his health. This may well have been the first indication of the illness that was to lead to his early death nine years later in 1895.

It was only a day trip to the seaside but he enjoyed swimming in the sea. On their return by train at Ely, Reginald got off and went to stay overnight to see Mary at Shippea Hill. First thing in the morning, Reginald said goodbye and went off to Cambridge with his cousin Dick. Reginald spent a few days there staying with the Vice Provost of King's, with whom he was still very much in contact since leaving the school three years before. It rained solidly all day. Reginald travelled back to Shippea Hill via Ely, having met up with Dick at Ely station; they found the Longs had forgotten to meet them. Why they did not wait for a train to Shippea Hill is not known, as on a very hot afternoon they walked the six miles to the farm. A bathe in the river cooled them down and then they all played more tennis in the evening. After a quiet Sunday, the family rode in a tumbrel[437] to Lakenheath for a picnic. He had a 'jolly' time particularly as

[436] Luke 13:6–8 when Jesus taught about giving time for fruitfulness in life to become evident.

[437] This was a two-wheeled open cart used on the farm.

he 'enjoyed himself very much with Mary'. His diary concluded with 'it was a lovely day'.

Innocent love was blossoming.

The next days continued with bathing and tennis. There followed a special day out when Reginald and five others[438] rowed in two boats to Ely on the Lark as described earlier. It was a beautiful summer's day. After mooring up at the quayside they had lunch in Ely and then visited the cathedral and went to the top for the stunning view of the surrounding Fens. The following day was spent on the river in the afternoon, too, with Mary, Alice and Will sailing. Mary and Alice had to go to choir practice in the evening, so Will and Reginald took the boat back.

There was another trip the next day to Lakenheath with Mary, Tattie, Alice and Will to the parish church to look at it in greater detail than their earlier visit and to sketch the font. The party split up after this with Will leaving them at Lakenheath, Tattie and Reginald going back to the farm by train to Shippea station, and Mary and Alice returning with the trap. Later that evening they went down to the river to pick bulrushes for Reginald to take home to his mother. He got wet throughout, but 'Mary came so I had a jolly time of it'.

The summer holiday on the farm with Mary came to an end when Reginald went to Cambridge early in the next morning, having said goodbye to everyone. Back home in St Ives, he said goodbye to his mother, sister Mabel, and brothers Ted and Tom who were off on holiday to stay with their cousins at Carleton Grange.

Reginald was busy during September before returning to school for his last year. He was revising and taking medical examinations in London, visiting a mental hospital and then attending his Grandmother Grove's funeral in Portsmouth. There were no letters written between them, but he did manage a very fleeting visit to see her before he left for school when he dropped in to give her a brooch as a present. He had bought the brooch when he had been up in London a couple of weeks before to sit his exams for the Institute of Apothecaries. He spent a few days in London afterwards and visited an exhibition in Olympia with his cousins. He said in his diary that the brooch was a 'jolly one'. He met up with her the day before he travelled back to school. He caught a train at St Ives at 6.15 in

[438] Tattie (surname unknown), Alice Long, Ethel Long, Mary Long, and Will (surname unknown).

the morning, arrived at Ely at 8.15, where he saw Ernest and Ted and gave them some things from home before riding the six miles to Shippea Hill on a bicycle. Unfortunately, when riding into Prickwillow he hit a pothole and went flying over his handlebars, cutting his head badly. Thankfully, he was able to get help from Revd Kingdon where he washed his wound and was given breakfast. He rode to the farm, saw Mary, gave her the brooch,[439] and then she accompanied him back to Ely. He got home about 6.30pm, having travelled 'as near to 50 miles as possible and fairly tired out'. Truly a labour of love.

Back at school, Reginald did not appear to be in a rush to write to Mary; he wrote to his brothers, as well as other friends like Major Dunn, but not to Mary. The first he mentions is when, at the beginning of November, he sent his photo to her.

Perhaps this was one wearing his top hat as a praepostor,[440] having been appointed earlier in the term. He was thrilled to get a letter back from her a few days later. But sending her his photograph somehow got back to his mother who spoke to him about it when he briefly saw her when he went to take scholarship exams for Corpus Christi College, Cambridge. In his words, she 'began rooting me about Mary and about sending her photo'. He wondered how she had found out!

But it did not put him off writing to his Aunt Elizabeth to ask if he could stay at Shippea Hill the following week, ostensibly so he could visit his brothers at Ely, as they were performing in their school's production of *The Sorcerer.*[441] But, of course, that meant seeing Mary again! His aunt agreed to his request. At the end of term, and after a few days at home, Reginald went by train with his mother and younger brother Tom to Ely for his other brother's speech day. Afterwards he travelled to Shippea Farm with his Uncle Hanslip and Aunt Elizabeth, and in the evening played crib[442] and chatted to Mary. He had brought his Christmas presents for her – Charles Dickens' well-known *A Christmas Carol* and less well-known *The Chimes*. She was very pleased, he said, with both.

The following day was frosty and he went skating along a flooded field next to the Lark for an hour and a half without the rest of the family; he

[439] In his accounts for September Reginald gave the price of the brooch at 2/6d (£15.72).

[440] Praepostors were prefects.

[441] *The Sorcerer* was Gilbert and Sullivan's third opera and was first performed in 1877.

[442] Cribbage: a card game generally for two players using a cribbage board to keep the score.

drove in the trap back to Ely with his cousin Dick to see the production of the play; both his parents were there, too, having stayed overnight at the old coaching inn, The Lamb,[443] in Ely.

Returning to the farm, he spent a few more days there; as the weather was initially still cold, he and cousins Hansie and Dick went to the same spot where he had skated the day before. Reginald got one leg very wet and the others less so, although the ice had a thick covering of snow. Rain then brought an end to this activity. Once they had dried out the evening was spent singing, talking playing games and music. The next day, Reginald went out with Hansie shooting on the farm, but he only got one shot at a pheasant and missed! He didn't say whether Hansie was more successful. Before being driven to catch the train at Ely for home, Mary gave him her photograph. Getting home at 5.30pm with the rest of his family, he managed to get a 'jolly card' off in the post to Mary.

Reginald thought he was the only one in his family to send any Christmas cards, and after Christmas complained that none of his relatives had sent him any, including Mary. She made it up when she sent one which arrived on 29 December which she had painted herself with the words inside 'better late than never'; Reginald thought the card 'splendid'. On New Year's Eve he sent her a card with a letter.

Mary and her sister had been invited by his mother to stay in the New Year, and they arrived on 12 January in the afternoon from Ely by train; Mary was not very well and had come to be 'doctored', as Reginald put it. She could not have been too unwell as they both went to a dance with the others that evening, and he danced with her as 'many times as we could arrange'.[444]

Their love for each other began to be a matter of concern for Reginald's mother and father, as they felt it was taking him from his studies. For his birthday she gave him 'a jolly Russia leather cigarette case'. He was particularly delighted that she had painted a bird on the outside and inside a spray of forget-me-nots. He joked that he did not think it was a love bird! Three days after celebrating his 18th birthday, on 16 January, a Sunday, when his mother had a bad cold and headache, and remained in bed all

[443] The Lamb was a coaching inn, near the cathedral, built in the 15th century. It is still in business today.

[444] The convention was that the ladies had dance lists onto which they put the names of gentlemen who asked them to dance.

day, she asked Reginald to see her privately in her bedroom after church. She told him she had noticed he was spending a lot of time with Mary. She told him that he 'always went everywhere where she did'. He kicked himself to think that no one would notice. He resolved to be more careful in future. He had wanted to spend the afternoon with Mary, but as a result of his mother's concern instead walked over to Hemingford on his own to visit his Uncle George. Unfortunately, his uncle was still in bed himself ill, so he could not see Reginald.

As long as Reginald and Mary were with others in the family their relationship was less likely to cause comment. The following day, all the junior members of the family, including his sister Mabel and Mary, went skating for two hours on a 'splendid' bit of ice halfway between the workhouse on the London Road across the bridge and the Woolpack pub. He was able to confide to Mary that he felt he had better not write to her next term, except on her birthday. He felt devastated that he would not hear from her and vice versa, but he did not want to get her talked about. Her response is not recorded. But a couple of days later she told him that while it was fine to write on her birthday, not to send a present. He was disappointed and hoped that she might change her mind. Before returning to school, he began to write an article for the School Magazine which he later was to dedicate to her. Keeping his resolve not to be alone with Mary, when he drove his mother in the pony trap over to Hemingford on 19 January to see his Uncle George to say goodbye to him and his aunt before going back to school, Mary accompanied them.

In the evening on their return to St Ives, there was a talk by a missionary in the Corn Exchange to which the family went. Somehow, Reginald snatched a few moments with Mary on her own and she told him not to send her a present on her birthday but it was all right to write. He replied that it was 'too bad of her not to let me write' once in the term but not to send a present. He hoped she would change her mind before she went home the next day. But it was not to be; Mary left for home on the 3.00pm train and, while she and Reginald spent some time after dinner talking, it was about 'nothing in particular'. The likelihood is that they were with others and so an intimate conversation was not possible.

Back at school, Mary was honoured by Reginald's 'Our Concert' article for the School Magazine mentioned earlier in this chapter. But letter-writing was put on hold, as was sending a present to her. He had promised not to write to her for her sake, but was unhappy at this, as it was such a long time to have no contact. Although she had told him he was on no account to send her a present otherwise it would be returned to him, he still resolved to get her as 'jolly' a one as he could find as well as afford, and chance having it returned.

During the Spring Term Reginald held back from writing as he had promised, but was delighted when Mary wrote in mid-March and sent him two photographs of herself for him to choose one. She had had them taken recently and asked him to send back the one she had previously, which she did not feel was very good. Reginald wanted to keep it. Her letter smelt of scent and of her fur lined hand warmer, and he wrote that 'she is a darling to write'. His heart was in a flutter. She also told him that her brother Dick had given up the idea of training in medicine, as he didn't like the thought of dissecting. He was now thinking of the Church as a calling, although Reginald commented that he couldn't see his cousin becoming a parson.[445]

Her letter had set his heart beating, but he felt he could not hope for another one before her birthday the following month. He started a long letter to her that evening which he finished the next day and posted off. In his diary he noted on 3 April that in the letter he received from home his mother had not enclosed any money, although he'd asked two weeks before for some. 'I wonder if they have any idea that I want to get Mary a birthday present and think they will stop me', he confided in his diary. 'It's foolish to think it but they have my birthday book at home and know when her birthday is and the Mater has often chaffed me about her.'

His father sent him a sovereign[446] a week later, and he went to try and find a present for Mary in the town. He was unsuccessful that day but next day in the afternoon after looking in vain for something pretty he bought the head of a girl on stained glass. He sent it off late in the afternoon with a long letter. Four days later she wrote to him a short note and thanked him 'for being polite enough to remember her birthday'. Was someone at home looking over her shoulder at her reply?

Home for the Easter holidays, after his epic walk from Uppingham to Huntingdon, he waited for a letter from her, fearing that he would not see her before going back for his last term. During the holiday he spent a week brass rubbing and visiting Long relatives near Carleton Grange. Taking a

---

[445] Dick Long started work to train as an auctioneer soon afterwards.

[446] A sovereign was a gold coin worth one pound (£126.81).

train back at Ely, he bumped into Uncle Hanslip, Mary's father, and Dick, her brother, for a second time. As he forlornly wrote, 'I had hoped to have seen Mary', but that was the nearest approach.

The next day at home he saw Kate Long, his cousin, and found out that 'Mary gets no better and still cannot walk or take much exercise'. This is the first mention he makes of her being ill which explains why they had not met in the holidays. However, he resolved to write to her in a few days' time and send her a copy of the Uppingham School Magazine with the article 'Our Concert' which he had dedicated to her. He also wanted to send her a copy of a 'jolly work' that he had come across when he had visited Cambridge. This was '*The Angel in the House*' which was a story set in a poetic form by Coventry Patmore. It had been first published in 1854 and later became very popular in the United States and England. It gave an account of Patmore's courtship of his wife Emily, whom he believed to be the 'perfect woman'. In time this term was used to describe the ideal wife and mother. Reginald wrote that 'it is simply splendid'.

He wrote to her 'in pencil' when he got to Huntingdon en route by train back to school; probably he used pencil as this was easier than using a pen in the station waiting room. He did not enclose the School Magazine, planning to send it separately. He did not mention 'The Angel in the House' in his letter. Reginald said that he was sorry they had not met during the holiday, and asked that she write to him in the next term.

Mary continued to be unwell as Reginald learnt from a letter his mother wrote to him a couple of weeks into the term. She was staying at Slepe House in St Ives so that Dr Grove could keep an eye on her. Reginald wished he was there and hoped he could see her in the summer holidays. She had not answered his letter from Huntingdon station, but he wrote back to his mother with a ruse. He asked for some cut flowers for his study as he felt that if 'they send them at all Mary will have to do it; I hope they fall into the trap'. It worked as Mary sent him a box of lilies of the valley a few weeks later.

Towards the end of May, Mary wrote again from St Ives where she was still staying. She asked him not to write to her there, but when she got back home when she would write again to him. In fact, she went to stay at a Mrs Ellis' in Norfolk, presumably as part of her recuperation.

The last edition of the School Magazine which he edited and had printed came out on 6 June; it contained an article which he'd written on brass rubbings and he sent a copy home, and kept one to send Mary later. He hadn't sent her yet a copy of the earlier volume in which 'Our

Concert' appeared, but had kept a copy to send with the latest edition. Mary wrote from Norfolk and asked him about an article she'd read in *Punch* magazine,[447] as she wasn't sure what it was a parody of. Reginald had no idea but his Housemaster, Revd Christian, was able to tell him that it was about 'The Devil's Walk' by Samuel Coleridge.[448] He copied part of the poem out and sent it to her in a letter that day; it was only a hasty note from her and he hoped it did not count as a letter as she had promised. She did write again, briefly just after The Queen's Jubilee celebrations with an 'awfully jolly letter' in Reginald's words. But sadly, she said not to answer it as she was going to stay with Augusta and Reginald and did not know her address. Who Augusta was is not known, but it was probably a friend rather than a relative, otherwise he would have known the address. He hoped she'd write from there before the end of term in a few weeks' time.

His last term at Uppingham ended on 29 July when he went home to St Ives. Next term he would go up to Sidney Sussex College, Cambridge.

His last diary entry was: 'Hear Mary is bad again, and will have to go away; hope I shall be able to see her again in a short time.'

Reginald's diaries for his first two years at university have not survived and so how long their romance lasted is not known. What is known is that Mary later fell in love and married a man called Ernest Bruges. They had two sons, Eric and William. By then, Reginald had fallen for a girl called Lizzie Parsons, the sister of one of his friends at Cambridge. Reginald wanted to become engaged but her father was against this, and the relationship cooled and ended. A year or two later, Reginald fell in love with Hilda, one of the daughters of a consultant professor, Thomas Stevenson, from Guy's Hospital. Reginald married Hilda in 1897. As detailed in Volume 3, they had ten children, one of whom was my mother.

Edward Thring, Reginald's Headmaster at Uppingham, wrote of his own marriage: 'I can only say I have found my marriage the most perfect earthly blessing, beyond my lover's hopes, even, and worth all.'[449]

Reginald and Hilda were to affirm this, too.

---

[447] *Punch* was weekly humorous magazine first published in 1841. It closed in 1992.

[448] Revd. Christian was partly correct in that Samuel Coleridge wrote *The Devil's Thoughts* in 1799. Later, in 1812, Percy Shelley published a poem called 'The Devil's Walk: A Ballad' as a continuation and this was a satirical attack on the British government of the day. Satan was portrayed as meeting members of the government.

[449] Parkin, George, *Life and Letters of Edward Thring* (Macmillan & Co Ltd, 1910), p. 53.

CHAPTER 9

In the Midst of Life

'To every man upon this earth death cometh soon or late...'[450]

Thomas Babington Macaulay (1800–59)

Macaulay's heroic poems were popular reading for Victorian schoolboys, with their themes of patriotism and daring deeds. Like other boys Reginald was familiar with, this story told about Horatius, the captain of the city gate and his two companions, who faced certain death defending Rome from the invading army of Etruscans.

Death was ever present in the Victorian period, with violent accidents occurring frequently, deadly epidemics that were spread in overcrowded housing conditions, as well as a high mortality rate at childbirth and in children. Thankfully, Reginald's mother was safely delivered in short succession of her five children, and none died in childhood. Besides the death of relatives and later the tragic death of a close boyhood friend, living in a doctor's household meant that Reginald was exposed directly to the fragility of life in Victorian times.

As a boy, Reginald noted the death of relatives as well as others quite factually. Perhaps this detachment reflected the attitude of his father as a doctor in discussing illness and death clinically. Young Reginald, with his youthful medical aspirations, may have adopted his father's professional detachment.

The 19th century saw significant advances in the treatment and the care of patients through the development of more professional medical training, nationally approved standards, new treatments and better nursing practice. Reginald's father was one of the first cohort of those trained rigorously under these new standards described in Volume 3. Additionally,

---

[450] From *the Lays of Ancient Rome* (Horatius) Stanza XXVII: 'Then out spake brave Horatius, The Captain of the Gate: 'To every man upon this earth Death cometh soon or late. And how can man die better Than facing fearful odds, For the ashes of his fathers, And the temples of his gods.'

Pasteur[451] and Koch[452] and others discovered the causes of a whole range of diseases; and then antisepsis and anaesthesia[453] enabled great strides to be made in surgery, and the improvement of hospital conditions and nursing impacted survival rates. While the discovery of diseases was an important breakthrough, curing them was more difficult, however, and compared to today, mortality rates were high.

Interestingly, in St Ives survival rates during the 1870s bucked the national trend. As described in Volume 3, the mortality rate[454] during the period 1870–77 averaged 17.5 per 1000, which was lower than occurred nationally, although infant mortality was, as reported by Dr Grove as Medical Officer of Health, 'still very high'. Compared with the 21st century the rate was massive.[455] Reginald's father would discuss these matters around the dinner table with his wife and guests; while Reginald as a young boy would have not understood much of the details of the subject of illness and death, he experienced an infant death close at hand when he was 11. This was when six-month-old Arthur Mann, the son of Dr Arthur Mann, the Organist at King's College Choir School, died in August 1880. So struck was he by this tragedy that Reginald kept the black-edged memorial card sent to him to commemorate the child's death until his own death 68 years later.[456]

ACCIDENTS

Accidents occurred frequently. There were no emergency services,[457] and Reginald's father, or his Medical Assistant, was often called to attend to

---

451 Louis Pasteur (1822–96) was a French biologist famous for his discoveries of the principles of vaccination, microbial fermentation and pasteurisation. He reduced the death rate from puerperal fever, and created the first vaccines for rabies and anthrax.

452 Robert Koch (1843–1910) was a German physician who contributed hugely to understanding of bacteriology and microbiology. In 1876 he researched the anthrax disease cycle and studied the bacteria that caused tuberculosis in 1882 and cholera in 1883.

453 The first operation in the UK under anaesthesia was performed by the Scottish surgeon Robert Lister in 1846. He used an ether inhalation and amputated a man's leg in 28 seconds.

454 Mortality rates are measured as the number of deaths within a population in a given period. The crude death rate is the number of deaths per thousand people.

455 The rate in 2017 was 9.1 deaths per 1000. Source: Mortality in the UK. House of Commons Briefing Paper January 2018.

456 Letter and memorial card 1880. Grove Family Archive.

457 In 1884 a horse-drawn ambulance service was created at the Liverpool Northern Hospital: it was the first in Britain. In June 1887 the St John Ambulance Brigade was set up to give first aid and ambulance services at public events in London.

those in need of emergency medical attention. These incidents were talked about at the family dinner table or, when he was at school, were mentioned in letters and local newspapers sent by his mother.[458]

Thankfully, many accidents were not fatal. In October 1884, just after Reginald had returned to school aged 15 during the Michaelmas Fair week in St Ives, a Mr Hight was knocked down by one of the fairground's 'swinging boats' on Market Hill. Walking through the throng of people at the fair some horses pulling carts were frightened by the noise of the organ and steam engine. As the horses reared up, Mr Hight was knocked into the path of the roundabout swings. Passers-by carried him to the Robin Hood pub nearby, where he was cared for until Dr Grove's assistant, Mr Haynes, had been called and examined him. Taken home, he remained under his care and made a good recovery:[459] another topic for discussion in the Grove household.

Reginald had just started at the University of Cambridge in October 1887 when his father was called out to another accident. A Mr F. J. Adams left his home in East Street one Thursday evening to go to the Literary Institute which was a short walk away. On his way he slipped and fell, trapping his leg underneath him. Two men heard his cries for help and managed to lift him and carry him in great pain to Mrs Hunt's house nearby. Reginald's father arrived quite quickly and found the leg broken in two places; his ankle was also dislocated. He arranged for a stretcher to be brought from his surgery, and Adams was then taken home. The newspaper account concluded that 'the patient is, we believe, progressing as well as can be expected'.[460]

Some accidents were more serious, however. Just before Reginald came home from his last term at school in June 1887 a two-year-old girl was playing in the road outside Slepe House when she was knocked down by a passing vehicle owned by Mr Butcher of Needingworth. The cart's wheel nearly went over her head, but instead took the skin off her scalp and she was unconscious for a couple of hours. Hearing the noise in the street, the staff from Slepe House rushed out, and the child was brought into the surgery

[458] His mother wrote at least once a week, sometimes more frequently when he was at boarding school.

[459] Norris Museum newspaper scrapbook. Newspaper not known.

[460] *Hunts County News* 22.10.87.

immediately. With Reginald's father's help the child made a good recovery.[461]

The next month another potential lethal accident happened to an old man and his young granddaughter, to which Dr Grove was called. A cattle dealer, Mr Matthews, was driving out of his home paddock with his three-year-old granddaughter when the horse was startled and bolted across the road. He grabbed the child in his arms before the cart collided with a lamp-post and fencing. Thrown out of the trap onto the ground, Matthews held her tight; thankfully, his quick actions protected her and she was unhurt. He was less fortunate himself as he hit his head and was knocked out. Taken back inside by his family, the old man was in deep shock. Dr Grove 'was in quick attendance', and the newspaper[462] said that it 'hoped his condition is favourable for recovery'. As there was no story in the press the following week, it seemed likely that this accident did not result in a fatality.

Interesting, a few years later when Reginald was helping out in his father's practice, he experienced a similar accident when, having just visited a patient, his horse shied coming out of the gateway into the road. He and his groom, Barker, were thrown out of their trap onto the road, and their chestnut horse's frantic actions snapped the shaft of the trap. Thankfully, he had 'nothing to show but a dirty pair of gloves and a little dirt on my hat. It was a most providential escape.'[463]

ACCIDENTAL DEATHS

But some accidents did sadly end in death. Sudden deaths were investigated formally by a Coroner and jury, and inquests were convened within a few days of the person's death and held in local pubs or hotels. Such was the public interest in the proceedings that they were reported in depth, sometimes verbatim by the local papers. Reginald's father was called to give evidence on a number of occasions and these incidents were the topic of conversation at home.

One such sad death happened in January 1871 when Reginald was only three. William Adams was a young man in St Ives 'beloved of all who knew him personally and respected by all he came into contact with'. One Monday he was at the market carrying on business for his father, who was

[461] *Hunts County News* 25.06.87.

[462] *Hunts County News* 09.07.87.

[463] Letter from Reginald Grove to Hilda Stevenson. 03.03.96. Grove Family Archive.

a brewer, chatting and laughing, and afterwards left at about 8.00pm to go home to Fenstanton, a village a couple of miles away. He was found dead the next day, having fallen down a flight of stairs.

A Coroner's inquest was held by Mr W. C. Mellor with 'a most respectable jury' at the George Inn in Fenstanton, which was about 150 yards from where Adams had lived with his father. Reginald's father's evidence was that he had known Adams well as his doctor, and he was not aware that he had suffered any complaint apart from him feeling a little dizzy a few weeks before. But when he had been called out by the family he found that his neck had been dislocated and he died from a fall downstairs. The staircase was a 'dangerous one', and he believed Adams 'had lost his footing and pitched down head foremost'. The jury 'at once returned a verdict of accidental death'. The death was a huge shock to the local community and when the news broke the words hanging on almost everyone's lips were 'poor William Adams'.[464] In a small market town like St Ives, where most people knew each other, the words of the Anglican funeral service that 'in the midst of life, we are in death'[465] would be a poignant reminder of that fact.

Reginald was seven when a three-year-old called Arthur Birchnell drowned in the river swimming with three friends one warm Monday evening in July 1876. While the water was fairly shallow opposite the parish church, it was much deeper in the middle which, at this spot, was also quite wide as the river swept round a bend towards the bridge at St Ives. In a youthful prank, Birchnell jumped onto the back of his friend, William Templeman, and both fell into the deeper water. Another of the boys called Green rushed in and pulled Templeman out, but he failed to get hold of Birchnell who remained submerged. Reginald's father was called and rushed over the bridge and along the Hemingford Meadow bank to where the drowned boy had been pulled out. He tried to resuscitate him using the 'Silvester Method',[466] but without success. The Coroner, a Mr C. B. Margetts, met at the Unicorn Hotel with a jury, heard the witness evidence, including the doctors', and then recorded a verdict of accidental

---

464 *The Huntington News* 21.01.87.

465 *Book of Common Prayer* (1662) according to the rites of the Church of England and said at the burial service just before the internment of the body in the grave.

466 This is a method of artificial respiration where the injured person is laid on his or her back and air is expelled from the lungs by pressing the arms over the chest and fresh air drawn in by pulling them above the head.

death.[467] Birchnell's mother, Hannah, had died in 1869 and so his father was left to mourn his son's death alone.

Another drowning happened some years later when 64-year-old William King, a wine and spirit merchant, took a short cut from Merryland to Bridge St down Woolpack Lane one Saturday evening. He missed the turning walking down the lane and fell into the river. Another local doctor, Dr Mence, was nearby and tried to revive him after he was pulled out. Tragically, he was dead. As King was a patient of Dr Grove's, Mence got a bystander to fetch him. In his evidence at the Coroner's hearing held at the Cow and Hare, off the Bullock Market, Reginald's father confirmed that Mence had done all he could to save him. But after being in the water over five minutes, Mence's delay in getting to him, and given his age and weak heart, it was not possible to save King who had been a patient for 25 years; he concluded that 'his habit was to walk quickly with his hands in his hands in his pockets, his sight was also defective'.[468]

Another sudden death occurred in the spring of 1878, when Reginald was nine, and involved 65-year-old Mr Paine who had been a groom to his father and lived in with the family at their home in the Bullock Market. His death by poisoning deeply affected the family, especially as it first appeared to be suicide.

The Coroner's inquest[469] was held at the Unicorn Hotel, another public house in the Bullock Market opposite the Grove family home. The jury having viewed the body, evidence was then given by Oliver Howard, 'a servant of Dr Grove' who lodged at the Paines'. Next was Mrs Paine and then Reginald's father. It became clear that Paine had taken some liniment medicine by mistake. This had been prescribed a year before by Reginald's father for Paine's son who had a sore toe. It contained belladonna made from the highly toxic deadly nightshade plant. The bottle was half full, clearly labelled poison, and had been left on a shelf next to another bottle bought from Mr Barton, the chemist, whose shop was in Bridge Street. The other bottle was a paregoric[470] for a cold.

Paine did not want his supper that night, as he said it would make him

---

467 *Cambridge Express* 08.07.76.

468 Newspaper and date unknown but report transcribed by the Norris Museum in a compilation of Coroner reports.

469 *Cambridge Express* 13.04.78.

470 A camphorated tincture of opium.

cough and he didn't want any beer for the same reason. He just took what he thought was his cough medicine and poured some into a wine glass with some water. He began to choke 'with some flying out of his mouth, nose and eyes'. He said that it 'was very hot and burnt his throat'. His wife told him not to make such a fuss over his medicine, put some water in the glass, and 'told him to take it steadily'. He drank it, but said it still burnt his throat. He sat for a while and then went off to bed; in the early hours he was in intense pain, feeling dry and tossing and turning in bed; he drank a jug of water and then began to ramble incoherently. Howard was woken up to get Dr Grove to come immediately. His assistant, Mr Wallace, was on duty that night and came and examined him. It was then that it was discovered what he had drunk by mistake. Wallace called for Dr Grove to come. By this time the Grove household were wide awake.

Reginald's father found Paine suffering from belladonna poisoning, unconscious, his face flushed and coughing violently. An emetic[471] was poured down his throat. It did not make him vomit, so they used a stomach pump instead. Paine was then filled with strong coffee and given a morphine injection to calm him. The two doctors stayed until 5.00am and he seemed a little better. Dr Grove returned at midday and found Paine recovering and coherent. But sadly, he was suffering from acute bronchitis and died the following day. The jury 'without hesitation returned as their verdict that the deceased died from accidentally taking poison, that the bronchitis supervening from the effects of that accident'. Afterwards, Mrs Paine, who the newspaper had reported had given evidence 'with great emotion and difficulty', was handed by the jury their fees![472] The fact that the Grove family knew Paine well, that the poison he took was prescribed by Dr Grove, and the painful manner of his death had a profound impact on everyone in the household.

Death by accidental poisoning was not uncommon, as lethal ingredients were used in a number of remedies available for sale through chemists or prescribed by doctors. A very similar incident occurred a few years later in a small village near Kingston upon Thames in Surrey. Interestingly, this was only three years after Reginald's Uncle Frank and his grandmother had left the Kingston area, so it is likely that they picked up the story from the national newspapers.

---

[471] Medicine to cause vomiting.

[472] *Hunts County Guardian* April 1878.

Samuel Jones, a retired seaman in his sixties who lived in New Malden, had been prescribed by his doctor a lotion to help ease the aches and pains of rheumatism. The lotion contained belladonna and aconite which were both highly poisonous. He bought a bottle of rum on Christmas Eve 1884 and put it on his mantelpiece above the fireplace, next to the bottle of lotion. He got up at 7.30am on Christmas Day and decided to celebrate with a small dram. He poured himself a drink into a glass and downed it, only then realising he'd taken the wrong bottle. Despite his doctor, Dr Edwin Child,[473] attending immediately and giving him emetics to vomit up the poison, this had little effect, and he used a stomach pump to remove the lethal potion. Tragically, Jones became delirious and died early the next morning. The inquest held a week later at the local Norbiton Park Hotel, chaired by the Coroner, found that his death was from 'misadventure'. Despite an antidote being given, the aconite was too strong a poison.[474]

Further details of newspaper reports of Coroner inquests attended by Reginald's father and Reginald are given in Volume 3.

A SUICIDE

Reginald only recounts one incident when he was at school of a tragic death. This was in March 1886 when he was 17, when he walked two and a half miles to the village of Glaston with two other friends, Reid[475] and Berry, to see where the incident had happened.[476] He often went walking with the latter around the surrounding villages to look at country churches.[477] Berry was to walk with him a year later at the end of term on their epic hike to Huntingdon, as described later. They deliberately went to Glaston out of ghoulish curiosity to see the 'haunted house … where a man hanged himself ten days previously'.

A man called James Liquorish had been walking near the Old Glaston Hall where he met with some boys from Uppingham School, and they

[473] Dr Child had a patient list of about 5,600 from New Malden and the surrounding area. Having trained at the Charing Cross Hospital, he set up practice in 1866 more or less at the same time as Reginald's father. He died in 1886.

[474] Gill, Robin, *The Village Voice* (New Malden History, February 2020), p. 8.

[475] William Reid was at Redgate, too, but tragically died in a drowning accident in Ceylon when he was 27.

[476] Henry Berry later became the captain of Redgate in Reginald's last year.

[477] The week before, he and Berry had visited Stockerston Church to look at old brasses which they found 'rather quaint' and 'more like a stable than any church I know'. 27.03.86 diary.

went into the ruins of the hall. Walker, Reginald's contemporary, believed that the boys were from Redgate, although Reginald never mentioned this; presumably he would have done if this had been the case.[478] The boys wanted to see the 'Haunted Room', which was known locally for having the occasional spectral sighting. The boys suddenly screamed in horror and ran from the building. Liquorish looked around and saw the decomposed remains of a man hanging by the neck from a door lintel. As Walker described it, the boys 'legged it homewards' and one of them did not recover from shock for some days. No wonder! The body was cut down after Liquorish went to get assistance. The body was presumed to have been there for a week or so. The man was identified as William Church, a 70-year-old former groom, and his flesh had been eaten by the bats and rats that infested the ruins.[479] Reginald's grandmother read about the incident in the newspapers, and, in writing to Reginald, hoped he had not been to the house, as mentioned in an earlier chapter.

SCHOOL FRIENDS

A surprising number of those who were at Uppingham with Reginald died in the 20 years after he left in 1887. Some were killed in accidents, but most from natural causes. 102 boys joined Uppingham from January to September 1883, of which 11 died[480] over the next 20 years, representing a mortality rate of 10.9%. As mentioned in Volume 2, the following died as a result of accidents:

> Ernest Brass November 1902 drowned in the Wilge River,[481] South Africa;
> Arthur Heald October 1892 in SS *Roumania* (sic).[482]

---

[478] Walker, Henry, *Memoirs Books 1 and 2* (1957) Uppingham School Archives. Handwritten and pages unnumbered.

[479] http://deathonmydoorstep.com/index.php/2018/03/04/leicestershire-rutland/.

[480] Uppingham School Roll 1824–1905.

[481] This river is a tributary of the Vaal River in Central South Africa. Brass served in the Anglo-Boer War in 1900 with the Special Services.

[482] The SS *Roumania* (sic) was sailing from Liverpool to Bombay and was wrecked in a heavy storm on the coast of Portugal with the loss of 113 lives, 55 of whom were passengers. Charles Heald was one of six British officers travelling with their wives. There were only seven survivors, one of whom 'was a white man and the rest Lascars. Most heroic attempts were made by husbands to save their wives, but without avail. The shore is strewn with the bodies of women and children.' Tragically, it was reported in the newspapers that the local Portuguese fishermen robbed the bodies washed up on the shore and stripped them of their clothes. The cargo, which floated ashore, was hidden away too. (Press Association Report 31 October 1882.)

William Reid September 1896 drowned in Ceylon.[483]

The following from natural causes:

William Abbott September 1890
Charles Blois December 1900 on voyage to Australia
Charles Evans February 1892
Francis Milman May 1891
William Campbell April 1906
Henry Rotherham November 1902
Joseph Fox-Tarrant October 1898
William Fox-Tarrant December 1883 (brother to the above).

When he was just 12 years old, Reginald wrote that the mother of one of the boys at King's Choir School, Berkeley, had died. This was in February 1881. Berkeley had been at home with her during term-time, so he must have remained at home while she was nearing her end. Berkeley wrote to him about her death and he replied with a letter of condolence. Reginald noted in his diary, without further comment, that Berkeley then returned to school from the Isle of Wight where he lived. His friend left King's before the end of the Spring Term and Reginald noted that in August he 'went away'. He does not mention him again; he could well have been taken out of school because of his mother's premature death. Two days after this he heard that Uncle Arthur, on his mother's side, had died. Quite factually he noted five days later that his mother had written to tell him that another uncle, James Mardall, married to Martha, one of her sisters had died as well.[484]

KATE GOLDIE

In January 1882, Kate (Catherine) Goldie, one of the daughters of the vicar of St Ives, died aged 22. The Revd Charles Goldie and his wife Harriet lived around the corner from the Groves in the large vicarage in Church Street, and the two families knew each other socially as well as from church. Reginald's father was the family doctor as well as being one of Goldie's churchwardens for some years. The Goldie family was large even by the standards of the time, with nine children,[485] all but one being

[483] Reid was a tea planter in Ceylon.

[484] Uncle James and Aunt Martha Mardall's life in Harpenden has been described earlier.

[485] National Census Records 1871.

daughters. John, their only son, who gained fame as a rower at Cambridge, was 30 when his sister died.[486] It was a Sunday and Reginald was at church at both the morning and the evening services. Kate died in the afternoon and her death must have been announced at the evening service. Besides noting her death, he wrote that it 'rained very hard in the afternoon and evening'. The age gap between them was large so it's understandable that the relationship was not close and he was closer to Kate's sister, Beatrice, who was a year older than him. Kate Goldie was buried five days later, on his birthday. He returned to King's that day and did not attend the funeral with the rest of his family.

REVD CHARLES GOLDIE

In January 1886, almost to the day of his own daughter's death, Revd Charles Goldie died.[487] It was a Monday, and the day before it had snowed hard but overnight began to thaw, Reginald observed. Goldie was only 61 and had been looked after by Dr Grove during his illness. Goldie had been the vicar of All Saints for most of Reginald's boyhood. Reginald turned 17 the following week and was packing up to visit his Long cousins at Shippea Hill; he was looking forward to seeing his sweetheart Mary again and taking part in the play they were putting on with others at nearby Prickwillow. Taking the train to Ely mid-morning, with his brother Ernest and their friend Will Langhorne, they were met by cousin Alice and Mary who then drove them by trap back to their farmhouse. Reginald had other things on his mind than the death of the vicar. He wrote that evening that it 'rained hard and thawed most of day so it was awfully dirty'. When the funeral took place, Reginald was still at Shippea Hill and Mary 'pressed me to stay'. He knew he should attend but love won the day. He returned to St Ives the next day, missing the funeral.

GRANDMOTHER GROVE

As described in an earlier chapter in September 1886, Reginald's paternal grandmother, Grandmother Grove, became ill and died in Southsea, Hampshire.

Reginald first heard about her illness soon after he got home from his

[486] John Goldie died at the relatively young age of 44 in April 1896. (Norris Museum newspaper cuttings.)

[487] Revd Charles Dashwood Goldie was the Vicar of St Ives 1866–86.

trip to London for his examinations with the Institute of Apothecaries. This was before he went back to Uppingham for his final year at school. He found out that his father had travelled to the south coast urgently to see her. His father returned late in the afternoon by train the next day, as she was a little better. Sadly, the next day a telegram arrived to say she had got worse, and his mother and father rushed off by train at midday to be with her. The next day, after his brothers Ernest and Ted went back to school, his father returned, but at 7.30pm a further telegram arrived to tell the household that, sadly, Grandmother Grove had died in the early evening at 6.30. She was 69. The news was transmitted quickly using the telegram service.[488] His mother returned the next day in the afternoon, but was 'not at all well'. Whether this was her grief or caused by something else, Reginald did not say.

The funeral was held three days after she had died, and she was buried in Kingston Cemetery, Portsmouth. Reginald left early that day, catching the 7.30am train for London. There was enough time to get to the Apothecaries Hall[489] in the City of London to see his exam results which were posted on the noticeboards: to his joy he found that he had passed. En route, fearing rain at the graveyard, he bought an umbrella and took the 11.30 train from Waterloo to Portsmouth arriving just after 2.30pm. Despite the sad reason for his trip, he enjoyed looking out of the train windows, seeing Arundel Castle and 'some splendid scenery'. On arrival, he and his father stayed with a relative of his grandmother's, a Mrs Haynes. He helped make a wreath for the service the next day.

Reginald had the honour, as the eldest grandson, of following the cortège with three others – his father, his Uncle Frank and Dr Guillemard. The latter, previously a Medical Assistant in his father's practice, lived in Southsea and knew the Grove family well.[490] He had set up practice there after leaving St Ives in 1884, and Grandma Grove was one of his patients, as Uncle Frank was later.

No other members of the family were present. After the ceremony, they had tea at a Mrs Haynes' where they were lodging. They then went across to Southsea for dinner in the evening.

---

[488] The first telegram service in Britain was launched by the Electric Telegraph Company two decades before nationalisation of the telegraphs in 1870.

[489] The Worshipful Society of Apothecaries is based at Apothecaries Hall, in Black Friars Lane in the City of London.

[490] He lived at 22 South Parade, Southsea.

The next day, before breakfast, Reginald went down to the docks and on-board HMS *Crocodile*. She had been built to transport of troops between the United Kingdom and the Indian subcontinent.[491] Mrs Haynes cooked him a hearty breakfast and then he went for a long walk over to Portsmouth and back; after lunch at Mrs Haynes, Reginald caught a train back at 2.00pm and got home at 7.15. It had been a long day and he went to bed early. In his diary he said nothing about how he felt about his grandmother's death. Returning for his last year at Uppingham two days later, no doubt he had other things on his mind.

JAMES SMITH

The tragic death by a heart attack of one of his father's patients clearly affected Reginald and many others in St Ives in the spring of 1887. 39-year-old James Allpress Smith had run a drapery business in Bridge Street for 13 years. He travelled on business to Bletchley station in Buckinghamshire one Monday evening, and as he walked down the platform, he suddenly collapsed and died. The stationmaster telegraphed Mr Starling, the stationmaster at St Ives, to tell him and he contacted some of Smith's closest friends and they then broke the news to Mrs Smith. This was how it was reported in the local press. But Reginald's account was different. His diary said that while playing whist in the evening the game was 'disturbed by the Pater having to go and break to Mrs Smith the fact that her husband, one of the leading tradesmen in the town had fallen down and died at Bletchley station'.

It is more likely that Smith's doctor was the one who asked to see his widow and tell her the tragic news. Dr Grove took the first train from St Ives the next day to Bletchley, taking Mr Blinkhorn, his assistant, with him. Knowing that his patient had had heart problems, and having expected the result for some time, he went to see if an inquest could be prevented. While Smith's body lay in one of the waiting rooms at the station, Dr Grove carried out a post-mortem examination. Meanwhile, Reginald had gone to Cambridge to visit the parents of his friend Bensly who had died. It had been a very difficult visit, so this new, unexpected death was a further emotional challenge for him.

[491] The ship had a single screw, a speed of 14 knots, one funnel, a barque-rig sail plan, three 4-pounder guns, and a white-painted hull. Her bow was a 'ram bow' which projected forward below the waterline.

Smith's body was placed in a 'shell'[492] and arrived at St Ives station by the 7.15pm train accompanied by Dr Grove.

The undertakers took the body from guard's van and carried it to Smith's house in Bridge Street. The *Hunts County News* reported that 'Universal signs of respect were shown and most blinds and shutters en route were closed. Smith was an active member and deacon of the Particular Baptist Church where he led a young man's bible class.' The report concluded that for 'his unassuming manner and kind disposition he was held in high esteem. He was ever ready in alleviating the distress of the poor and they have lost in him a true friend and helper.' The townsfolk respected his Christian example and 'the sympathy for the family is general throughout the town'.[493]

Later in the evening Reginald stayed up late to speak with his father after the latter had returned from a dinner at the Primrose League[494] in the town. Reginald 'waited up for him alone' and had a 'talk with him about everything in general and did not get to bed until 12.00pm [sic]'. There was much on his mind with the recent death of his young friend, the raw grief of his parents, and the sudden death of Allpress Smith at such a young age, leaving a widow. Reginald attended the funeral service in Smith's Particular Baptist Church in East Street. 'It was a very big one, nearly all the tradesmen in the town were there, as well as the shop assistants,' he commented in his diary.

EDWARD THRING

In his first term at Sidney Sussex College, Cambridge, in October 1887, the news reached him of the sudden death of Edward Thring, aged 65, his old Headmaster. There was no indication of any ill health; the day before he fell ill on Sunday 16 October he had enjoyed a family dinner. He then wrote his sermon for the following day based on the passage in Genesis 3:4–5, when Satan tempts Eve to eat from the fruit of the tree of good and evil. His diary entry ended: 'And now to bed, sermon finished, and a blessed feeling of Sunday coming'.

Thring had only said goodbye to Reginald two days before the end of the Summer Term. It had not been an easy meeting as Thring had told him that

---

[492] A shell was the inner section of a coffin placed inside the outer coffin. However, in this context the term was used to describe the temporary coffin used to transport the body home.

[493] *Hunts County News* 23.04.87.

[494] Founded in 1883, the Primrose League was a new political organisation for spreading Conservative Party principles – see Chapter 10.

> he intended to give me the Praepostor's Leaving Medal, but it was with misgivings as I had only done sufficient work here to satisfy an easy conscience: this is because I had not attended properly to his talks on divinity though he talked through nominally of [sic] all my work yet I knew he really meant divinity and to that I own to only have done sufficient work etc.[495]

As described in Volume 2, Thring gave him a little prayer book in parting, saying that 'in every temptation, at the very moment of temptation there was an inspiration to do right and very seldom was that inspiration present even in ten seconds afterwards'. Thring was referring to the passage in St Paul's First Letter to the Christians in Corinth,[496] and no doubt his intention was to remind Reginald that, in leaving the cloistered life at Uppingham, he would face the temptations of 'the world, the flesh and the Devil',[497] but would be strengthened against these. Sadly, the prayer book has not survived.

One Sunday at chapel, Thring was due to preach the sermon mentioned above but he fell ill during service. Skrine recalled that Thring's 'labouring voice ceased with the Collect; he resigned the book and walked down the nave, between wandering rows'.[498] Young, ten-year-old Henry Walker recounted many years later:

> I was present in Chapel when the Old Man, while reading the Ante Communion Service handed the book to Revd Christian and slowly and steadily looking very ill tottered down the aisle. Revd W. Campbell came out to assist him but was moved aside within a yard of me as I was kneeling at the end of the 2nd row below the Chair. Skelly Robinson, the School Porter opened the door and closed it behind the retreating figure of our beloved Headmaster and we saw him no more. He died on the Saturday following.[499]

On hearing the news of Thring's death, Reginald immediately wrote to his old Housemaster, Revd Christian, and asked if he and others at Cambridge

---

[495] Reginald wrote that 'But in everything else I think I have tried my best; of course, sometimes I have scamped [sic] work but usually I have done my best'.

[496] 1 Corinthians 10:13: 'There hath no temptation taken you but such as is common to man: but God is faithful, who will not suffer you to be tempted above that ye are able; but will with the temptation also make a way to escape, that ye may be able to bear it.' King James Version.

[497] Book of Common Prayer: The Litany.

[498] Skrine, J. H., *A Memory of Edward Thring* (Macmillan & Co 1889), p. 275.

[499] Walker, Henry, *Memoirs Books 1 and 2* (1957) Uppingham School Archives.

could attend the funeral service.[500] 'The sad news of Mr Thring's death has fallen very heavily on every OU up here'. Permission was given and he travelled from Cambridge with an Old Uppingham boy, Edward Weaver, with whom he was friends. While they were more or less the same age, Weaver had joined the Lower School in September 1882, moved to The Lodge and left at the same time as Reginald before going to Trinity College, Cambridge. Like Reginald he had been a praepostor.[501]

The funeral took place in the school chapel the Thursday afternoon after he died.

It was a dark and stormy October day. The local paper said that

> the weather itself was the most depressing character, rain falling the whole day, gusts of wind blowing, so that it seemed as though the very elements themselves were mourning the loss of a truly great man. The town of Uppingham was wrapped, as it were, in a shroud.[502]

Perhaps the thoughts of many who watched dwelt on words that Thring had written in one of his poems about the school's time at Borth, North Wales, in 1876:

> With sad, sad heart life did depart,
> A ghostly silence fell;
> With sad, sad heart they turned to depart,
> And–farewell, home, farewell.[503]

The school bell tolled. The coffin, draped with wreaths, was lit by the gas lights in the chapel where the boys, masters, their wives, Old Boys, school servants and town well-wishers sat in rows. Reginald was one of the 116 Old Boys and friends of Thring who attended.[504] Walker recalled in his memoirs as a boy in the Lower School that the schoolmasters and boys were 'all "stuck of a heap"; as the vulgar parlance has it'. He went on to say that for many of the staff Thring had done much of their thinking and ruled with a firm hand and his death left them fearful for the future. Walker remembered the funeral as being 'most impressive and there was a

---

500 Letter from William Reginald Grove to Revd Christian 24.10.87.

501 After Cambridge, Weaver became a barrister and later lived at Great Bookham, Surrey. (Uppingham School Roll.)

502 *Rutland, Oundle and Stamford Post* 28.10.87.

503 Thring, Edward, *Borth Lyrics* (John Hawthorne, 1881): 11 The Summons.

504 Ibid.

huge gathering'. He and the other boys lined the High Street as the coffin went by. Besides being dark and stormy, it was a cold day and Walker and the others wore two pairs of drawers and vests to ward off the cold in addition to an overcoat with a band of crêpe around their school caps which they wore for the rest of the afternoon. 'I felt like a trussed chicken', he commented.[505]

After the service finished, the procession to the churchyard was led by five senior boys, five abreast, followed by 'Gallery' boys, masters, five abreast, Trustees four abreast, who all walked before the coffin. On either side walked 16 bearers. After the coffin came Thring's family, the masters' families five abreast, then Old Boys, including Reginald, followed the cortège and then last of all by visitors and representatives from the town.

They went in driving rain to the churchyard by the Old School Room. Vast crowds lined the way and at the graveside 'O God, Our Help in Ages Past' was sung 'with sad feeling'. Each School House had sent a wreath, as had 'Trustees, Masters, Old Boys, Visitors, Townspeople, Clergy and Gentry of the town and district'. At the graveside, it was estimated that 2,000 mourners were present when his coffin was lowered into the grave.[506] There were too many wreaths to be put in the vault.

It was a sad, bleak, solemn occasion. But for Thring, the words from Psalm 16 spoke the truth:

> You make known to me the path of life [author's emphasis]; you will fill me with joy in your presence, with eternal pleasures at your right hand.[507]

GRIEF AND MOURNING

The 1890s 'witnessed the golden age of the Victorian funeral'.[508] Towards the end of the century funerals had become more and more elaborate. For the middle class the hearse was often open glass with the carriage covered in black crêpe and surrounded by flowers. Perhaps four horses with black plumes would pull the hearse preceded by paid 'mutes' dressed in black shawls and drapes over their tall silk hats who were then followed by the mourners, also dressed in black.

---

[505] Walker, Henry, *Memoirs Books 1 and 2* (1957) Uppingham School Archives.

[506] *Rutland, Oundle and Stamford Post.*

[507] Psalm 16:11.

[508] Arthur Bigge writing to Arthur Ponsonby and cited by A. N. Wilson, *The Victorians*, p. 279.

Elaborate mourning rituals were traditional during this period and generally lasted for more than a year. Paying a call to the bereaved widow was customary. Mrs Beeton's *Book of Household Management* recommended that a lady

> should send in her card, and if her friends be able to receive her, the visitor's manner and conversation should be subdued and in harmony with the character of her visit. Courtesy would dictate that a mourning card should be used, and that visitors, in paying condoling visits, should be dressed in black, either silk or plain-coloured apparel. Sympathy with the affliction of the family, is thus expressed, and these attentions are, in such cases, pleasing and soothing.[509]

Public mourning left a considerable impact on impressionable children. It was customary for a widow to wear black for two years before moving to grey or lavender for a further six months. The five-year period of mourning by Queen Victoria for her husband Albert was unusual, but reflected her deep grief at his death. Mourning brought social isolation as no invitations to dinner could be accepted or visits made to the homes of social acquaintances. By convention, a dead child was mourned by parents for a year, as was the period for the death of a parent. This would have been the case when Reginald's grandmother died in 1886. Letters had black borders to signify mourning: there are a number of these letters written to Reginald after he left school from grieving relatives. To help those who mourned, and show respect to the dead person, there was much ritual and formality, which began at the moment of death, which took place in most instances at home. The body remained in the house until the funeral. The blinds were drawn and remained close until the funeral, which generally was arranged within a few days. Sometimes, plaster casts were taken of the person's face or their hand, although Reginald never mentioned this happening.

Until 1885, when it was made legal to carry out cremations, all funerals were by burial. The move was partly prompted to stop the spread of diseases, but there was also the convenience for mourners not standing at

---

[509] Beeton, Mrs, *Book of Household Management* (Ward, Lock & Co., London, 1907 edition), p. 20.

a graveside (as happened with Thring) in 'pouring rain'.[510]

Until the funeral took place, in middle-class households rigid etiquette then fell into place; a member of the family wrote invitations to all those they thought should attend; very often women were not expected to attend due, it was felt, to their weaker sensibilities; Queen Victoria, for instance, did not attend her husband's funeral. It appears that in the funerals Reginald knew about, women did attend, as this became more common as the century progressed. Black-edged notepaper was used for the invitations.

At Grandma Grove's funeral there were only four family mourners – all men. At the funeral of Reginald's father, described in Volume 3, there were many more and, as already mentioned above, there were 2,000 at Edward Thring's funeral committal at the graveside.

The simplest funeral listed in Cassell's 1869 *Household Guide*[511] cost £3 5s (£412). This provided a carriage, a horse, a coachman, pall-bearers, an attendant with a hatband, an elm-lined coffin, a pall and items for mourners to wear or 'mourner's fittings' – gloves, scarves and mourning-bands which were lent to the mourners by the undertaker. This was probably the type of funeral arranged for Grandmother Grove.

The Revd Goldie's funeral would have cost much more. For £53 9s (£6,721) an undertaker would provide a hearse, four horses, two coaches for the family mourners with four hours each, 23 plumes of ostrich feathers, velvet coverings for the carriages and horses. The coffin had a padded mattress, lined with fine linen, and a pillow. There was lead casing within the oak coffin which had an inscription and brass handles, and was covered by a silk velvet pall. Those attendants supplied by the undertaker

---

[510] The Cremation Society of England promoted cremation and it built a furnace in 1879 on land bought near Woking, Surrey, but strong local protests prompted the Home Secretary to refuse to allow cremations to proceed without parliamentary approval. The Society continued to campaign to change public opinion, and following a legal pronouncement that cremation was legal in 1884, informed the public it was prepared to proceed with the cremation of 'anyone so requesting it'. The first cremation was carried out at Woking in March 1885.
(https://www.goldencharter.co.uk/news-and-info/2018/a-short-history-of-cremation-in-the-uk/ 01.08.20.)

[511] *Cassell's Household Guide to every department of practical life: being a complete encyclopaedia of domestic and social economy. Volume 1* (Cassell, Petter and Galpin, 1869).

were two mutes,[512] 14 men and the coachmen.

Generally, the mourners did not return to the house with the family. Memorial cards were sent out afterwards to those who were unable to attend giving details of the person's name, age, date of death and where the grave was located.

'In the midst of life, we are in death'.

512 Mutes were those who lead the procession. Sometimes they were children which added extra pathos. In Charles Dickens' *Oliver Twist*, young Oliver was taken on by the undertaker Mr Sowerberry for children's funerals. Sowerberry tells his wife: 'There's an expression of melancholy in his face, my dear, which is very interesting. He would make a delightful mute, my love… I don't mean a regular mute to attend grown-up people, my dear, but only for children's practice. It would be very new to have a mute in proportion, my dear.'

CHAPTER 10

Public Service in St Ives

'non nobis solum nati sumus' [513] ('not for ourselves alone are we born')
Cicero

At Uppingham Reginald became well versed in the classics. Cicero's dictum was one of the Latin pieces he construed[514] for his Headmaster, Edward Thring – as was the Latin motto adopted by the St Ives Town Council in 1874 when the town was incorporated as a borough: *sudore non sopore* ('by sweat not by sleep'). This was a slight pun on the word 'sleep', as the old English name for the town was 'Slepe'! It was also Oliver Cromwell's motto.

His father's example of public service, the teaching he received at school, as well as a core element of his Christian faith, all contributed to Reginald's adult life of service formed in his early years.

A few years after Reginald's death in 1948 a tablet was placed under the window in the south aisle of St Ives' All Saints parish church in memory of Reginald and his wife Hilda. Carved into the Portland stone was the inscription '...who in their time gave faithful service to this church and town'.[515] His was a lifetime of public service learnt at an early age from his father. As Reginald's father became more established in his medical practice, he gained the respect of those in the town, and his life of public service developed. Dr Grove served as a model for his son.

Medical general practice was hard work, particularly with seven days a

---

[513] Marcus Tullius Cicero, *De Officiis* 1:22.

[514] This meant preparing a set passage in advance and then, in class, or in a small group, orally translating it.

[515] The full inscription reads: 'In loving memory of William Reginald Grove physician b.1869 d.1948 and of his wife Clara Hilda Justice of the Peace b.1872 d.1954 who in their time gave faithful service to this church and town.' The plaque cost £49. Above the plaque is a stained-glass window depicting St William, St Gregory and St Richard. The lettering below each window state reads: 'To the Glory of God and in memory of Dr Grove [Reginald's father]: Of the Lord a faithful servant to the people a beloved physician; from 1852 to 1895 churchwarden of this parish aged 57 years' (600B 958/78.) NB: The wording is incorrect as Dr Grove only arrived in St Ives in 1865. (Registers and Records at the Cambridgeshire County Record Office, Huntingdon.)

week, 24 hours per day service being provided. But, despite this, in rural areas like St Ives, it was possible to become involved in the community as well as pursue a variety of leisure activities. In the obituary written when his father died, Dr Grove's many commitments were highlighted – from his role as medical officer of health to being a churchwarden for many years (see Volume 3).

Reginald's role model was that of his father serving the local community.

POLITICS

From Reginald's diary entries there is only occasional mention of national or international events – the turmoil of Home Rule or the 'Scramble for Africa', or the colonial wars around the world that Britain fought did not feature. Local politics were commented on, but only as background to other matters.

Reginald's father did not get deeply involved in politics but he was passionate that St Ives should take advantage of the opportunity to become a recognised municipal borough in its own right like Huntingdon and Godmanchester.[516] This status accorded with the growth of its booming cattle market which attracted business from across the country, as well as the rail freight and passenger travel across the country. Dr Grove's motivation was that public health could be improved, especially through better town drainage, which could be funded through more revenue from increased rates levied on businesses and residential properties.[517]

A petition signed by hundreds of 'inhabitant householders' from St Ives was drawn up, including Reginald's father, in 1873, and sent to The Queen asking for the Privy Council to grant a Charter of Incorporation. This was under the same act that Godmanchester had been awarded municipal status. Not all were in favour in St Ives, as a counter petition, which had 75 signatures from other inhabitants, was sent in. Those against the idea were largely from south of the town, as some areas of the town, including south of the river, would not be covered. Those in favour won the day and in 1874, 11 years after Dr Grove came to the town, a new Charter was granted. The bells of All Saints were pealed in celebration,

---

[516] Huntingdon's status dates back to the Middle Ages and the town was recognised as the county capital; Godmanchester, which was much smaller than St Ives, gained its municipality via the Municipal Corporations Act 1835.

[517] Little, Bryan, and Werba, Herbert, *St Ives in Huntingdonshire* (1974).

no doubt fascinating five-year-old Reginald who was living a few hundred yards away from the church.

How those who sat on the town council should be appointed was the next challenge. A list of local government voters was prepared based on property qualifications, and in October 1874 a public meeting was held to consider how the elections should be carried out. The Vicar, Revd Yate Fosbrooke, and Reginald's father proposed that the new town council should be appointed 'by amicable arrangement'. This suggestion did not find favour and an election was eventually held with 25 candidates from the Liberal and Conservative parties standing for the 12 seats. The Returning Officer was a solicitor, Mr Green, and Dr Grove acted as his deputy and did not stand for election[518]. George Newton Day, a solicitor from the family firm whose offices were in the Bullock Market near the Grove medical practice, was appointed the borough's first town clerk. Day had drawn up the original petition that went to the Privy Council.

Reginald's father played no further role in local politics, although he was a staunch Tory, supporting Benjamin Disraeli who was Prime Minister from 1874 to 1880, and who died in 1881 aged 76. Unlike some other constituencies, after 1868 Huntingdon elected one just one Member of Parliament[519] who was often unopposed.[520] Where there was a contest, turnouts were high – in 1873 83%, and in 1885 80%. Throughout the 1870s and 1880s Huntingdonshire was represented by a Conservative with a very small electorate of around 1000 having the vote. Edward Montagu (Viscount Hinchingbrooke) was the Member of Parliament from 1876 to 1884 until he was elevated to the House of Lords as the Earl of Sandwich. A by-election held then saw Robert Peel, son of Sir Robert Peel, who had led the Conservative Party and been Prime Minister twice, elected by just nine votes against the Liberal Party candidate Charles Veasey. This changed in the general election of 1886 when the first Liberal won the seat.

Dr Grove was a Conservative, as was his brother Frank. But unlike Frank, he was a member of the local Primrose League and attended their meetings held in St Ives.[521] The League had been founded in 1883 after

518 Undated talk about St Ives given by Jane Grove, called 'Old St Ives'.

519 The last election when two members were returned to Parliament was 1868. Whether Dr Grove was on the electoral roll then is not known. At the time the electorate numbered 383 in 1865 and 976 in 1868.

520 1865 and 1868.

521 Norris Museum press cuttings 1796–1914, 21.04.88.

Disraeli's death to spread the principles of Conservatism across the country with ordinary people; as the primrose was known as Disraeli's favourite flower, the League adopted it as their emblem.

Sometimes the Primrose League meetings were purely social as when, in his last year at school during the Christmas holidays, Reginald went to a 'smoking concert' held in the Corn Exchange in Market Hill. These social gatherings were popular at the time, being 'men-only' evenings when men would smoke and discuss politics while listening to live music or singing. On this occasion there was a good crowd, there were some comic songs sung, and 'towards the end some of them began to be very "merry"'. The liquor had obviously flowed freely! Captain Fellowes, future MP, magistrate and Governor of the St Ives National School, 'made a good speech'. Reginald was rather pleased to be introduced to him afterwards.[522] Ailwyn Fellowes was elected to the Ramsey constituency (sometimes called North Hunts) in a by-election. Although Reginald was in his last term at Uppingham and followed the election results closely, he missed the drama at the count in Market Hill. Edwin Saint, a local businessman in the building trade, was a keen supporter of Fellowes. As he helped Lady de Ramsey [Fellowes' sister-in-law] and Mrs Fellowes leave the count in the Corn Exchange 'either through a fall or a cowardly blow, he had his skull fractured and paralysis developed'.[523]

While Reginald did not become active in local politics, he supported the League's aims and was enrolled as a Knight Harbinger[524] of the League in April 1889.[525] In that year there were 54,580 such Knights belonging to the League and total membership was over 672,000. The membership numbers varied considerably across the country. As a percentage of the

[522] Captain Fellowes gave a rousing speech at the opening ceremony of the new St Ives Market in October 1886. He lived at 'The How' which was a rather imposing house on the Ramsey Road.

[523] *Huntingdonshire Post* 22.12.1916, 'Death of Mr Edwin J. Saint'.

[524] The solemn oath sworn by a Knight Harbinger of the League (an honorific title given to a member) stated that 'I declare on my honour and faith that I will devote my best ability to the maintenance of religion, of the estates of the realm, and of the imperial ascendancy of the British Empire; and that, consistently with my allegiance to the sovereign of these realms, I will promote with discretion and fidelity, the above objects, being those of the Primrose League.' The League was closed down in 2004 after 121 years' existence. Its remaining funds of £70,000 were given to the Conservative Party. (https://en.wikipedia.org/wiki/Primrose_League 19.03.19.)

[525] Diploma of Knighthood 12.04.89 Number B84784. Grove Family Archive.

population Huntingdonshire was 2.8%, Cambridgeshire 1.8% and Rutland 8.2%, the highest in any county.[526] In general the Primrose League was best represented in regions where the Conservative Party was active, although its strength in the East Midlands, as exemplified in Rutland, demonstrated how it took root in areas which were generally Liberal and nonconformist in character.

Father and son had the same political affiliations. The lines in Gilbert and Sullivan's 1883 opera, *Iolanthe*, that political loyalties were often passed from one generation to another, was true in the Grove family:

> I often think it's comical,
> How Nature always does contrive,
> That every boy and every gal
> That's born into the world alive,
> Is either a little Liberal
> Or else a little Conservative.[527]

While Dr Grove was a Conservative, Edward Thring, Reginald's Headmaster, described himself thus: 'if I call myself anything I call myself a Radical Conservative, as all my heart is for change, and all my heart and head for a change that shall not pull down but gradually build up – for growth that is'.[528] Thring was somewhat of a maverick in his religious views, too, as detailed in Volume 2.

Thring's influence on Reginald's faith was considerable, but in his politics is less clear. Reginald had a passing interest in local and national politics mentioning national events such as the death of Benjamin Disraeli in April 1881, the Conservative politician who served twice as Prime Minister,[529] and Alexander II Czar of Russia being assassinated the month before in St Petersburg. Clearly the adults with whom he mixed talked much of these events. General Gordon's death in Khartoum in February 1885 was another event that was much talked about. Reginald was older then and Gordon's death was the top story in all the newspapers. It shook

[526] In Huntingdonshire there were 1637 members in 1888 against a population of 57,761 (National Census 1891) Diana Sheets https://core.ac.uk/download/pdf/4818363.pdf 1986.

[527] Iolanthe 11. Sir William Gilbert (1836–1922) wrote the words and Sir Arthur Sullivan (1842–1900) composed the music of 14 light operas. *Iolanthe*, a comic opera, poked fun at English law and the House of Lords.

[528] Parkin, George, *Edward Thring: Life, Diary and Letters* (1910), p. 326.

[529] Reginald referred to him as the Earl of Beaconsfield, which was his correct title.

the nation. At Uppingham a service was held in his memory, such was Gordon's public stature.

The general election in November 1885, held when Reginald was 16, was a significant one nationally and a topic of great discussion at school. It was the first general election when the franchise was extended, as well as limiting the number of parliamentary seats to one for each constituency. While the extension of the franchise did not yet apply to women, it meant that the majority of adult men (aged over 21) could vote. Because of these radical changes, the outcome of the election was uncertain. In the Huntingdon constituency the number of registered electors increased from 1,052 in 1880 to 5,665 in 1885.

Reginald mentioned the upcoming election the day before polling began, noting the current state of the two parties – Liberals and Conservatives – both holding 84 seats. On election day, 27 November 1885, the town was 'shut up a great deal'. Unlike elections today with the results known within 24 hours of the end of polling, in this election the results were not evident immediately.[530] Reginald kept a record of the changing results, and by 30 November the Liberals led by William Gladstone had a majority of 12.[531] More results were known the following day, with Reginald recording that the Liberals were 20 seats ahead of the Conservatives (180 vs 160). By the time all the results were in it was found that, while Gladstone's Liberals had won the most seats, the Irish Nationalists held the balance of power.

At home, Reginald found that for the first time ever, Huntingdonshire had returned a Liberal as the Member of Parliament – Thomas Coote,[532] whom Dr Grove knew well and who was probably one of his patients. His majority against his Conservative rival, George Montagu, the Earl of Sandwich's son, was 146, with the former polling 2,354 votes against Montagu's 2,208. It was a huge upset for the Conservatives in the Huntingdon constituency.

---

[530] On this occasion polling took place on a rolling basis across the country from 24th November until 18th December. Polling day at Uppingham was on 27th November.

[531] Although Reginald did not mention it, this election saw the first socialist party take part with the Social Democratic Federation field three candidates. None were successful.

[532] Coote's father, also called Thomas, was a corn merchant. With the development of the railways he saw the opportunity of buying and selling coal and became a coal merchant, as well as a director of one of the local railway companies which built him his offices in Station Road, St Ives. His son Thomas (1850–1939) ran Coote and Sons Ltd. He lived at Ambury House in Huntingdon. The company merged with F. Warren & Co Ltd in 1908 to form Coote & Warren Ltd, and continued to buy and sell coal in bulk and transport it by rail until the 1960s when the business closed.

While only his father had the vote in the Grove family, the result was one that generated much discussion in the family.

Politics continued to interest Reginald and he particularly commented on a debate held some months later at Uppingham in the schoolroom with the motion that 'the Conservative Party has no policy'. He thought it was 'the best debate we had for some time'. The motion was lost 48 to 27. The local papers were sent to him both at King's and Uppingham, and his diary references showed that he kept abreast of political events.

The question of whether Ireland should be granted 'home rule'[533] was one that divided the Liberal Party in a similar way to how the issue of the United Kingdom's relationship with the European Union divided the nation in the 21st century. Such was the divide within the Liberal Party over Home Rule that a further election was held the next year in July when Reginald was 17. On this occasion, Coote's short tenure was ended when Arthur Smith-Barry[534] won the South Huntingdon parliamentary seat[535] back from the Liberals by beating them with a 161 majority. Reginald's interest in local politics was such that he made a specific diary entry about the result.

MILITARY SERVICE

In April 1860 in Huntingdon a volunteer detachment was formed called the 1st Hunts Rifle Volunteer Corps; it was also known in a shortened form as the Hunts Rifle Volunteers. This volunteer movement grew out of the local militia, when voluntary service was introduced in 1850. In the late-1850s Anglo-French relations deteriorated after both countries had been close allies against Russia in the Crimean War (1853–56). There was a real fear of an invasion of Britain becoming a reality. The British Army was fully stretched after the Indian Mutiny (1857–58) and, as a result, a popular movement led to the establishment of the Volunteer Force across the country. Much later this became the Territorial Army which played such an important role at the beginning of the First World War in Belgium

---

533 Self-government from the Westminster parliament.

534 Arthur Smith-Barry was an Irish landowner who was one of the two representatives for County Cork in Ireland in 1867, a seat he held until 1874. He was returned to parliament in the general election of 1886 and represented Huntingdonshire until 1900. In 1902 he was made 1st Baron Barrymore and sat in the House of Lords.

535 Craig, F. W. S., *British Parliamentary Election Results, 1885–1918*. Aldershot: Parliamentary Research Services (1989), p. 299.

and Northern France.

Reginald's father learnt about the new force two years after its formation when he moved to Huntingdon in 1862. He was set on serving his Queen and Country through his medical training. A detachment was set up in St Ives besides the one in Huntingdon. In 1872 the 1st Hunts Corps were included in the 1st Battalion of the Cambridgeshire Rifle Volunteer, and in 1876 the Corps moved its main location from Huntingdon to St Neots. In September that year Reginald's father was commissioned as an assistant surgeon in the Volunteer Force. He was 38.

Joining the military on a part-time basis was not uncommon during this period and serving became common among doctors through the Volunteer movement. Like others who joined, he had a deep commitment and passion about the importance of public service and most viewed it as a serious duty.[536] 4–7% of GPs held military appointments in the period 1860–99.[537] Friday evenings were set aside for drilling and other training. These took place in the Corn Exchange, as well as at the National School.[538] Reginald sometimes went with his father to watch.

Reginald also accompanied his father to Volunteer inspections. There was one on the evening of Tuesday 21 June 1881 when Reginald was 12; this was probably a practice before the St Ives Volunteers went to Cambridge for another inspection the following Tuesday. This was the anniversary of The Queen's Coronation and a special event held in her honour. Reginald did not go with his father on this occasion.

Some general practitioners served in colonial wars, like the Boxer Rebellion, and of course the First and Second Anglo-Boer Wars. Assistant Surgeon Grove, however, was not called up to war.

The commandant of the force was Lt W. A. Watts in 1885,[539] but prior to this it was a Major Dunn, who was a friend of the family. There are no public records or newspaper reports about Dunn, but he played an important role in the St Ives Corps. One Easter holiday Reginald travelled back on the train from Cambridge on a Friday afternoon with him and then went on to watch Dunn drill the Volunteers at the weekly meeting. After the formal part of the evening activity had ended, the men played

---

536 Digby, Anne, *The Evolution of British General Practice 1850–1948*, p. 86.

537 Anne Digby, *The Evolution of British General Practice*, p. 80.

538 *St Ives Business Register* 1885.

539 *St Ives Business Register* 1885.

whist while Reginald looked on. Dunn certainly took an interest in Reginald and was a regular letter-writer to him at school.[540] In June 1885, Reginald had a 'jolly long letter' from him, enclosing a very welcome postal order for a sovereign (£132). Later that month, Dunn visited him at Uppingham, arriving at noon and staying until 5.00pm. He lunched at Redgate and Reginald 'took him about and showed him all over the school'. Their correspondence and friendship continued, and in June the following year he enclosed 10/- (£63.25) with his letter which Reginald was delighted to receive, noting in his diary: 'always be thankful for small mercies, especially ten bob[541]'. The depth of their friendship was shown when Dunn was one of the three chosen to be sent the School Magazine in which Reginald's special article 'Our Concert' was published in February 1887. The other two were his father and his good friend Bensly.[542]

While Reginald was a small boy, the St Ives detachment held its annual supper in November 1876 at the White Horse Hotel,[543] which was 'exceedingly well patronised not only by members of the Corps but by the local gentry'.[544] The innkeeper, a Mr Thornton, excelled himself in decorating the room where an excellent meal was served up. It was clear from what was reported that Reginald's father had been suggesting to local young men, no doubt his patients, to join up in the year following his commission. The next year, in late-November, another supper was held, this time in the Corn Exchange[545] in Market Hill which was used in the evenings for a variety of functions, including the Volunteer drills on Friday evenings. Given that 160 attended, as reported in the press, a larger venue was clearly needed.[546] The local newspaper reported that the town's dignitaries were present in force – the Mayor, last year's Mayor, a number of Aldermen from the town council, the vicar and a nonconformist minister. Colonel Heathcote presided over the occasion and numerous toasts were made: 'The Queen', 'The Prince and Princess of Wales', 'the Army, Navy

[540] Diary 12.07.85.

[541] Ten bob was a colloquial term for 10 shillings which was half the value of one pound.

[542] Later he sent a copy to his Uncle Frank.

[543] It is not certain whether this was incorrectly reported in the local newspaper and was in fact the White Hart Hotel in Market Hill, a well-known coaching inn which still stands today.

[544] *Cambridge Express* 11.11.76.

[545] The Corn Exchange was built in 1864 and used during the day as a venue for the sale of grain, as its name implies. At other times it was hired out for a variety of meetings.

[546] *Cambridge Express* 08.12.77.

and Reserves Forces', 'the Bishop and Clergy of the Diocese and Ministers of all Denominations', and finally 'The First Hunts R.V.C.' The National Anthem was sung, there were more toasts proposed,[547] followed by 'some other unimportant toasts'.

Speeches were made by Colonel Heathcote encouraging those present who had not enrolled to do so, and thanking at the same time Acting Assistant Surgeon Grove for his hard work during the year in recruiting new Volunteers. Reginald's father replied that what was needed was not just prizes and money, important though these were, 'but the sympathy of the employers of labour and their influence with those under them to get them to join'. He looked forward that by the next annual supper 'they would have a full company'. Loud cheers greeted this statement! The meeting ended, after ten major toasts had been proposed, at about 11 o'clock. Given the amount of alcohol consumed, it was a merry evening by all accounts.

An incident was reported in the local press in January 1887 which Reginald read when the paper was sent to him at school. It was reported that a fight had broken out in the town between some soldiers from Huntingdon who had been drinking and who set upon some local lads on their way home – presumably by train. 'The soldiers ultimately got the worst of it – 21 days' hard labour!' Reginald wrote in his diary. Such incidents did not endear the St Ives locals to the military.

Besides weekly Friday evening meetings, the reservists went once a year in mid-July on a training annual camp held under canvas. These camps were held a few weeks before crops were harvested so as not to disrupt this essential task. Reginald never mentioned where the camps were held, apart from his last year at school, but it appears they may have been at different locations in East Anglia. He had a letter at King's from his father in July 1882 when Assistant Surgeon Grove and the Volunteer detachment were at camp. In July 1883 Reginald described how he travelled with his father by train with the company on his way to spend some of his summer holiday on his Uncle Hanslip and Aunt Elizabeth's farm near Ely at Shippea Hill. After he got off the train, the Volunteers travelled on to the camp probably somewhere in Suffolk for a week's outdoor training. In

[547] The other toasts were to: 'The Town and Trade of St Ives'; 'The Mayor and Corporation'; 'The Visitors'; 'The Subscribers and Donors of Prizes'; and lastly 'The Health of Col. Heathcote and the Chairman of the Meeting'.

1885 his father wrote while at camp, as did Major Dunn. Reginald's diary made no mention of his father being at camp in the summer of 1886, but in July 1887 Dr Grove and the volunteers were in camp in Lowestoft on the Norfolk coast. He noted in his diary of July 1890, when at Cambridge University, going to the station one Saturday morning to see his father and the volunteers on their way to camp that summer[548]. With his father's increasing ill health, this may well have been his last summer camp.

After his commission in 1880 the Corps became 'J' company of the new 1st Cambridgeshire Rifle Volunteers. They were led by Captain the Honourable Octavius Duncombe,[549] late of the 1st Life Guards,[550] Lieutenant John Heathcote, junior, and Ensign William Theed. It was commanded by the Earl of Sandwich, and its soldiers wore dark green uniforms, allegedly the 'colour of the county'.

In April 1889 Dr Grove, aged 51, was commissioned[551] as a Surgeon Major in the medical reserve and continued to hold this rank until his death. But later in 1889 'J' company was disbanded. He became the only volunteer from St Ives in the county left. He was bitterly disappointed at the demise of the volunteers and next year set up a public meeting in the Corn Exchange in Market Hill. Such was his enthusiasm that sufficient men wanted to enrol. Sadly, 'no gentleman could be prevailed upon to take the post of officer and nothing came of the effort'.[552] Before he died, he was awarded the Long Service Medal granted by Parliament to reservists. A Volunteer Corps was formed before the First World War, called the Hunts Cyclist Battalion Territorial Force, which met in a Drill Hall in Bull Lane under the instruction of Sergeant Joseph Buck, and was commanded by Lieutenant G. L. Day, the son of the well-respected solicitor and town clerk George Dennis Day.[553]

Dr Grove would have been delighted at its formation.

At many public schools the formation of a cadet corps became quite common in the late-19th century, but Edward Thring, Reginald's Headmaster, was not in favour of them. Back in the 1850s when Thring

---

548 Diary 19.07.90.

549 His father, also called Octavius, was a well-known Tory politician, who died in 1879.

550 The 1st Life Guards were part of the Household Cavalry. Interestingly, they did not take part in the Charge of the Light Brigade during the Crimean War.

551 On 18 April 1889 on the same day as the Corps was formed 29 years before.

552 Obituary, *Hunts County News* 28.12.85.

553 Lt Day was killed in the First World War.

had only been Headmaster for a few years, the weaknesses in the British military capability, together with the scare of a possible invasion by the French already mentioned, resulted in a call by Lord Elcho for public schools to introduce military drill. This led to a meeting held in London in 1860 for public school heads to discuss the formation of cadet corps. Uppingham was not represented but later cadet corps were started at Rossall School (where Reginald had sat for a scholarship before going to Uppingham), Eton, Rugby, Winchester, Harrow and Marlborough; eventually, upwards of 30 schools formed corps.[554]

The move to establish these corps was driven by those who saw imperialism needing military power as essential for the growth and stability of the British Empire.[555] The horror of the 1857 Indian Mutiny, despite the passing of a little less than 30 years, was still fresh in living memory. But Thring was wary of any form of outside control, as his constant battles with the governing body of the school bore witness. This may well have caused him to resist, allowing the British Army to gain a foothold in the school.[556]

The corps formed by other schools were led by masters assisted by one or more 'sergeants' who had previously served in the Army and took up posts, often as the school porter. These non-commissioned officers (NCOs) had responsibility, under a Master, for teaching drilling, boxing, fencing and shooting. Rifle Corps were established separately and the establishment of the National Rifle Association's competitions, held originally at Wimbledon and later at Bisley, for schools to compete for the Ashburton Shield (first held in 1860) did much to make shooting popular. But it never reached the same status as other sports at these schools. Like Dr Grove's Volunteers, annual camps formed an important activity for the corps.

---

554 Tozer, Malcolm, *The Ideal of Manliness: The Legacy of Thring's Uppingham* (Sunnyrest Books, 2015), p. 285.

555 Thring favoured the concept of imperial federation rather than imperial aggression which was an idea emanating from the Christian Socialist philosophy. Imperial federation was expounded by a good friend of Thring's (and his later biographer), the Canadian Sir George Parkin. Thring's brother, Henry Thring, later Lord Thring, also did much to develop a written constitution for the Australian and Canadian colonies based on the concept of federation. The Dominion of Canada was first formed in 1867 for the then provinces of Canada, Quebec, Nova Scotia and New Brunswick. Full sovereignty was only given in 1931 under the Statute of Westminster.

556 Tozer, Malcolm, *The Ideal of Manliness: The Legacy of Thring's Uppingham* (2015) p. 287.

But at Uppingham no corps was established, despite the fact that in the list of teaching staff at Uppingham in 1859 a 'Sergeant Major Ellis' was shown for 'Drilling etc'.[557] It appears that Ellis never actually arrived at the school, as his name was deleted in ink from the printed list; in Thring's own handwriting his name was replaced by a Herr Beisiegel as someone to teach fencing and gymnastics[558]. Thring was not in favour of these corps and was largely out of step with the approach taken by other schools. This led to the comment in the School Magazine, written by a boy who called himself 'Volunteer', to say that 'a Rifle Corps was an institution common in every other public school'.[559] A 'drilling class' was introduced the next year,[560] but it did not last long and was not without its critics, one of whom, an Old Boy, wrote that that he hoped to see the school playing cricket at Lord's sometime in the future but it would not happen if a boy was 'playing at soldiers in a fine uniform … when he ought to be learning to catch a ball'.[561]

There were other attempts to introduce a Rifle Corps in 1876 and also in 1885 during Reginald's time due to the uproar at General Gordon's death in the Sudan. Another writer, calling himself 'Martial Spirit', led a jingoistic call to arms some months later: 'Of what importance are games when compared to the glorious occupation of learning how to fight for their homes, country and freedom?'[562] Reginald made no comment about this in his diary, but in fairness he only began to comment on the articles in the School Magazine in his last year when he was editing them and contributing a few articles himself!

Thring's unwillingness to follow the example of other schools may well have been because it did not fit with his concept of manliness which was central to his educational philosophy as explained in Volume 2.

Uppingham formed a cadet corps in April 1889 after Thring's death when Dr Selwyn replaced him. Membership was voluntary at the start, but the popularity of the initiative was demonstrated by the fact that a third of

---

557 Tozer, Malcolm, *Edward Thring's Theory, Practice and Legacy* (Cambridge Scholars Publishing, 2019), p. 61.

558 Ibid, citing a letter from Herr Beisiegel to Edward Selwyn, Thring's successor as Headmaster 22.05.1902.

559 Uppingham School Magazine May 1863 p. 41.

560 Ibid, May 1864 p. 192.

561 Ibid, November 1863 p. 278.

562 Ibid, December 1885 p. 372.

the boys joined by the end of the first term.[563] When Reginald paid a visit to his old school in his third year at Cambridge, he saw 'a detachment of the new volunteers of the school going off to drill; rather wished they had been on in my day'.[564]

Whether the lack of a school cadet force was partly why Reginald did not follow his father into the Volunteers[565] is not known. However, as mentioned earlier, his brother Ernest joined the Royal Artillery,[566] and his friend Frederic Warren, mentioned in an earlier chapter, was commissioned as a lieutenant in the 4th (Hunts) Volunteer Battalion, the Bedfordshire Regiment in 1908.[567]

One of Reginald's nephews, a second son of his sister Mabel, Lieutenant Rex Wilder, was killed fighting in November 1914[568] during the first few months of the war. He was aged 20 and part of the Suffolk Regiment.[569] Like other tragic deaths in that war, it devastated the Grove family.

CHURCHWARDEN DUTIES

Reginald's father and mother were faithful members of All Saints Church from the time they set up home together after their marriage in 1868. From the beginning they took an active part in church life. In May 1868 Dr Grove was appointed to the committee which was set up to run the Church Institute. This was a new initiative to encourage reading and companionship for men and boys. The daily newspapers (*The Times, Standard Telegraph, The Churchman* and *The Guardian*) were available at the Institute, plus two local papers and the *Illustrated News, Punch, Fun*

563 Tozer, Malcolm, *Edward Thring's Theory, Practice and Legacy* (2019), p. 232.

564 Diary 18.06.90

565 The Volunteers became known as the Territorial Army in 1908, and played an important role in the early few months of the First World War when they distinguished themselves as part of the British Expeditionary Force (BEF) later dubbed 'a contemptible little army' by the Kaiser – hence the nickname 'Old Contemptibles' which they bore with pride.

566 Ernest served in the Anglo-Boer War in Royal Artillery and was awarded the Distinguished Service Order (DSO). Just after the outbreak of the First World War he was a major with the 79th (Howitzer) Battery based in Jhansi, India. He was promoted to the rank of Colonel later (Norris Museum press cuttings November 1914.)

567 *The London Gazette* 10 November 1908.

568 It is likely that he was part of the 1/4th Battalion of the Suffolks which landed at Le Havre as part of the Jullundur Brigade of the 3rd (Lahore) Division in November 1914 for service on the Western Front. He died on 19 November 1914.

569 Norris Museum press cuttings 7758.

and the *Hunts News*. Around 100 books were available in the library. There was an annual membership of £1 (£126.81) for honorary members', 10/- (£63.25) for ordinary members and 6/- (£38.00) for boys 14–18.[570] In March, Dr Grove was appointed to a committee to obtain 'subscriptions' (gifts and grants) for the restoration of the church spire.[571]

His father was one of the two churchwardens, and served from 1881 to 1895, although he had been approached about becoming one ten years previously. In an Anglican church, the role of churchwarden dates back to the 16th century. Their main duties were to keep order and peace in the church and the churchyard, and they carried staves as a mark of their office. These staves are now ceremonial but in the 19th century they were used as a deterrent for dogs or other animals getting into the church itself. They had a legal responsibility for all the property and movable goods belonging to a parish church. The Vicar tended to leave the day-to-day maintenance of church buildings and contents to the churchwardens.[572] In 1886, Dr Grove and his colleague warden were responsible for the organ being moved and the vestry being enlarged under the then Vicar, Revd Luke Paget.[573]

Usually there were two wardens appointed each year, one as the Vicar's Warden and the other as the Parish Warden;[574] the former was appointed by the Vicar and the latter elected by the congregation at a Vestry Meeting. These meetings could be contentious as described in a later chapter. In April 1876 Reginald's father was nominated by Revd Charles Goldie to be his Warden. The Vestry meeting was a difficult one held in the Corn Exchange in the evening. Mr Read Adams had carried out the role of Parish Warden since 1867 and had been the first Mayor of St Ives in 1874. The meeting drew a large crowd as everyone knew that a 'contest was eminent' and both sides had marshalled their supporters. A Mr Wallingford proposed that Read was elected again. He obviously felt that Read would act as a brake on Goldie's determination to move the church towards the High Church tradition. Read however seemed not want to stand again. The contention

570 *St Ives All Saints Parish Magazine* May 1868.

571 Vestry meeting minutes, All Saints St Ives Parish Records 1847–1937.

572 In 1876 at the vestry meeting there was concern expressed that Mr Read, as People's Warden, together with the Vicar, had approved work to be carried out by a Mr Jarvis to put up four new stone pinnacles for the tower. Unfortunately, they paid him £14 (£1,775) in advance and he then died. The £14 had to be written off.

573 Norris, p. 21.

574 Sometimes known as the People's Warden.

about Goldie's High Church views was brought out into the open as Wallingford stated his reasons with conviction for nominating Adams.

Adams, however, seemed not to want to stand again. He was beginning to regret the increasing unpleasantness of the meeting as it proceeded as was Reginald's father Dr Grove. Amid an uproar he said, 'it was the misfortune of this parish to have a Ritualistic clergyman and he would show what this meant'. He went on to say that 'they desired to Romanise the Church'. The meeting broke into further uproar as the local newspaper graphically reported.[575] The Vicar tried to head off this line of argument but Wallingford began to read from a pamphlet that he had brought. This resulted in 'howls and shouts' from some at the meeting. The Vicar managed to restore some order, and Adam's nomination was seconded by a Mr J. Hankin.

A Mr C. Greene then spoke and said that he had met with Adams ten days before and he said that he did not want to stand again, as he was not in good health. As a result, a Mr T. King was approached to stand. He was a businessman and a 'Churchman' who would carry out his duties diligently. A Mr Matthews seconded this nomination. Adams then spoke up for the first time to say that despite his health he should continue, and cited his deep concern at some practices – a young girl of 15 had been given a book at confessional, which he held up, which contained in his view 'the most indecent rubbish', which he then quoted amid more uproar. A Mr Goodman then spoke, although he admitted he did not often attend church. But he believed that some of the practices in the church were 'illegal and contumacious'[576] and asked a Mr King whether he would stand and oppose these. King said he would stand, and if elected he would do his duty as a 'thorough Protestant despite some saying he was the Vicar's tool'. Dr Grove was now caught up in an embarrassing and raucous public argument.

A vote took place to elect either Adams or King. There were some scuffles but eventually a show of hands was obtained, with Adams getting the most votes. A secret ballot was then demanded which took place at 8.00pm. Meanwhile, Reginald's father became increasingly uncomfortable about his position. Adams gained 289 votes and King 182, so Adams continued in the post. Meanwhile, Dr Grove told the Vicar he was not willing to be the other warden. Interestingly, Goldie then nominated his

575 *Cambridge Express* 22.04.76.

576 Rebellious or insubordinate.

groom, Mr Whiteman. Employed by Goldie, he would do as the Vicar instructed. The evening was further marred by a 'band of roughs' who roamed the streets and broke some windows.

Not an edifying evening by any stretch of the imagination.

Reginald's father later became the Vicar's warden in April 1881, taking over from Whiteman, Goldie's groom. The then Mayor, Thomas Knights JP, was the other warden who stepped down when Dr Grove was appointed. He continued to serve as the Vicar's warden for Revd Dashwood Goldie, Luke Paget[577] and Edward Tottenham until February 1895, when he stepped down due to ill health and George Brownlow took over.[578]

He served in other roles, too; in September 1885 Reginald accompanied him to a parochial church meeting about the Harvest Festival which his father chaired. Reginald sometimes helped his father in his duties; for instance, during his school holidays in April 1886 he helped 'the Pater to copy some church notices with Cyclostyle'.[579] Later in the holidays he went with his father to Over to 'get some books on church matters'; and then the next day he accompanied him to a vestry meeting.

Sadly, after the ruckus of the warden's election in 1876, there were difficulties of another sort within All Saints. An unfortunate incident occurred when Reginald was at Cambridge just before his return before Christmas. It illustrated one of the more unusual duties of churchwardens concerning the allocation of seating in the church pews, as well as the custom of pew rents[580] themselves. As reported in December 1888 in the local newspaper, it was headed 'A Scene in the Parish Church':[581]

> What is happily a most unusual occurrence took place in the Parish Church on Sunday evening last. The doors were kept closed until a quarter past six,

---

[577] *Hunts County Guardian* April 1887.

[578] All Saints Church St Ives Parish Register 1847–1937.

[579] A Cyclostyle machine was an early type of duplicator.

[580] During the 19th century pews in many churches and chapels were often set aside for specific individuals or their families for which an annual rent was paid. In some churches, the individuals had paid for them to be built and this cost, in a newly built church, went to the building costs. Many pews were handed down through families from one generation to the next. They could often be the cause of dispute. The custom was a source of controversy in the 1840s and 1850s, especially in the Church of England. The legal status of pew rents was, in many cases, very questionable and by the 1860s and 1870s many churches influenced by the Tractarian movement became 'free and open churches', having done away with pew rentals. (http://anglicanhistory.org/misc/freechurch/fowler_pews1844.html 29.03.19.)

[581] Norris Museum press cuttings 1796–1914.

by which time a crowd of worshippers had gathered in the church yard. To explain what followed we should state that sixteen years[582] ago Miss Giddins, living in the Cow and Hare Yard[583] gave up her usual seat in the Church, at the request of the Churchwardens (Messrs Ansley and Read Adams) to accommodate two elderly ladies, and sanctioned by the Vicar, she was allocated another seat. This she has retained and occupied almost without intermission ever since, the longest period of absence being five weeks, which she spent in pursuit of her occupation as nurse.

After about fifteen months since the seat was allocated to Mr. F. Ruston, since which time the Churchwardens have made strenuous efforts to induce Miss Giddins to cease occupying the pew. As, however, there was ample room for both Miss Giddins and the Ruston family, she stoutly refused to give up her seat, although the Churchwardens assured her they had absolute control of the sittings. The affair culminated on Sunday evening when the Churchwardens (Messrs W. R. Grove and Knights) occupied the pew in company with two of the ringers. When Miss Giddins arrived, she asked to be allowed to pass into her seat but was told to 'go and sit somewhere else – you shan't come here anymore'.

Some other conversation passed between her and the Churchwardens, to the great surprise of the congregation, and Miss Giddins remained standing in the aisle for some time. Ultimately, Mr Day of Bridge Street who occupies a pew near, came and asked her to sit there, his kind invitation she reluctantly accepted, and Mr and Mrs Day thereupon left the church. The affair caused an amount of painful excitement. It may be stated that Miss Giddins had offered to give up the pew provided another regular sitting was found for her, which was refused. It is stated that legal proceedings are likely to follow, as the Churchwardens have instructed a solicitor who has communicated with Miss Giddins. Of course, as in every question, it is well to hear both sides and we are pleased to give the following statement by the Churchwardens: The doors of the Church are never open until 6.15. Miss Giddins was requested to vacate her one sitting previous to Mr Rushton being allotted the whole pew, to which she was entitled for himself and his family, another sitting being provided for Miss Giddins.

This she accepted, but afterwards refused to occupy; another sitting was offered to her but in spite of kindly advice by the Vicar and Churchwardens, she persistently occupied the sitting. Last week legal advice was taken by the

---

582 1872 before both current Churchwardens were in the post.

583 The Cow and Hare Inn was in the Bullock Market (now No 6 The Broadway). It was a popular meeting place on Sunday nights for dealers for the Monday market. It closed as a pub in the 1960s. The Cow and Hare Passage remains to this day and leads to East Street.

> Churchwardens and Miss Giddins was written to by the lawyer, who stated to her that the seating was entirely in control of the Churchwardens and that they would gladly find her an equally comfortable and suitable sitting and hoping that she would accept it and prevent any further unpleasant steps being taken. The Churchwardens regret having compelled to take the steps they have done. Miss Giddins, however, has her remedy in referring the matter to the Bishop whose decision would be final.

A sad story. Nothing further was reported in the press, so Miss Giddins must have given up her campaign to sit in 'her pew'.

Fanny Giddins was born in 1849 in Hemingford Grey, a few miles from St Ives upstream. At the time of this incident she was 39 and, as the newspaper reported, lived in one of the lodgings in Cow and Hare Yard,[584] off the Bullock Market on her own. She was a 'sick' nurse and domestic servant who probably looked after the elderly or those in need of nursing care.[585] She was not one of the nurses who were starting to be professionally trained in nursing schools. Today, her job would be called a Care Assistant. Four years before the incident she was working as a dressmaker in West Street, and advertised her services in the *St Ives Business Directory*, so it looks as if there had been a significant change of her personal circumstances.[586] There were nine other dressmakers offering their services in St Ives, so market competition may have forced Fanny to look for other work.[587]

Although a working woman, she was a person determined to face up to the local establishment for what she believed were her rights, despite the

---

[584] National Census 1891 and 1901.

[585] In her book on household management, previously cited, Mrs Beeton described the qualities of a sick nurse as being a 'good temper, compassion for suffering, sympathy with sufferers, which most women worthy of the name possess, neat-handedness, quiet manners, love of order, and cleanliness'. Generally, they were anything but this before the nursing reforms in the mid-19th century were introduced. In *The Old Curiosity Shop*, written in 1841, Dickens described those who looked after Little Nell's grandfather as 'strangers who made of it a greedy trade, and who, in the intervals of their attendance upon the sick man, huddled together with ghastly good-fellowship, and ate and drank and made merry, for disease and death were their ordinary household gods…'

[586] *St Ives Business Directory* 1885.

[587] *The St Ives Business Directory 1885* lists the following as dress makers, besides Fanny Giddins, two of whom worked in West Street as Fanny did: Maria Lee, The Quay; Alice Lowings, Carlisle Terrace; Hannah Marriott, Bullock Market; Jane Norris, West Street; Sarah Owen, Orchard Terrace; Rebecca Porter, The Quadrant; Alice Thornell, Barnes Walk; Rebecca Alderton, Crown Place; and Elizabeth Cooper, West Street.

threat of legal action being taken by the churchwardens. But the might of the establishment was too great and she had no resources to fight a legal action. Only the Day family came out of this in a good light by giving up their pew for her. It was a sad day for the local church.

Giddins was a common surname in the area and she was related to the family which owned a boathouse in Hemingford Grey next to the parish church, as well as a boat repair business. Their boathouse was frequently a subject for the artists[588] who flocked to paint the Ouse and the villages in Huntingdonshire towards the end of the 19th century. This business continued well into the next century. By 1901 Fanny had moved to Prospect Place in St Ives and was still single. It seems likely that she died in 1916 aged 68.

[588] Henry John King (1855–1924) was one of the early artist visitors and his oil canvas of the church and Giddins boathouse called 'On the Ouse, Hemingford Grey' is a classic of the period. (*Artists along the Ouse 1880–1930* by Bridget Flanagan, 2010, p. 39.)

Part 2

Relaxation

***

CHAPTER 11

Messing about in Boats

'Here Ouse, slow winding through a level plain, of spacious meads with cattle sprinkled o'er, conducts the eye along his sinuous course delighted.'
William Cowper – *The Task*[589]

Kenneth Grahame wrote the classic children's story, *The Wind in the Willows,* in 1908. He was 49 and Reginald was ten years younger. The book told the delightful story of the exploits of Ratty, Mole, Badger and Toad against the Edwardian backdrop of an English river – the Thames in Berkshire near where Grahame lived.

Ratty loved 'simply messing about in boats'. And so did Reginald, whose garden at his home in his early years stretched down to the Great Ouse. And East Anglia had plenty of Fenlands rivers – the Great Ouse, the Old West, the Cam and the Lark, which all flowed into The Wash.

Reginald loved the river. It had

> a strange, indefinable smell, scent of reeds and peaty waters, of sallows and meadowsweet, of rotten lily pads – and of fish. That smell of freshwater fish which is penetrating, ineluctable, indefinable. An old, strange, blended smell, a smell as old as Time, compounded of scents that belonged to an untamed, undrained England, the England of the Saxons.[590]

This was the Fens.

Another son of St Ives, the poet Theodore Watts-Dunton, who loved the river at St Ives and its meadows, described a sunset on the Ouse:

> More mellow falls the light and still more mellow
> Around the boat, as we two glide along
> 'Tween grassy banks she loves where, tall and strong,
> The buttercups stand gleaming, smiling, yellow.

---

[589] Cowper, William, *The Task Book One (*1785), lines 163–66.

[590] J. Wentworth Day writing in 1954 in his *History of the Fens.* He lived in Wicken, a village on the edge of Wicken Fen, the only part of the original Fens not drained. It is now managed by the National Trust.

She knows the nightingales of 'Portobello';
Love makes her know each bird! In all that throng
No voice seems like another: soul is song,
And never nightingale was like its fellow;
For, whether born in breast of Love's own bird,
Singing its passion in those islet bowers
Whose sunset-coloured maze of leaves and flowers
The rosy river's glowing arms engird,
Or born in human souls – twin souls like ours –
Song leaps from deeps unplumbed by spoken word.[591]

Watts-Dunton wrote another poem, 'A Star Sonnet', which some believed was a description of the Thames above Kew. Another St Ivian, Herbert Norris, disagreed[592] and said that

> every one familiar with Hemingford Meadow will see that it describes the Ouse backwater near Porto Bello,[593] where the author as a young man was constantly seen on summer evenings listening from a canoe to the blackcaps and nightingales of The Thicket.[594]

Norris enthused, too, but in prose:

> There is, as far as I know, nothing like the Ouse elsewhere in England. I do not mean that our river surpasses or even equals in picturesqueness such rivers as the Wye, the Severn, the Thames but that its beauty is unique. There is not to be seen anywhere else so wide and stately a stream moving so slowly and yet so clearly. Consequently, there is no other river which reflects with such beauty the scenery of clouds floating overhead.[595]

He thought that this was due to the stream moving over a flat bottom consisting of gravel.

The garden of Reginald's first home in St Ives' Bullock Market sloped

[591] Douglas, James, *Theodore Watts-Dunton* (1904) p. 28.

[592] Ibid, p. 29.

[593] This is the name given to the north bank of the river beyond The Thicket (see note below) and Nobles Field upstream between St Ives and the Hemingfords where the river widens for a short distance. The origin of the name is a mystery. It is spelt both as one word as well as two words on occasions.

[594] The Thicket was, and still is, a footpath surrounded by trees that runs upstream from All Saints Church on the north of the Great Ouse towards the Hemingfords.

[595] Norris, Herbert, *A History of St Ives* (1889).

down to the banks of the Great Ouse. On the opposite side was Hemingford Meadow. The description of the scene given by James Douglas remains the same today:

> It is a level tract of land on the banks of the Ouse, consisting of deposits of alluvium from the overflowings of the river. In summer it is clothed with gay flowers, and in winter, during floods and frosts, it is used as a skating-ground, for St Ives, being on the border of the Fens, is a famous skating centre. On the opposite bank of the meadow is The Thicket, of which I am able to give a lovely picture.[596]

His description was a backcloth to his biography of Theodore Watts-Dunton who, in his home, had a number of watercolour paintings of the Ouse executed by one of the well-known Fraser brothers.

And when the Grove family moved to Slepe House in Cromwell Terrace, the river was only half a mile away. While at school in Cambridge, the Cam was nearby and much time was spent bathing at Sheep's Green and enjoying the annual college boat races. While visiting his cousins on their farm in Cambridgeshire during his school holidays, Reginald enjoyed trips on the River Lark nearby.

DARK, SATANIC MILLS

The irony was that until the decline of the commercial river trade and some local industries like brick making in the 1870s, the river at St Ives was polluted like so many others across the country.

Public concern mounted at the state of the nation's rivers. It came to a head with what became called the 'Great Stink' in the summer of 1858 in London. The extremely hot weather exacerbated the smell of untreated human and industrial waste flowing down the river. Combined with an extended spell of dry weather, the level of the Thames dropped and raw effluent from the sewers remained on the mudbanks. Members of both Houses of Parliament were outraged.[597] Queen Victoria and Prince Albert attempted to take a pleasure cruise on the Thames, but returned to shore within a few minutes because the smell was so terrible. The problem had

---

596 Douglas, ibid, p. 29.

597 *Punch* magazine commented that 'The one absorbing topic in both Houses of Parliament … was the Conspiracy to Poison question. Of the guilt of that old offender, Father Thames, there was the most ample evidence'.

been mounting for some years, with an ageing and inadequate sewer system that emptied directly into the Thames.

Rivers served as a water source for both domestic and industrial use. Factories and workshops increased with the rise of manufacturing across the country and were often built next to rivers and canals for transport purposes. Like today, rivers were also the depositories of sewage from cities and towns which lay on their banks.

The 1867 Royal Commission on the Pollution of Rivers stated that rivers were 'polluted in proportion to the extent of local manufacturers'. While it might be assumed that it was the newer industrial northern and Midlands cities which were the culprits, towns like Oxford, Windsor and Cambridge were dumping their untreated sewage into their rivers: Oxford into the Isis and Cherwell, Windsor and Kingston into the Thames upstream from London, and Cambridge into the River Cam.

At Kingston, 'the daily discharge of the sewage of several thousands of persons renders the banks and the streams in the vicinity disgusting to the sight and frequently offensive to the smell.'[598] Indeed, Cambridge was described in the 1880s 'as an undrained, river polluted cesspool city'.[599] The sewage disposal for Magdalene College, for instance, consisted of privies which butted out over the river with the contents falling straight into the Cam above Jesus lock.

An amusing story of a visit to Cambridge by Queen Victoria was told by the Master of Trinity College, Dr William Whewell.[600] As she looked down from the college bridge over the Backs she asked, 'What are those pieces of paper floating down the river?' to which his quick thinking reply was: 'Those, ma'am, are notices that bathing is forbidden'.[601] He need not have spared her the details of the lavatory paper drifting down the Cam, as she was well aware what was strewn on the riverbanks of the Thames and the resulting smell that wafted up in the summer to Windsor Castle!

It was in the Cam that Reginald learnt to swim while at King's, although the bathing places were on the upper river, on Sheep's Green and Coe Fen before the main town's drains and sewers fed into the river. Only two of the

---

598 *Endangered Lives*. Anthony S. Wohl quoting Parliamentary Papers RCRP1867 First Report.

599 Ibid, quoting *Transactions of the Sanitary Institute of Great Britain VI* (1884–85).

600 As Whewell died in 1866, her visit must have taken place sometime before this; he died as a result of a fall from riding his horse.

601 Raverat, chapter 2.

seventeen Cambridge colleges abutted the river end on and both of these, St John's and Queen's were upstream of the main town.

Major dangers to public health through contaminated drinking water were from cholera and typhoid.[602] A report for a parliamentary committee in 1895 highlighted that for the previous 30 years the dangers had been known of drainage of fields manured by human waste being carried into the water supplies of towns and villages. This led to outbreaks of waterborne typhoid.[603]

...A NOXIOUS AND POISONOUS GAS

Towns upstream of St Ives were Huntingdon, St Neots and Bedford, and they used the river for waste disposal which caused contamination. There was a serious typhoid outbreak in St Neots in 1865 as the contents of latrines (known as 'night soil') were used to manure the surrounding arable fields. Twenty inhabitants died having drunk water from the brook that ran through the area into which the fields of three farms drained.[604] And the contaminated water was carried downstream to St Ives.

Pollution came also from other waste going into the Ouse in St Ives itself. In 1854 two millers, Potto Brown and Henry Goodman, built a new steam mill on the south bank of the river at St Ives a few hundred yards downstream from the bridge. Their corn mill still stands today, minus its original tall chimney, and it has been converted to luxury flats. Potto Brown[605] was well known for his business acumen. Grain for milling arrived in carts by road, as well as by river. A large wharf was built for his fleet of barges and these were also used to deliver up the river to other mills. Once the new railway line to Godmanchester was built, Potto Brown could import grain and coal by rail; interestingly, he had his own railway sidings. There was another steam mill built on the Low Road, Fenstanton.

---

[602] A major typhoid outbreak from contaminated drinking water occurred at Uppingham six years before Reginald went to the school, which resulted in the school evacuating to Borth in North Wales.

[603] *British Medical Journal*, Waterborne Typhoid 1858–1893 published 20.06.95.

[604] Ibid.

[605] Potto Brown, born in 1797, came from a Quaker family and was a formidable and influential local resident. He lived in Houghton (where a bronze bust of him stands in the village square). He was a Presbyterian and philanthropist. One of his sons, Bateman Brown, became Mayor of St Ives, only the second nonconformist to hold the position since the time of Oliver Cromwell. Brown snr set up British schools in Houghton and St Ives, and donated £3,000 to build the Free Church in St Ives in 1864 and £1,000 to the cost of Huntingdon Free Church.

All these mills disposed of their waste into the river.

There were brickworks to the east of the town, along where The Thicket is now. In the 19th century this track was busy with carts carrying bricks, coal and other materials brought in barges and used in brick construction. Besides the dust and dirt, the open kilns belched sulphurous smoke. Limestone was also burnt to make the lime for mortar. There were brick limekilns in the yard of the Dolphin Hotel on the south side of the river near the bridge at the time that the many-arched New Bridges causeway was constructed in 1822.

While the Bullock Market, Bridge Street and Market Hill were cobbled, other roads were not, and seepage of industrial waste eventually found its way into the river. St Ives had another industry, too – making candles, which were produced in the premises of two grocers called Nix and Wasdale in the Bullock Market near Reginald's first home. The production of tallow candles and dips, used to light homes before gas was installed later in the century, produced noxious smells. Fat was rendered down into tallow which was then used for either rush lights or candles or perhaps soap. Other local businesses prepared and dyed leather in Bull Lane, as well as Water Lane. Industrial waste generally ended up in the river, as did the effluence from the small workshops on the river front; storage areas used for malt, corn, brewing and coal were sometimes flooded and materials were swept away downstream.

Additionally, of course, livestock which grazed on the meadows along the riverbank drank from the Ouse and their faeces eventually seeped or were washed into the river. And in St Ives the livestock brought to market were led to drink and be washed in the shallows where the roadway sloped down into the water at The Waits at the end of the Bullock Market. Animal waste matter went directly into the river.

Reginald's father, as the newly appointed Medical Officer for St Ives, wrote in a report in 1873 that

> The drains are in a bad state and there are no traps (grills) to the drains. The river opposite The Waits is in a poor condition. A large quantity of waste of all kind is discharged into it. It remains in the vicinity and mingles with decaying vegetable matter which in hot weather emits a noxious and poisonous gas.[606]

---

[606] Mary Carter, *19th Century St Ives*, p. 84. Newspaper source not given.

Despite all this, the river was no bar for those who worshipped in the numerous chapels in St Ives, and were publicly baptised as believers in the river. This generally happened after the morning service on Sundays when all the worshippers went down to the Quay; there the minister went down into the water from one of the slipways used for washing horses. A crowd would gather to watch – summer or winter, as the person being baptised followed the minister into the water after hymns were sung and prayers said. The water was shallow enough for participants to stand before being totally immersed.[607] Whether anyone caught any infection from these baptisms is not recorded.

SIMPLY MESSING ABOUT IN BOATS

When the commercial river traffic started to decline with the building of the station at St Ives in 1847, the Ouse began gradually to be used for leisure; the same applied to the Cam.

Dr Grove kept a close eye on the purity of the water, and by the 1880s when Reginald was 12 or 13, he allowed him to row, sail, swim and fish in the river. In the winter he went walking along the riverbank or skating.

The switch to leisure occurred as the middle classes in mid-Victorian England began to have the time and means to enjoy gentle outdoor leisure activities. Playing tennis as well as boating then became very popular. The general public began to enjoy river jaunts for their own leisure, especially on Sunday afternoons in the summer after morning worship. The widespread popularity of river pastimes was described by Jerome K. Jerome in his book *Three Men in a Boat*, published in 1889. While the setting of the story was the Thames upstream of Kingston, the essence of the book captured the pleasure of river pastimes. The advent of trains from London to places like Henley then meant that the river at weekends was less than tranquil.

Reginald's diary is full of days spent on the river messing around in rowing boats and sailing dinghies. Sometimes he went downstream towards the villages of Holywell and Earith, but more often upstream to the Hemingfords and sometimes further to Huntingdon which was four miles from St Ives. In September 1882 he rowed nearly to Huntingdon and then the next morning he rowed downstream, reaching Overcote, five miles from St Ives, where the ferry crossed the river at the 18th-century

[607] Mary Carter, *19th Century St Ives*, p. 79.

Pike and Eel Inn.[608]

After coming back on the first day of his summer holidays in 1885 when he was 16, he 'went out on the boat that Papa has got us for the holidays, found it leaked, and took it to Hemingford to be done up, left it there and went to see Uncle and Aunt George and others'. He probably took the boat to Giddins Boat House in Hemingford Grey. In the afternoon, he 'went to fetch the back with Ted and Arnie Ulph' and on the way broke a rowlock. Often his days out on the river were with his brothers, like Ted, or his sister Mabel, or friends like Arnie who lived next door to Slepe House. The following day, in the afternoon, he 'took the boat back to be mended and while it was being done went and had a bathe'. A day later he wanted to take Miss Reynell, the sister of his old Headmaster at King's, out on the river for a row. She was staying with them at the time. Unfortunately, 'the river was very low and the boat was on dry land so took her for a walk up The Thicket'. He was able to take her out in his boat a couple of days later, and they collected some water lilies at Battcock's Island.

During that August, despite spending some time away in Cambridge, Reginald went out in his boat on 14 separate days. On a few days he also went swimming from the boat. Sometimes he swam with other boys, like his friend Cyril Goodman, at the St Ives staunch downstream of the town. Here they could dive off the stone structure into deep water. His other spring and summer holidays were spent in a similar way, boating and fishing.

FISHING

Fishing was a regular pastime during his school holidays. The Ouse teemed with fish – roach, perch, pike, dace, chub, gudgeon, pike and of course eels. Fenmen and women viewed eels as a great delicacy. His diary had a number of entries describing how he went fishing, generally with someone else. For instance, aged 13, he spent a morning fishing in the holiday with Herbert Strange, but neither caught anything. In September 1885, aged 16, he went fishing with his Uncle Frank, who was staying with them, and he caught two perch.

For those who enjoyed the new sport of angling, the St Ives and District Fish Preservation and Angling Society was founded in 1881, as described in Chapter 4.

---

[608] The inn still stands today. As a boy in the 1950s I remember the large bell on the Over bank to call for someone from the inn to operate the ferry. The bell and the ferry has long since gone.

Writing in 1885, William Glover recalled his days as a chorister at Trinity College some 50 years previously.[609] He was an enthusiastic angler like Reginald. This is his delightful account:

> How enchanting it is to lie basking on the bank of a river in genial summer time, when all is still, except the warblers in the trees, and a gentle murmur from the stream. The dashing, cheery thrush pours forth his confident notes in a bold and full-voiced melody, spreading his pert and almost upright tail as if he, too, would be a peacock if he could and yet retain his musical powers. Then a small member of the weasel tribe steals out in the stillness to inspect, with the utmost caution, a large dead pike...

Glover went on to describe more of this idyllic scene he remembered from his boyhood:

> In quiet portions of the stream, when you have long been silent, a scarecrow-looking heron may perhaps be seen, standing on his long, skeleton legs, intently calculating all the chances of the fishing question: whether he can seize with certainty a particular fish, whether anyone will interrupt him in the attempt and whether he can return to a favourable rising ground suitable for a fresh flight to other scenes of piratical depredations ... after a long silence, a little red-brown rat may perch herself on a small sluice-gate, looking like a large, fat mouse, with a long, thick coat and sparkling, beady eyes, earnestly studying the enormous biped on the bank.[610]

This was fishing at its best.

ROWING

While at King's, Reginald was introduced to the delights of competitive rowing which took place at the university during the May Races each spring. The years might have passed since Glover wrote about them but what happened at the races had not changed when Reginald went with the others boys to watch 'the bumps' on the River Cam on a number of occasions[611].

---

[609] Glover, William, *The Memoirs of a Cambridge Chorister*, pp. 23–27.

[610] Ibid, pp. 76–78.

[611] Because the river Cam is quite narrow, races were (and still are) held below Jesus lock where each boat starts from a fixed distance from each other at the same time. The aim is to bump the boat in front before being bumped by the boat behind. If neither happens, the crew are said to 'row over'.

As Glover explained:

> as the Cambridge boats are many and the river narrow, it would require much ingenuity to place twenty or thirty boats abreast, in order to compete, in such a stream; they are therefore reasonably required to pass one after the other in Indian file and 'bump' each other if they can.
>
> I have now to attempt a description of one of the most popular amusements known to the people of Cambridge, namely the exciting art of boat racing. The scheme must be witnessed to be properly appreciated. You see before you an enormous crowd of struggling spectators, reckless of everything but the terrific contest which is taking place. Excited rowers attempting the possible and endeavouring to conceal for a given time the frenzy within. Enthusiastic friends and admirers urging on the rowers to still more impossible feats. Hundreds of volunteer instructors rushing to and fro like so many restless and panting shepherds' dogs, anxious to do a great deal more than enough in the grand and glorious cause. If all these advisors could have their way, victory would be secure and everybody satisfied; at least, so thought the volunteers.

Reginald did not write as effusively in his diary as Glover did, but there is no doubt that events like the 'bumps' laid the ground for his interest in rowing when he went up to Cambridge as an undergraduate at Sidney Sussex College. Glover continued:

> Shouts, screams, yells and other alarming sounds rend the air; saints, male and female, are openly invoked, in spite of all doctrinal teaching to the contrary with frankness and familiarity suggesting long, intimate acquaintance. 'Now go Catherine, look alive; the Maudlen [sic] fellows are after you'. 'Go it, Johns, take care of Corpus', 'Emmanuel's aground'. Magdalene's done for and been 'bumped' three times already.
>
> If you could hear for the first time the sounds which are really uttered and which create neither surprise nor indignation in the minds of the residents; if you could realise all the excitement, tumult, and enthusiasm displayed at these boat races you would be inclined to suppose that all Cambridge had frantically broken loose and resolved with one mind, if not with one voice, to take part, with unlimited freedom of action, in the ever popular drama of Nautical Bedlam.

Interestingly, a report in the Uppingham School Magazine from 'T.W.S.', an Old Boy at Oxford, when Reginald was at King's and watching the Cambridge races, commented that there was much less cheering the crews on at Oxford, but more about 'mechanical inventions, such as bells and rattles, are gradually taking the place of the human voice'.[612]

As described in Chapter 4 the St Ives Rowing Club was formed and both Reginald's father and he were enthusiastic and active members.

STEAM LAUNCHES

While sailing and rowing were the main activity, Reginald had the opportunity in the spring of 1886 to crew a steam launch[613] which belonged to his Uncle George. On this occasion, the launch was moored at Ely, so he went by train there, met his uncle and a Mr Hunt, and then 'had a splendid trip round by the Old West[614] river to Earith, got up to Hemingford at 4.30pm – a splendid run'. This was just under 30 miles by water.

Other family friends owned boats which Reginald was invited to be a passenger on. The Ulph family next door owned a boat called 'The Green', and Reginald went out on it on a number of occasions. He never described what sort of craft it was, but it was unlikely to have been powered by steam, otherwise he would have said so. Sometimes his trips on The Green were on a Sunday afternoon; he and Miss Ulph went on the river in the autumn of 1882. Three weeks later the Ulph family and Reginald all went out on the boat in the afternoon; Reginald arrived back in time for the evening service at the parish church. The Ulphs, being Nonconformists, attended the Free Church in Market Hill.[615] He and the Warren boys, who were with him at Uppingham, and a cousin of theirs, went out during the Easter holidays in 'a splendid new boat of Minson's[616] the tailor'.

LEISURE TRIPS

After the commercial traffic declined, sections of the waterway between locks gradually fell into disrepair. But leisure boating took off. Upstream at Huntingdon, St Neots and Bedford boating facilities were set up, but the only boats generally seen above St Ives were canoes, punts and skiffs.

---

612 Uppingham School Magazine June 1880. No 138.

613 Steam launches were popular as pleasure craft and besides the engine fired by coal, often had a canopy to protect against the sun or rain.

614 This stretch of the Ouse meanders seven miles from Cottenham Lode Junction to Earith. The distance from Earith to Ely is about 15 miles.

615 Diary 24.09.82.

616 William Minson lived in Bridge Street, had five children and was a tailor. Clearly his business was prosperous to own a boat which was much more than a rowing boat, although not powered by steam.

These could be hauled around the locks on the rollers provided. By the 1880s rowing boats, punts, skiffs and canoes could be hired in the summer for trips along the river.

Trips on the river by groups of people now became popular from St Ives upstream. In September 1874 the Church Institute, which his father helped found, held a 'Water Party' with a barge to carry the excursionists; dancing followed a tea with a brass band playing the music.[617] Reginald was only five at the time, but when he was 13 he described in September 1882 a trip up to 'Mr Ballcock's[618] [sic] island, about 60 went'. Trips like this became very popular. When the weather was balmy in the summer water parties were organised by the nonconformist chapels in the town, or the parish church or Temperance Society.[619] Potto Brown and Henry Goodman lent a large lighter and a horse to tow it the three miles to the island. J. Kemp Foster, writing in a local paper[620] a few years later, described the sort of trip mentioned by Reginald:

> During my school days the most appreciated outings offered the public were the picnics arranged up and down the river. The favourite resort was Battcock's Island at Hemingford Grey[621] and it would be difficult to imagine a better spot for the purpose. The parties usually numbered about a hundred and quite half the charm consisted in the journey to and from the island.
>
> A towpath followed the course of the river as it gently wound its way along the huge flood meadow to the Hemingfords. The meadows provided rich pasture for cattle.

---

617 *St Ives* by Bryan Little and Herbert Werba, p. 40.

618 This was Battcock's (not Ballcocks) Island, which was a narrow island opposite the village of Hemingford Abbots separated by two channels; the east side lay opposite Houghton Meadows. It was a small, wooded area of about an acre. The island was owned by Mr Battcock. Edmund Wimperis, in his article for *The Leisure Hour* (1895) cited under the Artist's Colony below called Battcock 'the squire of the neighbourhood'. He said that on it Battcock 'on it he turned his sheep which had to conveyed backwards and forwards in a punt'. He and Dr Grove were good friends and Reginald often visited the Battcock family during school holidays. Mr Battcock was one of the many mourners who attended Dr Grove's funeral in 1896. It is likely he was a patient of Dr Grove, too.

619 The temperance movement began in the 1830s across England to counter the acute rise of alcoholism. In 1847 the Band of Hope was founded in Leeds, with the stated aim of saving working-class children from the dangers of drinking. Those who joined had to promise to abstain from all liquors of an intoxicating quality, whether ale, porter, wine or ardent spirits, except as medicine.

620 *Hunts County News* 26 June 1909. Reminiscences of J. Kemp Foster

621 The island was actually further up the river at Hemingford Abbots.

'The usual method of conveyance,' Foster continued, 'was by a huge lighter, most lent by Messrs Brown and Goodman and towed by a horse the whole distance'. The Temperance Society and the churches and the chapels organised many of these outings as well as other associations. One of the most charming features of these outings was the sociable nature that marked them. At these gatherings the enjoyments of fishing etc to cultivate rare appetites for tea were augmented by the delights of music, chiefly on the return journey:

> On a moonlit night it was picturesque in the extreme to be a member of a returning boatload. The silent swish of the moving boat, with periodical lapping of the water by the alternatively dipping and tightening of the tow-rope, proved a capital accompaniment to the feast of song. And those at home waiting the return of friends found the music thus sent across the water more entertaining even than the Hemingford bells[622] on a beautiful summer evening. The picnic excursions generally started from Mr John Bullard's ozier yard at 2 o'clock and returned in the evening between 9 and 10 o'clock.

What a delightful way for St Ivians to start the week!

In 1890 the first water carnival at St Ives was organised. This comprised a procession of lighted boats from the bridge downstream to the railway bridge[623] while a band played on the quay decorated with Chinese lanterns.[624]

Such was Foster's love of the English river. Such was Reginald's. Such is mine. It was a love shared by Edward Thring, his Headmaster at Uppingham. When he was studying as a young man at King's College, Cambridge, he wrote in his poem, 'To a River':

> Companion of my boyhood,
> My manhood's living friend
> I fain would know thy rising
> I fain would know thy end.[625]

---

[622] St James Parish Church at Hemingford Grey lay alongside the river and further upstream there was another at Hemingford Abbots. Both had fine peals of bells, although the steeple of the former had been knocked down in a gale in 1741 and the spire only partially rebuilt.

[623] The Huntington & St Ives GN & GE Joint Railway branch line crossed the river at two points – just above St Ives Staunch on the Fenstanton Road and then upstream just before the Hemingford Lock.

[624] Flanagan, Bridget, *Artists along the Ouse*, p. 32.

[625] Thring, Edward, 'To a river' *Index Rerum* (a collection of jottings) Cited by Malcolm Tozer, *Edward Thring's Theory, Practice and Legacy* (2019), p. 77.

THE ARTISTS' COLONY

By the time Reginald was in his teens, St Ives and the surrounding area was becoming a destination for a number of artists who came to paint the river scenes for which St Ives became well known. Train travel made their journey easy.

The first of these artists, George Gordon Fraser,[626] arrived in 1881.

Besides the ease of travel by train to St Ives, the attraction of the river for these artists lay in its rustic and decaying charm. One of them, Edmund Wimperis, who was the Vice-President of the Royal Institute of Painters in Water Colours, wrote an article for *The Leisure Hour* in 1895 called 'Favourite Sketching Grounds – the Hemingfords'.[627] It captures the delight of the river which Reginald so enjoyed:

> It was in the early part of 1890 that my friend Keeley Halswelle told me he had heard of a new sketching ground, which he described to him as being full of subjects that would suit us both. It was the river Ouse between St Ives and Huntingdon. The traffic on the river, once no doubt considerable, had fallen off so much that as a means of mercantile communication it was almost disused. It still possessed, however, all the appearance of a navigable river stream, such as a towing path, with its bridges.
>
> Locks and fords and these in what to an artist was their most servable form – that is to say somewhat neglected, decayed and overgrown. There were fertile meads and rustic villages with here and there a church tower or spire half hidden by lofty trees or mirrored in placid pools. Then again, the condition of the banks was anything but trim and we should find all the beautiful weeds in undisturbed perfection; while the surface of the water had a wealth of water lilies, arrowheads, reeds, and flags in full luxuriance. So, we decided to go on an exploring expedition, though some misgivings, born of fruitless quests in previous years.

Their patience was rewarded, for he went on to say:

> On a certain morning in May we took the train to St Ives and started to walk by the river bank to Huntingdon, a distance of five miles. We crossed by a very picturesque bridge in the town itself a charming picture, and pursued the path on the left hand bank of the river and very shortly

[626] George Gordon Fraser (1859–95) was one of the well-known family of artists originally from Scotland which included Arthur Anderson Fraser, Gilbert Baird Fraser and Garden William Fraser. Reginald's eldest son, William, who was also a doctor, married Helen Fraser whose father was Gilbert Baird Fraser (1865–1947). They named their son, my cousin, William Baird.

[627] Flanagan, Bridget, *Artists along the Ouse*, p. 97.

> reached knight's mill, the surroundings of which would furnish a number of subjects for the pencil. Perhaps the best of all is the old lock, with its footbridge and its foreground of weeds and decaying timbers. Passing over the footbridge we came to a long reach of river, bordered on the one side by wide meadows, interspersed with fantastic and gnarled pollard willows, under whose shade cattle and sheep rest and on the other side shaded by lofty trees, which the tower and churchyard of Hemingford Grey reflected in a broad expanse of water. Sketched from the river this forms a very favourable representation of rural England. A little further on the village appears and a wide street slopes to the water's edge with boats moored at the bottom of the gardens and all the incidents of rural life.
>
> Here carters come down to water their horses, and the pleasure seekers to row[628] or fish or strollers to enjoy a pleasant walk along the bank to the next village of Hemingford Abbots. Continuing on the towing path for some little distance we find ourselves opposite an island[629] made by the separation of the main stream into two channels, on this our first sight of it, this island, well foliaged and willow fringed as it is, did not present any striking features, but as we passed on we caught a glimpse of the spire of Hemingford Abbots[630] rising above the trees, which looked very promising.

And so they continued their walk to Huntingdon.

Towards the end of the 19th century, St Ives began to realise, like many country towns, that it had numerous attractions to offer those who lived in the growing urban metropolis. The walkers who stayed with Mrs Honeybourne, mentioned by Reginald on New Year's Day 1881, may well have been such tourists.

With the river used mainly for recreation, bathing as well as boating became an issue; in 1892, while Reginald was ending his medical training, the Council at St Ives addressed a worrying issue of what was termed 'indecent' bathing. This was individuals or perhaps groups of boys,

---

628 As mentioned in the last chapter, the Giddins family owned a boat business at Hemingford Grey a few hundred yards upstream from the church. It had workshops which were knocked down to create a new purpose-built boathouse in 1905. It did an excellent trade in the summer hiring out rowing boats, punts and skiffs.

629 This was Battcock's Island opposite Houghton Meadow.

630 Reginald's youngest surviving son, David Stevenson Grove (1905–86), retired in 1969 with his wife Mollie (née Turner) to live in Hemingford Abbots, in the shadow of St Margaret's Parish Church at 'Riverside' in Church Lane, the garden of which slopes down to the river. David's wife survived him and died in 1992, when the property was sold.

stripping off and swimming off the bank at Hemingford Meadow in the same way that boys did in the Cam. It was decided to select a site where swimming could be more controlled, but it was not until 1913 that public swimming baths were built on Holt Island near the parish church.

Reginald's role in this is described in Volume 3.

Whether the river was sluggish and slow as in the summer, or deadly quiet and iced over in the winter, or a raging flood in the spring, it was etched into his heart. Like Kenneth Grahame's Ratty in *The Wind in the Willows*, Reginald knew that there was nothing, absolutely nothing that could compare with an English river. The sparkle, the ripple, the smell, the scents and the sounds of the river – it was Ratty's world. It was Reginald's world too.

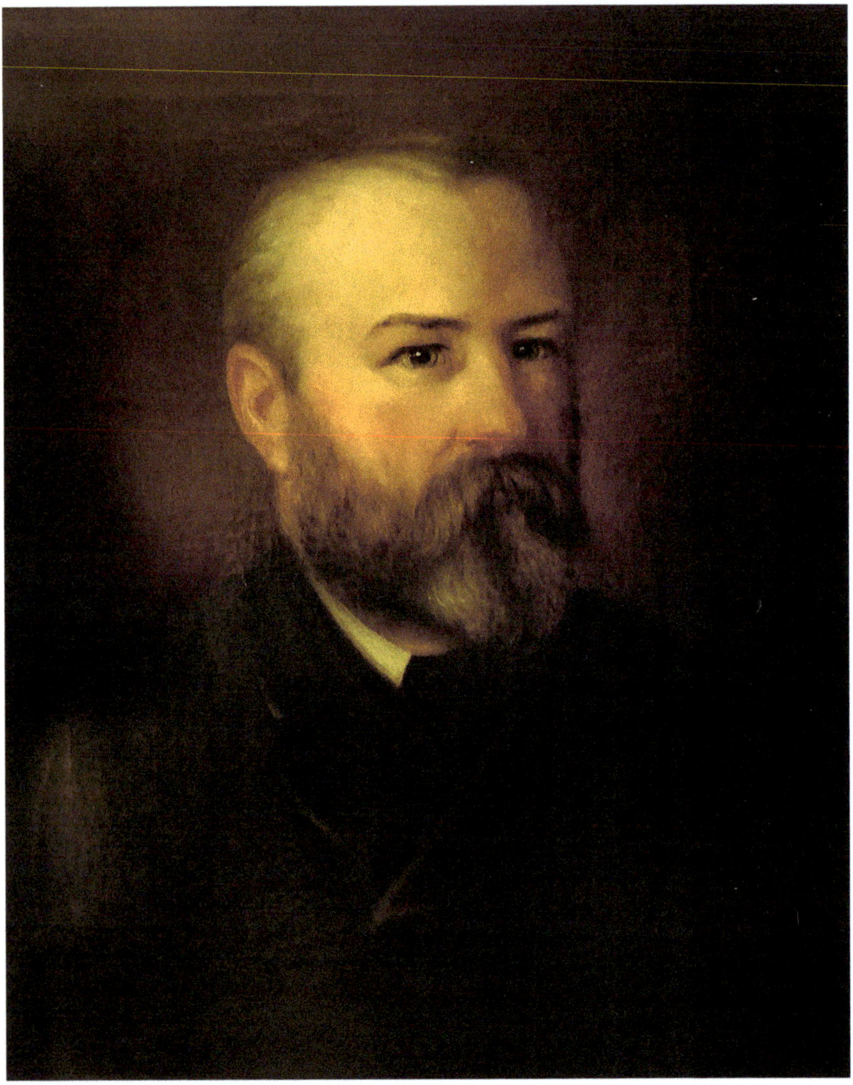

Dr William Richard Grove (1838–1895) aged about 50.
This portrait is one of a pair, by an unknown artist, and originally hung at Slepe House. It is now in the possession of one of his great, great grandsons.
COURTESY OF BILL AND ROSALIND GROVE

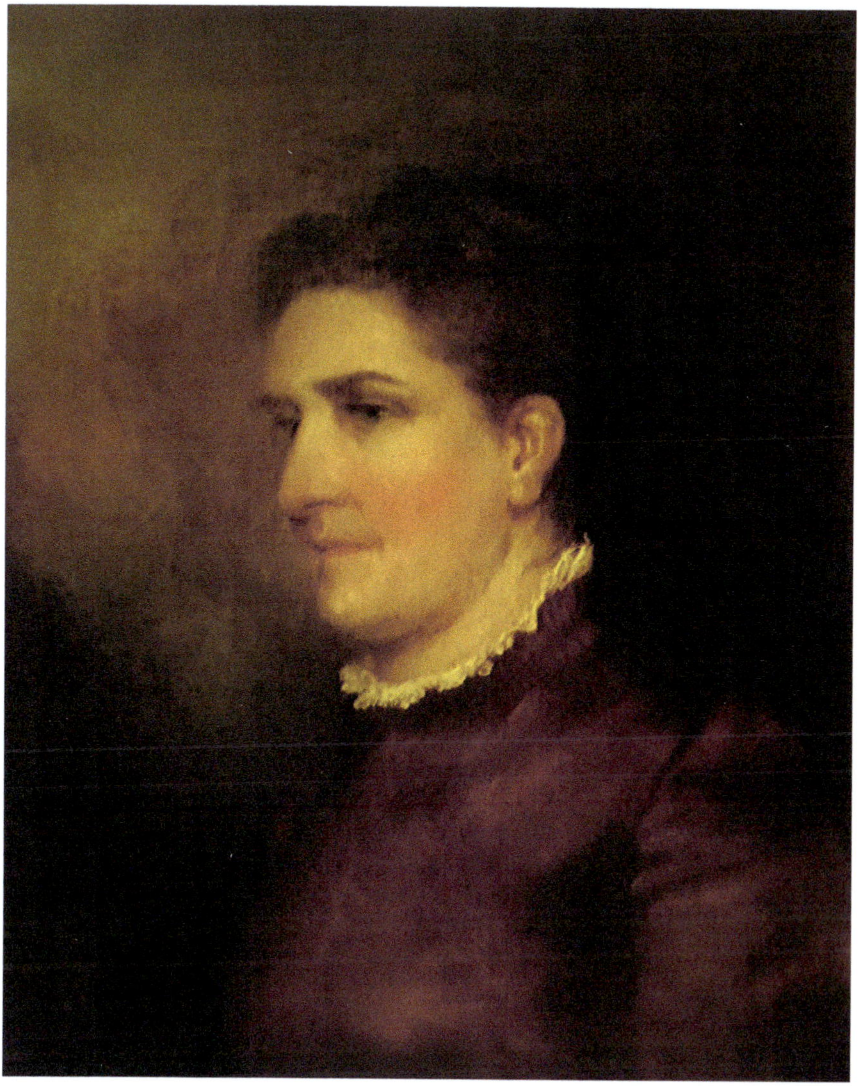

Maria Grove, née Long (1844–1930) aged about 50.
Like her husband's portrait, it is one of a pair, hung beside her husband's.
COURTESY OF BILL AND ROSALIND GROVE

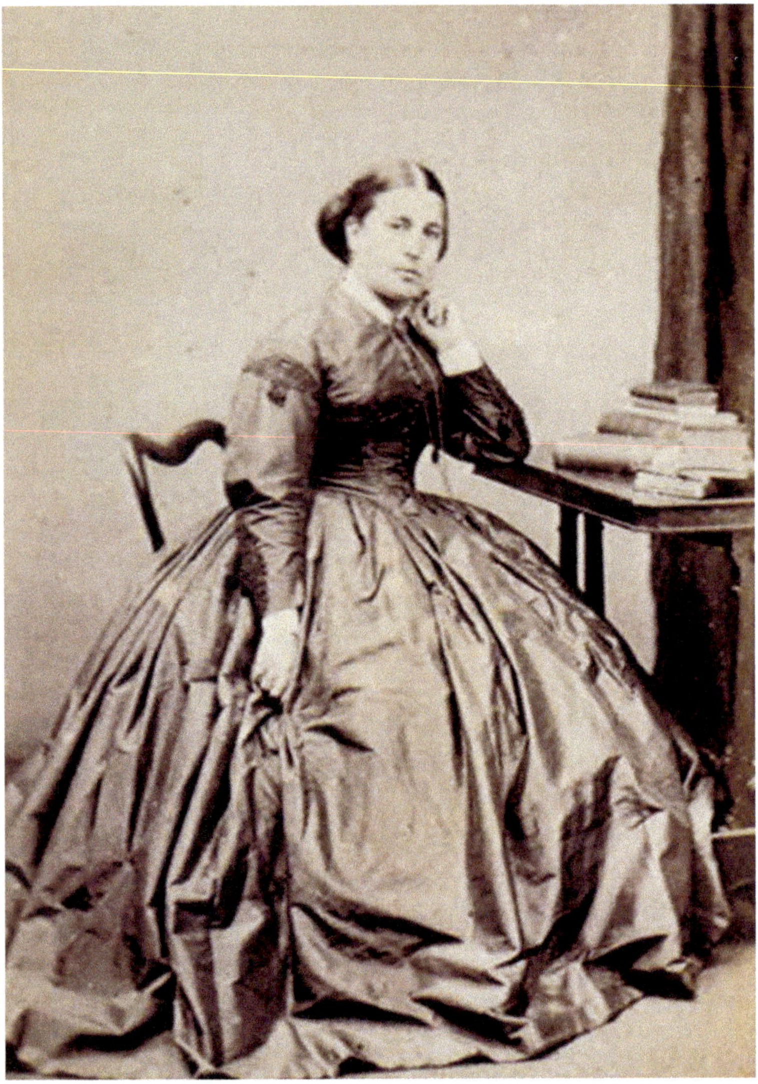

Martha Mardall (1832–1912), née Long, one of Reginald's aunts in her mid 30s judging from her crinoline dress. The daughter of a farmer, she ran a successful brewery in Harpenden, Hertfordshire taking it on after the death of her husband. When she sold the brewery it had 37 tied public houses.

PHOTO PUBLIC DOMAIN

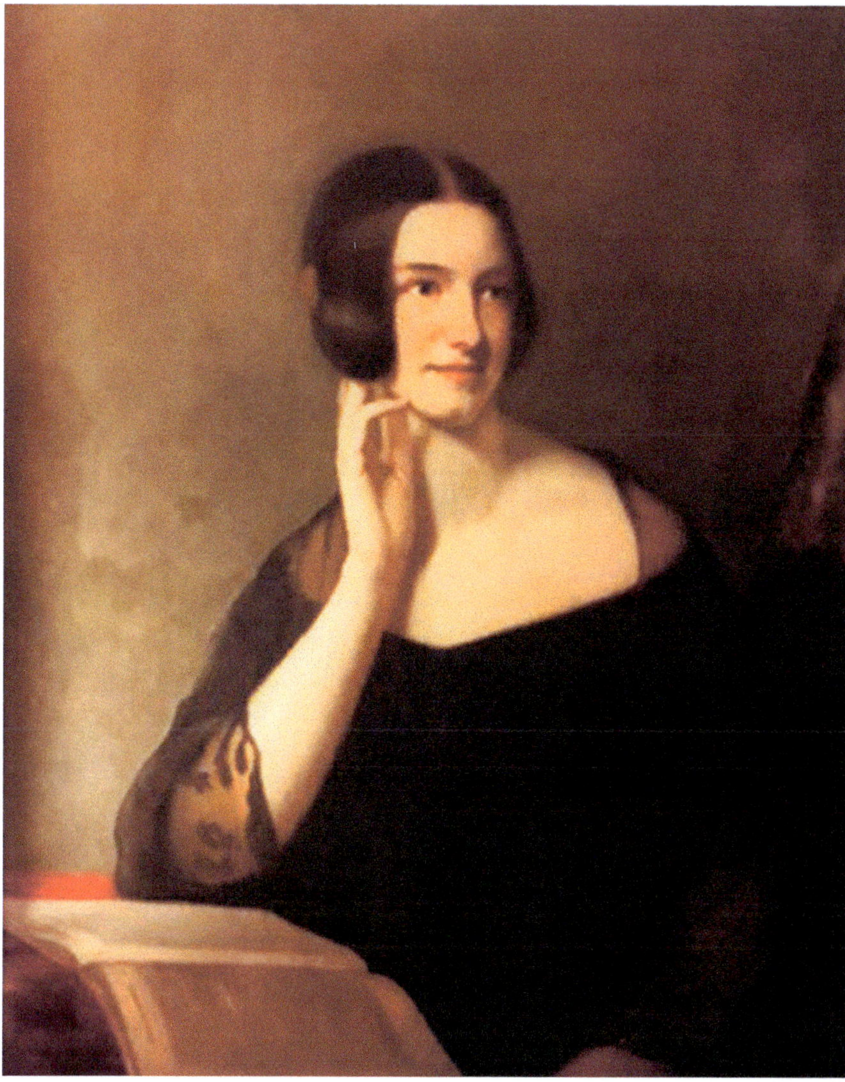

Georgiana Grove, née Barnes (1817–1886) aged about 20 but widowed when she was 24. The artist is unknown. The daughter of a pawnbroker, she took over this business while bringing up her two sons, Reginald's father and his uncle Frank.

COURTESY OF JOHN AND CHERRIE GROVE

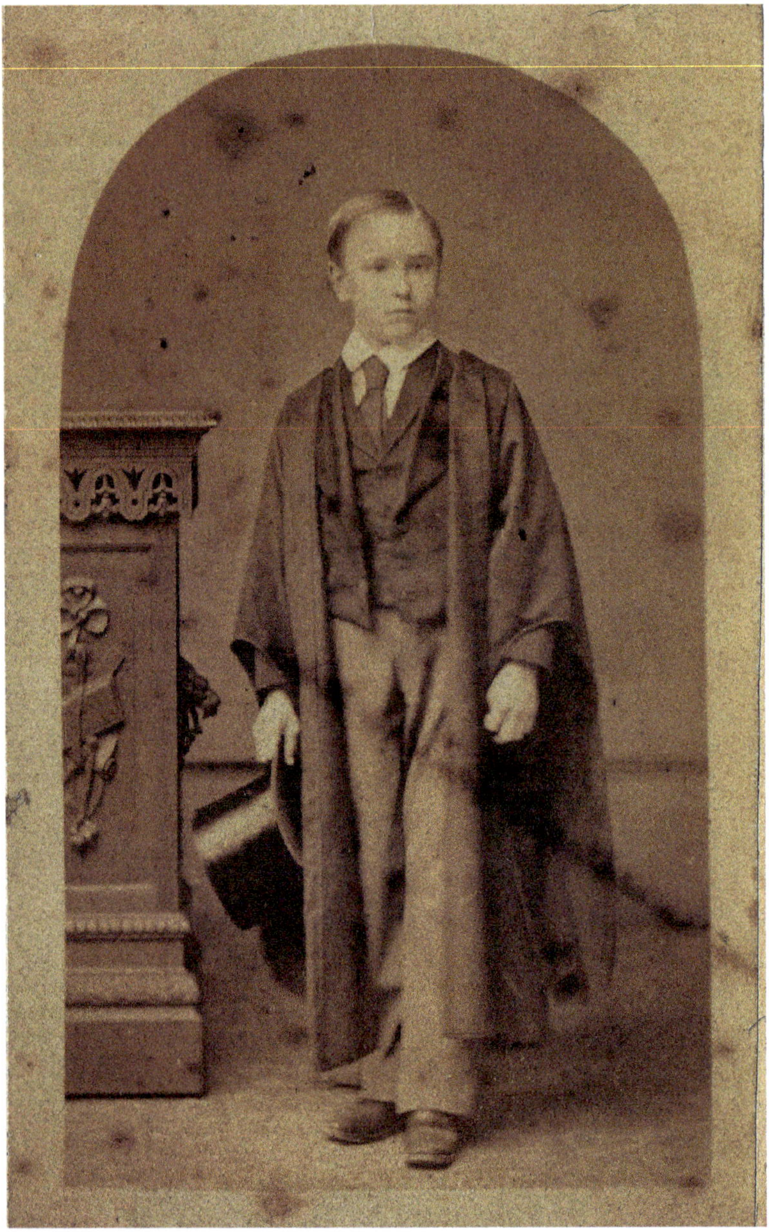

Reginald aged 9 after he joined the chapel choir of King's College, Cambridge in 1878.

GROVE FAMILY ARCHIVE

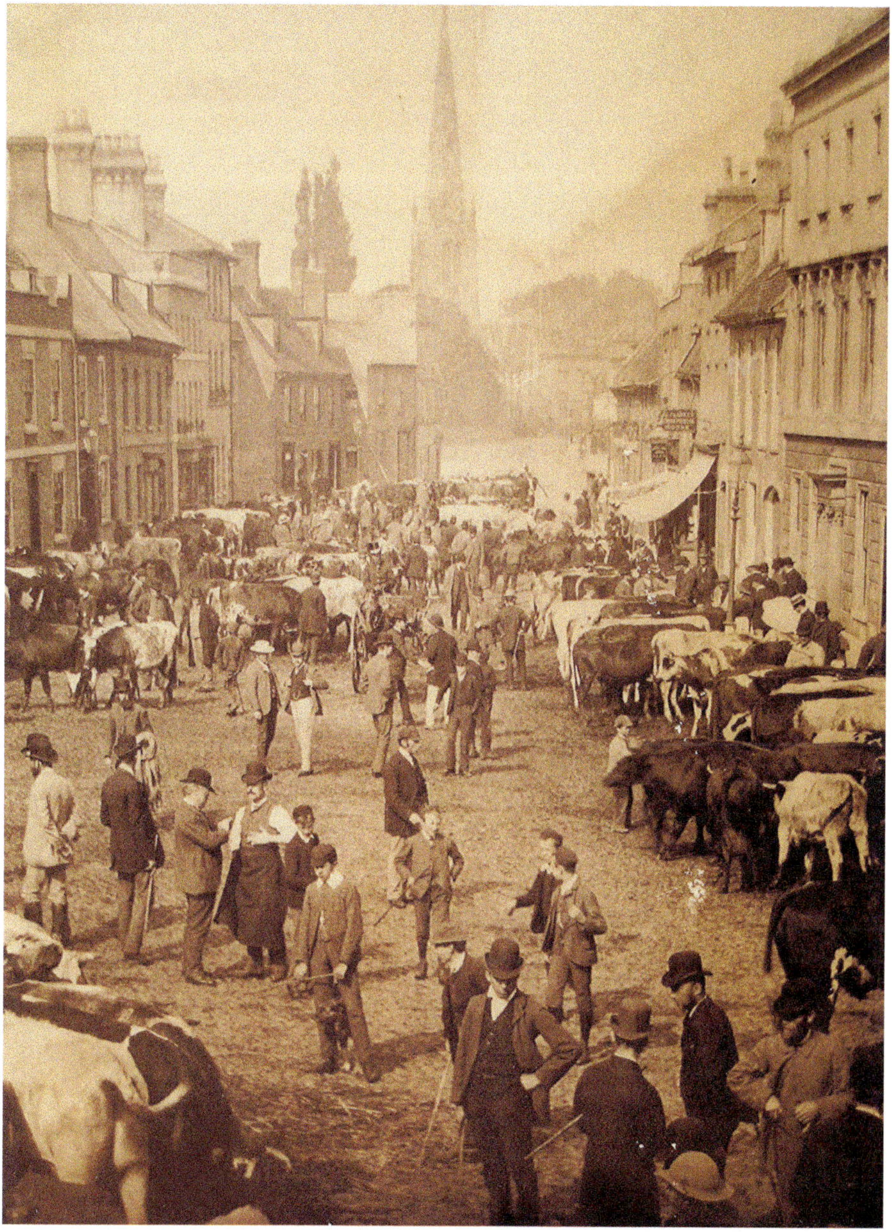

The Bullock Market, St Ives in 1886, just before the market moved. Reginald's first home at No 33, is on the left-hand side, set back a little from the road.
COURTESY OF THE NORRIS MUSEUM

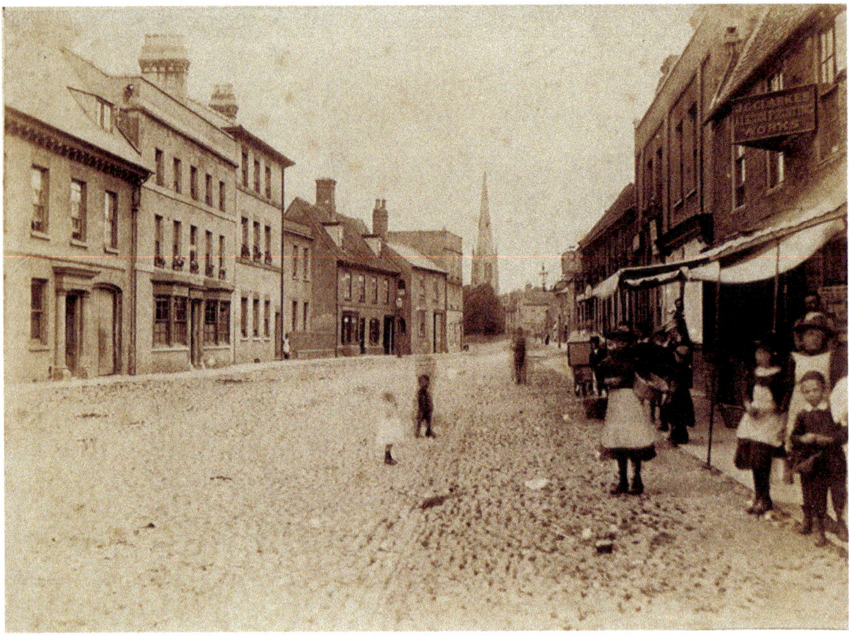

The Bullock Market, in the late 1880s after the weekly livestock had moved to its new, larger site near the railway station. Reginald's house is on the left hand-side, where the small girl in a white pinafore is standing.

COURTESY OF THE NORRIS MUSEUM

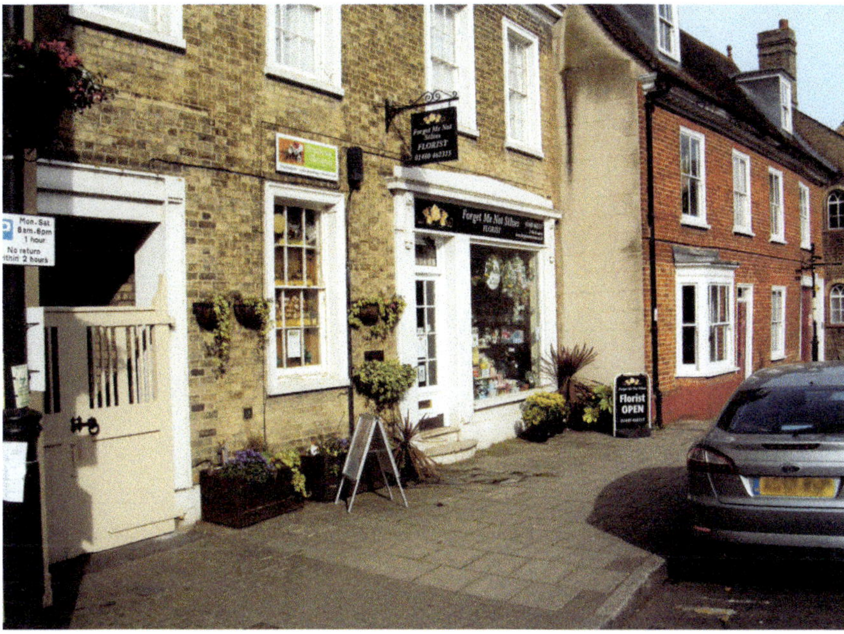

Number 33, The Broadway (as the Bullock Market was renamed) at the present-day showing Reginald's first home until 1881. The surgery was on the first floor. The entrance for the horse and trap is on the left. The original iron railings at the front, which stopped cattle reaching the front door, have long gone.

AUTHOR'S PHOTOGRAPH

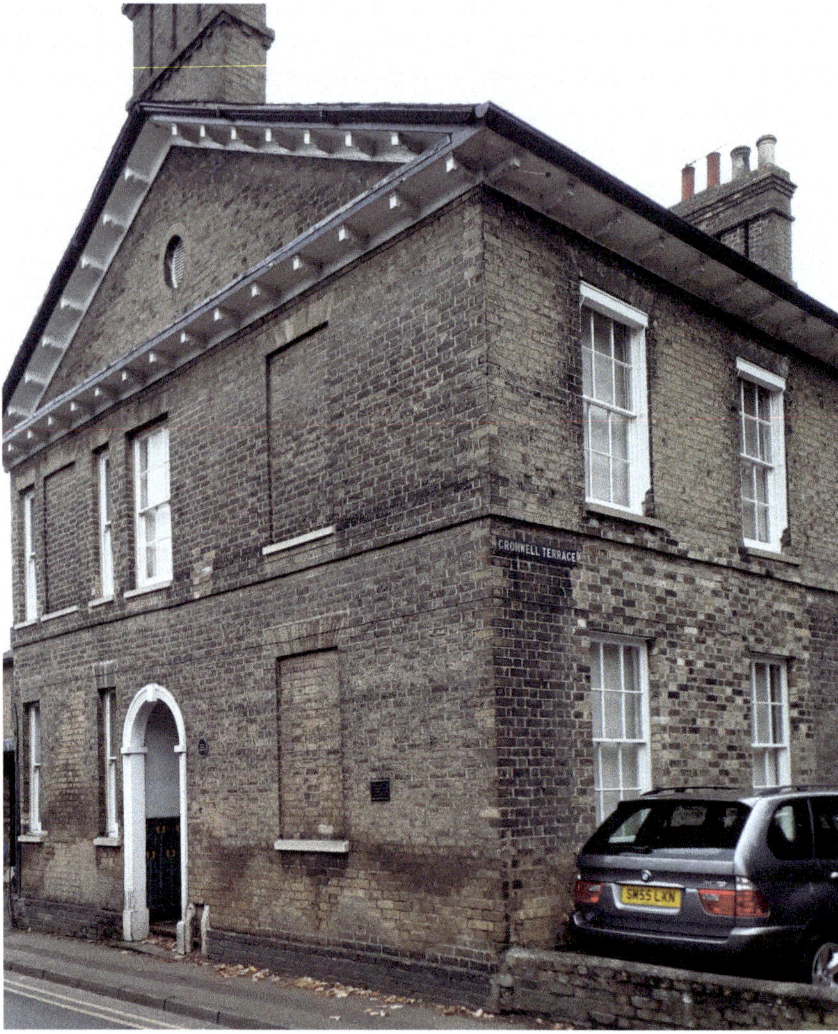

Slepe House in Cromwell Place, Reginald's home from 1881 which was used as his father's surgery. It continues to be used for this purpose today and is known as the Grove Medical Centre. The name commemorates the three generations of Grove doctors who practiced from the building for 85 years.
AUTHOR'S PHOTOGRAPH

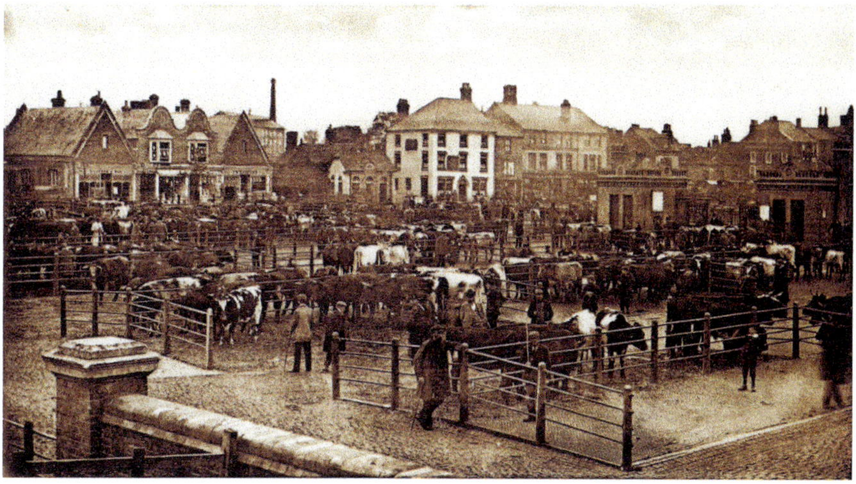

The new cattle market in the late 1880's after the Grove family had moved to Slepe House. The photo was taken from the garden of the houses in Cromwell Terrace which backed on to the market.

COURTESY OF THE NORRIS MUSEUM

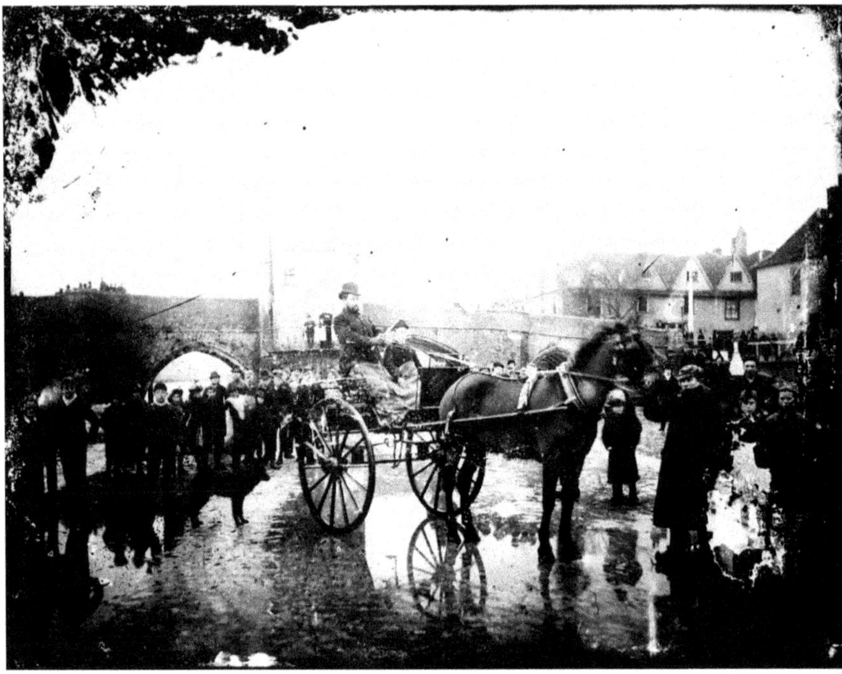

The Great Ouse at St Ives bridge during the very hard winter of 1891 showing skating.

COURTESY OF THE NORRIS MUSEUM

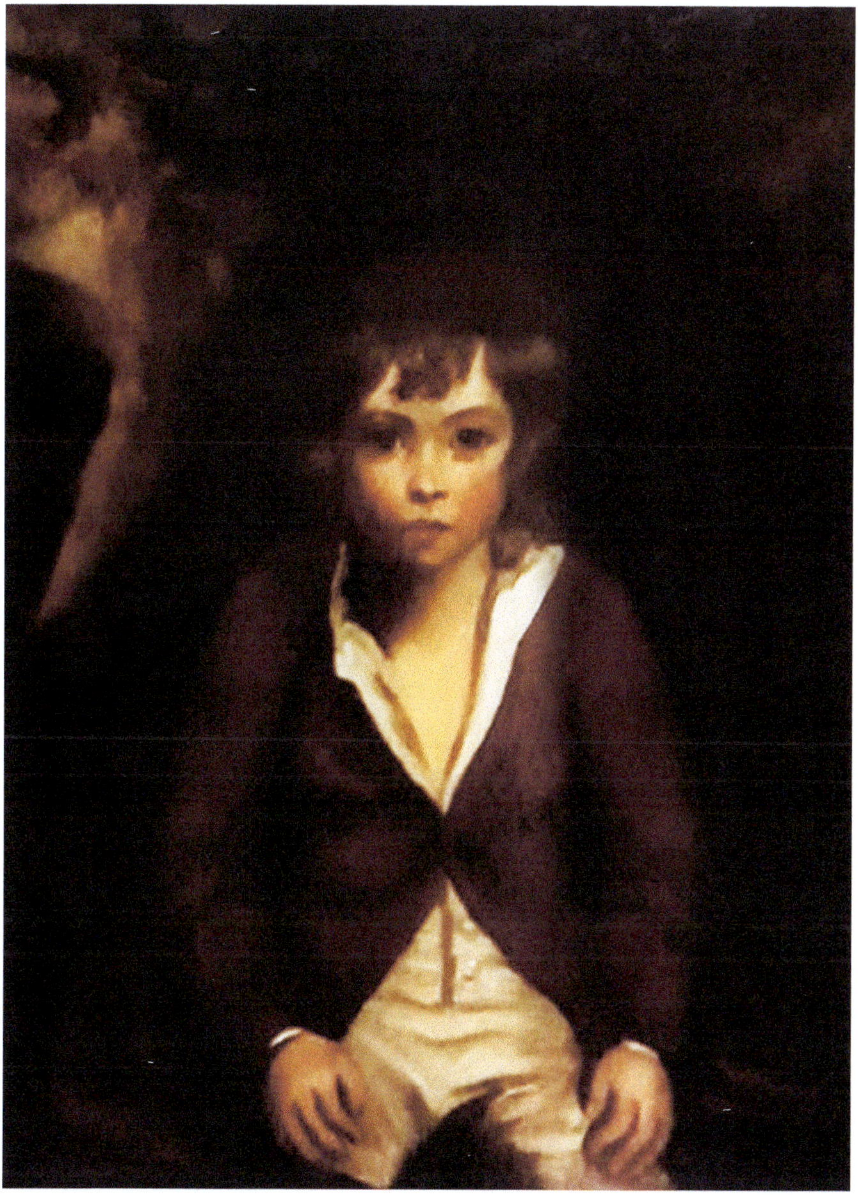

'Master Bunbury' is a copy of an oil by Joshua Reynolds. Master Bunbury was Reynolds' godson, Henry Edward Bunbury. The copy was produced by C. Davy of Newman Street, off Oxford, St, London. It hung at Slepe House and the original is in the Philadelphia Museum of Art.

AUTHOR'S PHOTOGRAPH

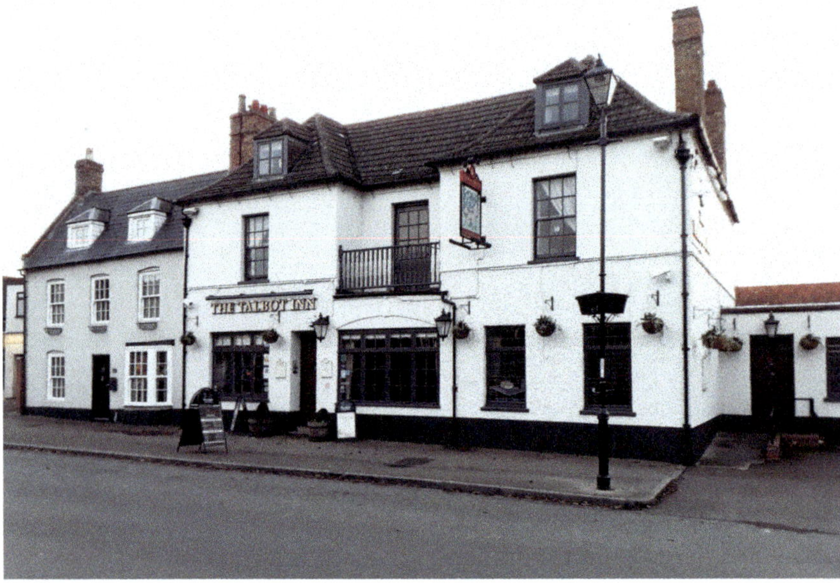

The Talbot Inn at Stilton, in the centre of the long village street. It was one of the inns that Reginald and his friend Berry stopped during their walk from Uppingham to Huntingdon in April 1887. It still stands today. Reginald said it was (then) 'an awful hole'.

AUTHOR'S PHOTOGRAPH

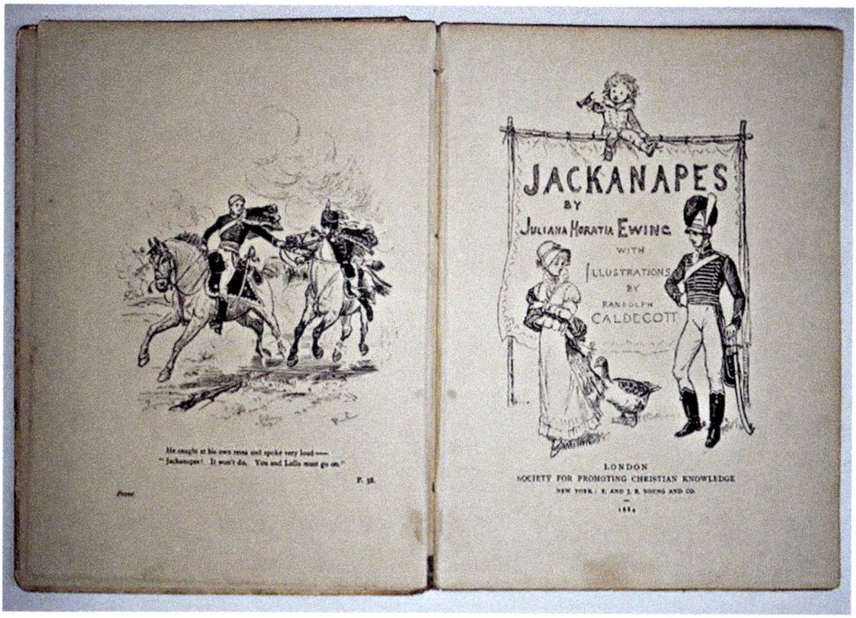

Jackanapes *by Julia Horatia Ewing, a friend of Edward Thring. This heroic story became very popular and this edition was bought by Reginald in 1884, the year of its publication. His signature is in the front cover.*

GROVE FAMILY ARCHIVE

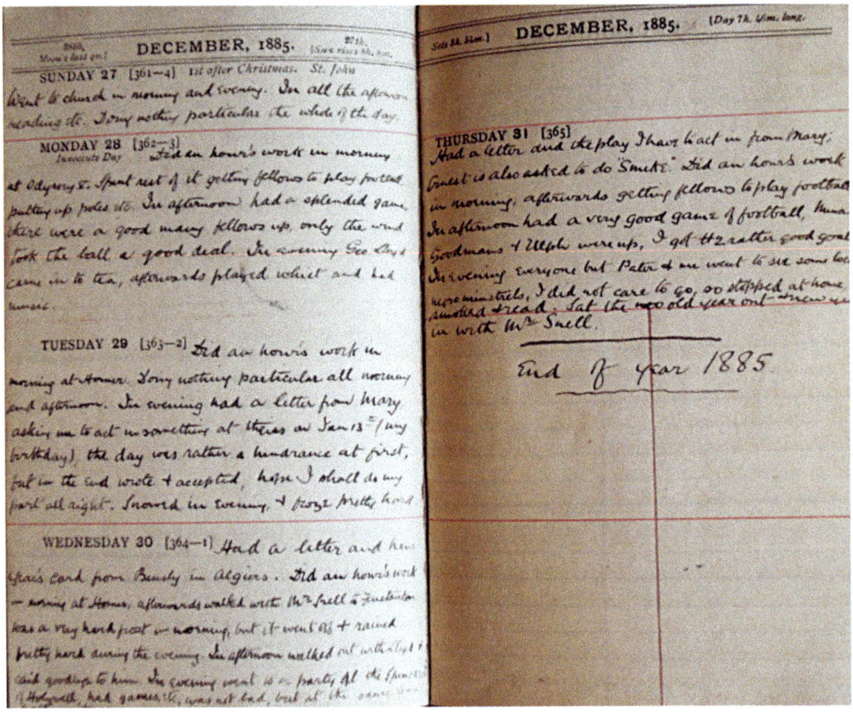
DECEMBER, 1885.

SUNDAY 27 [361—4] 1st after Christmas. St. John

Went to church in morning and evening. In all the afternoon reading &c. Doing nothing particular the whole of the day.

MONDAY 28 [362—3] Innocents Day. Did an hour's work in morning at Odyssey &c. Spent rest of it getting fellows to play football putting up poles &c. In afternoon had a splendid game, there were a good many fellows up, only the wind took the ball a good deal. In evening Geo Lloyd came in to tea, afterwards played whist and had music.

TUESDAY 29 [363—2] Did an hour's work in morning at Homer. Doing nothing particular all morning and afternoon. In evening had a letter from Mary asking me to act in something at theirs on Jan 13th (my birthday) the day was rather a hindrance at first, but in the end wrote & accepted, hope I shall do my part all right. Snowed in evening, & froze pretty hard.

WEDNESDAY 30 [364—1] Had a letter and New Year's card from Bunky in Algiers. Did an hour's work in morning at Homer, afterwards walked with Mr Snell to … was a very hard frost in morning, but it went off & rained pretty hard during the evening. In afternoon walked out with … said goodbye to him. In evening went to a party at the … of Holywell, had games &c, was not bad, but at the same …

DECEMBER, 1885.

THURSDAY 31 [365] Had a letter and the play I have to act in from Mary, Ernest is also asked to do "Smike". Did an hour's work in morning, afterwards getting fellows to play football. In afternoon had a very good game of football, … Goodmans & Ulph were up, I got two rather good goals. In evening everyone but Pater & me went to see some local negro minstrels, I did not care to go, so stopped at home smoked & read. Sat the old year out & new year in with Mr Snell.

End of year 1885

Reginald's diary showing the entries he made in December 1885. His diary for that year was a Pettitt's Annual Diary, sized 6 x 4in, which included an Almanac. It cost one shilling or £6.30 at today's value.

AUTHOR'S PHOTOGRAPH

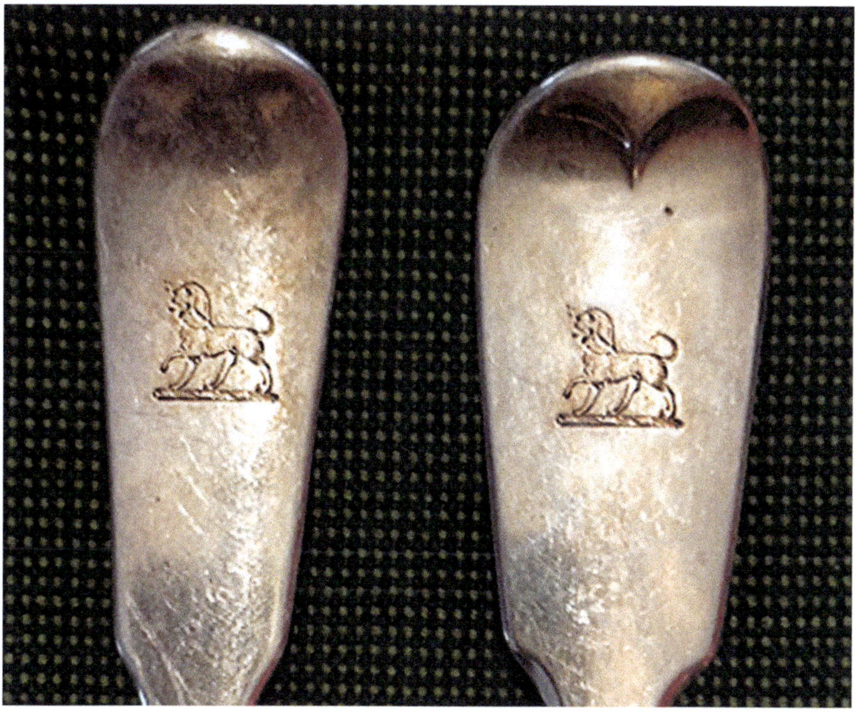

The Grove Crest displayed on the family cutlery.
The image is that of a dog, possibly a mastiff. The heraldic pose
is 'talbot passant sa collared'.

COURTESY OF JOHN AND CHERRIE GROVE

CHAPTER 12

Pastimes

'... had an awfully jolly evening, really far and away the best we have had; danced with Mary as many times as we could both arrange and I am actually at last able to dance the waltz with certain partners; kept it up until 9.00pm.'

Reginald Grove, 11 January 1887

TOYS AND GAMES

Neither Reginald nor his parents left any record of his early childhood, so the experience of other children from middle-class households during this period is our only clue for the toys and games that entertained him as a child.

Most children played with simple toys – large boxes of plain, wooden bricks made make-believe docks, stations, forts, towers and houses. In her memories of a Victorian childhood, Molly Hughes described living in London in the 1870s and playing with a box of thin and flat bricks with dovetailed edges. This enabled her and her family to build long walls around imaginary cities. In addition, 24 wooden painted French and British soldiers carried out battles across her playroom floor. Then, in another game of make-believe, her whole room became the sea with a chair upside down acting as *The Great Eastern* ocean liner which laid an Atlantic cable.[631] The ship was an iron sailing steamship designed by Isambard Kingdom Brunel. It was well known, even for a child like Molly Hughes, for carrying out this task in 1866, having been taken off the transatlantic passenger route.

Besides wooden soldiers, painted lead[632] soldiers were popular, too, especially with boys, and Reginald would have been no exception. Both boys and girls also played with painted wooden animals. Wooden indoor skittles[633] were popular. With the growing use of vulcanised rubber from

[631] Hughes, Molly, *A Victorian Family: 1870–1900* (Guild Publishing, 1990), p. 1.

[632] The danger from lead-based paint poisoning was not known until 100 years later.

[633] From the 1860s new inks and dyes became available and printing technology made it possible for toys to be painted in bright colours easily.

1839 onwards, outside games using rubber balls, catapults and wind-up toys like small boats became commonplace. Living in the Bullock Market until he was 13, with the garden sloping down to the river, this would have been an ideal place for Reginald to sail a wind-up boat.

Rocking horses and hobby horses were popular, too, and encouraged an escape into the world of imagination; the stables and the garden would have been an ideal location for a hobby horse. Hoops (bowled down a street with a stick) and whipping tops (wooden spun by a length of cord around it, pulled sharply and kept spinning by whipping it) were toys that Reginald would have been familiar with before he went to boarding school.

However, in general, parents wanted toys that were instructive for their children. A book by T. W. Erle called *Science in the Nursery*,[634] published in 1884, promoted this approach and was popular with middle-class parents in the same way that some toys with an educational purpose are favoured today. Whether Reginald had toys like these is not recorded, but it is clear later that he became interested in science as a foundation for what became his love of medicine. All kinds of moving mechanical toys were manufactured and sold. Those that have survived are a delight to see in action. Puppets, model theatres and doll's houses were also a means of stimulating the imagination of children – think of the meticulous detail given to the design and contents of doll's houses.[635] The Victoria and Albert Museum of Childhood in Bethnal Green, London, has a remarkable collection of over 100 delightful doll's houses.

BOYHOOD GAMES

Games that are still popular today with children were played in the Victorian period. With the start of his diaries aged 12 a clearer picture emerges of his entertainment. For instance, he played five stones and jacks,[636] and marbles at King's Choir School when it was wet outside. Marbles had grown in popularity from the 1850s when the glass balls found in fizzy drink bottles

---

[634] *Erle, Thomas William, Science in the Nursery: or, Children's Toys and What They Teach.* (Griffith, Farran & Co. London, 1884).

[635] A unique doll's house made for Reginald's future wife, Hilda, in the 1870s has been handed down through the family and is in my possession. It will be passed on to the next generation to enjoy.

[636] Five stones and Jacks are similar and played with five small objects (ten for jacks) and a small ball and the ball is bounced as the objects are thrown up and caught.

became widely used.[637] That same afternoon he played 'Spanish fly'. This was a form of leapfrog.[638] Bagatelle was another game he played over the Christmas holidays in January 1883 with two of his cousins, Willie and Hugh Mardall, who were visiting at the time.

Games played in the playground, such as tag, Grandma's Footsteps and What's the Time, Mr Wolf?, are still popular today, as is hide and seek, which the boys at King's enjoyed just before Christmas 1883. The school building provided many little nooks and crannies in which to hide. In the autumn, the line of chestnut trees lining the drive from West Road in Cambridge to the main entrance at King's provided piles of conkers; it was a favourite game for boys during this and later periods.

As he grew into adulthood there were a number of board and card games played. Cribbage, chess and whist were games that he played as he grew older, as was a card game called 'Boston'. Another card game he was introduced to and enjoyed was called 'Spin' just before his 18th birthday. The aim was to group four cards of the same suit together to try to get a high score. He played it a few weeks later with his father. It is still played today.

A card trick that he learnt when he and the family went for supper at a Mrs Kinder's on New Year's Day 1887 was called 'Banjo'. This is a sleight of hand coin trick still used by magicians today. On occasions he played chess with other boys when he was at King's in the Vice Provost's rooms in the college. Tea was an added treat.

In his last holiday before he left Uppingham aged 18, he played a new game with his father called 'Reversi'. Reversi was a strategy board game for two players on an uncheckered board,[639] and had only been invented three years previously. The aim of the game was to have the majority of disks turned to display one of the colours when the last playable empty square was filled.

As he grew older, he began playing billiards when he was home from

---

637 The glass ball used as a stopper in the bottleneck could be extracted by smashing the bottle to use as a marble. The temperance movement encouraged carbonated drinks as an alternative to alcohol.

638 This is a game of leapfrog in which the leader (jumping first) then sets feats for the others to perform. Any player who failed the feat then took his or her place at the back.

639 There are 64 identical game pieces called disks or discs, light on one side and dark on the other. Players take turns placing disks on the board with their assigned colour facing up. The game was invented in 1883 and gained considerable popularity in England at the end of the 19th century. The game's first reliable mention was in the 21 August 1886 edition of *The Saturday Review.*

school for the holidays. His home did not have one, so he went to the Literary Institute in St Ives where billiards were played. In the Easter holidays in 1885 he played with his father's Medical Assistant, a Mr Haynes. Eighteen months later, in the Christmas holidays in 1886 he went to the Institute in the afternoon to while away the time with a game, but found it too crowded to play.

PARLOUR GAMES, MUSICAL CONCERTS, ENTERTAINMENT AND AMATEUR DRAMATICS

Flickering gas light made reading difficult in the winter evenings, so parlour games, musical evenings and amateur dramatics played an important part in family entertainment. Without television, radio, computers or smartphones, middle-class families made their own entertainment in the evenings, especially at the weekends when social gatherings were generally held. After dinner, families would 'withdraw' to the withdrawing or (drawing) room for evening entertainment.

Parlour games were very popular during the late-1800s and early 1900s, as the period saw an increase in leisure time before the radio and television age. Friday and Saturday evenings were most popular for social gatherings, and along with parlour games would include light meals, music and a chance for young people to meet in a chaperoned environment. It was in this environment that Reginald met and began to court his sweetheart, Mary.

Some of the era's parlour games are still known today like Blind Man's Bluff, and some have evolved into 21st-century board games such as Balderdash. But many parlour games familiar to Reginald are no longer known or played, such as 'Old Man', 'Bull's Warning', 'Spin', 'Proverbs' and 'Stool of Repentance'.[640] But charades, which he and his family often played, especially with his Long cousins, is, of course, well known today. When he was 14 he went next door to a party held by the Ulph family with his cousin Willie Mardall, who had been staying after Christmas, and

[640] This parlour game was sometimes called 'accusations'. Those playing sat in a circle around a stool and one of the group (called the 'victim') left and those remaining wrote things about him or her about their character, appearance etc. When the 'victim' came back they sat on the stool and the players then read out what had been said them. They were then asked 'who said that about you?' A correct guess meant they could return to the circle and the person who made the accusation left the room as the victim. If, the 'victim' did not give the correct answer, they left the room again.

everyone played charades. Such was the fun that they did not get home until 11.00pm. But as in any family the moods of individuals affected everyone else.

On one occasion towards the end of the Christmas holidays Reginald's close friend Arnie Ulph was invited for supper. Reginald's mother had a headache and his father was in a bad mood. They all played word games and 'spin' it, but it was not a successful evening.

Families also created their own musical entertainment, and within the Grove family a number played instruments; Reginald played the flute and his father the violin, as did his sweetheart Mary. Reginald had been playing since at least 1883 when he was 14 at King's.

Often a family would settle around the piano to play classical as well as popular pieces; in fact, it was almost mandatory to have a piano and the Groves were no exception. If no one could play the piano, then there was the pianola instead.[641] In the new year of 1885 the Groves had a musical evening together when his father and Mary played violin and he played flute. A couple of years later in the new year Reginald with his mother, father and sweetheart Mary went to the Ulphs' next door for a 'sort of musical at home'. It turned out to be more of a concert than anything else. His father played the flute in three musical pieces, and Margie Ulph played the violin and also sang a song called 'The Brook'[642] (a well-known poem by Lord Tennyson) which had been set to music. The piano accompaniment exactly represented the 'babbling brook' in his view. Reginald judged the evening a great success, partly because the Ulph family were 'so musical', but also because their other friends were there: Mr Kinder, Mr and Mrs Twiberville, Miss Hudson and Miss Day contributed, too. All were from the Free Church at St Ives of which the Ulphs were members. Reginald commented that 'nearly all the dissenters enjoyed it', which seemed to indicate, on his part, a sense of 'them and us'.

Informal concerts were often put on to entertain others. Aged 13, in his Christmas holidays, he sang at one that was held one evening in the Literary Institute in St Ives – he sang four times and was encored on three

[641] With this instrument, separate pieces of equipment were placed next to the pianola to begin with. These had wooden fingers which lay over the keys and as punched paper roll was pulled around the mechanism, the wooden fingers pulled down and played the keys like human fingers. Later the equipment was built into the piano itself – either to play normally or set to auto. There were lots of popular tunes available.

[642] 'Brook Song' was composed by W. F. Sudds for the piano (Op. 118).

occasions! A few days later he travelled by train to Longstanton, a village on the line to Cambridge. The Herbert family lived there whom the Groves knew, and Reginald sang two solos at a concert as well as taking part in 'a dialogue'. He did not mention what the subject was or character he played, but this was a device used for two people to talk about a subject of interest to an audience; the sketches of Laurel and Hardy were a development of this in the early days of the cinema 40 years later. Over the Christmas holidays that year he sang two 'sacred' songs at concert put on by the St Ives Boat Club.

During the Easter holidays in 1885, Reginald mentioned going to the school at Brampton, near Huntingdon, with his mother, brother Ernest and Mabel where some theatricals were put on in the afternoon. He did not give any further details, but sometimes singing concerts were put on as entertainment for those less well off. During the new year of 1887 the All Saints' curate, Revd Pollock, arranged for a concert to be held at the nearby village of Woodhurst to raise funds for those in need in the parish. Reginald was one of a group of young men from St Ives recruited to sing 'glees'. These were parlour and folk songs, together with ditties normally sung a cappella in close harmony.[643] This was a style of singing that he had been involved in before – while he was at King's Choir School he went to a musical concert performed in the college where the boys sang two glees.

The main song performed at Woodhurst was called 'O who will o'er the downs so free'.[644] One of the group was meant to sing tenor, but in the end he did not turn up so Reginald had to 'raise my beautiful voice' in his place. The group was pretty dysfunctional, as when they assembled for the (horse-drawn) bus to take them to Woodhurst, four and a half miles away, 'two of them showed their caddishness by refusing to go at the last minute; however, we got on very well without them'. By the time they arrived, just after the concert had started, there were five singers in the glee. His brother Ted (then aged 15) sang a solo without going flat, and there were several 'good comic songs, readings and recitations', including Reginald's

[643] 'Glee Club' was a name dating back to the 18th century and originated from Harrow School. Glee Clubs had been established at Harvard and Yale universities by the mid-19th century.

[644] This is a love song which contains the memorable lines in the first verse: 'Her father he has lock'd the door, Her mother keeps the key, But neither door nor bolt shall part My own true love from me'. It was written and composed by Robert Lucas Pearsall (1795–1856) in four parts.

own recitation of the 'Owl Critic' poem.[645] It had eight verses, all of which he had memorised. He said the whole evening was a great success, except financially, as he was 'afraid that the poor will not get very much as the expenses were large and the receipts [ticket sales] small'. Afterwards, the performers and some of the audience went over the road to the local public house and enjoyed what Reginald called tea. They got home at about 11.30pm.

The following day, a Friday, Reginald, his sister Mabel and brother Ted went to another concert hosted by the Looker family when they were driven over by Mason, the family groom, in their brougham. There was a rehearsal during the afternoon and then the concert began – again a success according to Reginald. 'The Tinkling Duo' glee was good, and a very pretty duet called 'The Sleigh Race'. The performers had tied bells to their wrists for dramatic effect, and at certain points there was a chorus of 'Yo ho' from the other performers with a crack of the whip produced by two straps! Mabel joined with Grace Looker to play a duet, and his brother Ted sang the song he sang the previous day without getting very flat. The recitation of the 'Owl Critic' was Reginald's party piece again and he thought 'that it pleased the audience'. This was a family concert rather than a public one, and supper was served afterwards.

Reginald rather liked one of the guests, a Miss Harrison who was the daughter of the new vicar of Wyton, a nearby village. She was 'rather a nice girl', he felt. Mabel stayed the night, but he and Ted walked home and got back about 11.30pm. This was not the first time he sang in a glee, as a month earlier, just before he broke up for the holidays, the boys put on a concert at his house at Uppingham for Christmas, to which 60 came. He wrote down the programme in the back of his diary. The evening started with a piano piece played by a Miss Eliot, which was the overture from the comic opera *The Caliph of Baghdad* by François-Adrien Boieldieu. Who Miss Eliot was is not known, but perhaps she was part of the Redgate household run by Mrs Christian.

This was to be followed by a short play called *The Heir at Law*, which was comedy in five acts. Written in 1797 by George Colman, it was very

[645] This poem, subtitled 'a lesson for fault finders', was written by American author James Thomas Fields (1817–81).

popular during the 19th century, and its main character was Dr Pangloss:[646] Reginald played this character. There were a number of rehearsals for the play. The boys in the glee practised the day before in the morning, accompanied by Miss Eliot on the piano. There were two altos, two tenors (of which Reginald was one) and two basses. Besides the parlour songs they were to sing two school songs ('The Fives Song' and 'The Return') and some 'part songs', ending with the Uppingham School song called 'Farewell'. The last verse ended with the rousing lines:

> Brook no farewell,
> The good old days live on,
> Thy shall not forget,
> Shall not, shall not.[647]

The hall was decorated with evergreens and magic lanterns to give it a festive feel, and Reginald wrote the programmes[648] out, as it was not possible for some reason to use a Cyclostyle.[649] The evening was a great success, not least because Reginald felt, with unaccustomed hubris, that the glees were 'splendid chiefly due, ipse dixit[650], to the tenor'! In the end, there were 53 who sat down to supper and enjoyed the evening's entertainment. 'Certainly, the best praepostor's holiday since I came here'.

SOCIAL ACTIVITIES

Just before his 17th birthday Reginald experienced the not uncommon fear and embarrassment of a young man not being able to dance. One evening he and others in his family were invited for tea and supper by the Copley family whom they knew well; Mr Copley was a solicitor and the family lived a few hundred yards from Slepe House in Market Hill. The house is still used by a firm of solicitors practising under the name 'Copleys'.

After they had eaten, the guests got up for an impromptu dance with someone playing the piano; but the gauche Reginald squirmed with embarrassment: 'like a fool I would not'. He was not the only one, as

---

[646] While this character has the same name as the character in *Candide*, written by Voltaire, they are not the same.

[647] *Uppingham School Songs and Borth Lyrics* by Edward Thring. Edited by his daughter Sarah Thring and published by T. Fisher Unwin (1906).

[648] He copied out the programme in full into his diary.

[649] This was a machine often used to make duplicate copies using stencils.

[650] Latin: 'I say it mself'.

three others went with him upstairs to play 'nap'. After supper had been served the dancing resumed, but Reginald was too embarrassed to join in. Watching from the side he thought that a 'good part of those who did dance knew no more about it than I did'. The evening wore on with Reginald sitting on the side lines and he did not get home until 2.00am, feeling that 'I have made myself an awful ass'. Wanting the earth to swallow him up through embarrassment, this was a painful experience, especially as other young people in the gathering had enjoyed themselves.

Dancing was, for the young in St Ives, an activity which occurred at Christmas when families invited one another to their homes for parlour games, musical evenings and dancing. For adults, there were of course public balls held during the year for special occasions for charity or military celebrations. There were also public balls held in places like Assembly Rooms in large cities, and entrance was by paid ticket. There is no mention in his diaries that his parents went to anything similar.

The usual form of etiquette at a dance was for a gentleman to ask a lady for a dance and for her to record his invitation on the programme handed to each guest. The behaviour required by middle- and upper-class society at balls was detailed in publications like Hogg's *Habits of Good Society*.[651] This publication dealt with balls,[652] rather than small, private dances, but the general principles of genteel behaviour applied to both.

His mother, understanding his gaucheness, arranged dancing lessons for him during the Christmas holidays of 1886, with a Mrs Barley managing to rent two rooms in No 6 Cromwell Terrace next to Slepe House. One room upstairs was used for dancing, and the other on the ground floor for sitting during a break. There was a large group of 24 young people assembled, all eager to mix with one another. Apart from the fun of dancing and holding each other in their arms, a dance was an accepted way for young people to meet together in a chaperoned environment.

The first dance he was taught was the Valse step,[653] and the lesson was gruelling, beginning at 4.30pm and finishing at 9.00. 'It was', he felt, a 'very jolly evening indeed if it was not for the horrid Valse'. This dance is generally accepted as being an easy step for beginners to learn, so Reginald

[651] *Habits of Good Society: A handbook of Etiquette* (James Hogg and Sons, London, 1859).

[652] The chapter on balls began: 'Balls are the paradise of daughters, the purgatory of chaperons and the pandemonium of paterfamilias'! *Habits of Good Society* p. 330.

[653] This is the French term for a waltz.

was just expressing the difficulty of learning anything new – especially involving co-ordination and balance. After Christmas he spent some days in Cambridge sitting examinations for a scholarship, and his next lesson was on his return. He came back by train just after 4.00pm and had to change immediately for the dancing lesson at No 6 next door. He found a lot of young people from St Ives' middle-class families there whom he knew – the Warrens, Goodmans and the Battcocks. Despite finding the Valse difficult to master he had a very 'jolly evening'. This was even after Mrs Barley had been 'kind enough to tell me I was a "Muff"'. Nevertheless, he was extremely glad his mother was arranging the lessons, as he knew it was for his benefit and he got the chance to draw close to young ladies, even though he had 'two left feet'.

He practised dancing the waltz (as he then described it, rather than the Valse) with his sister Mabel and felt that he had made 'great improvements', as he wanted to surprise Mrs Barley the next day, just before his 18th birthday on 13 January. His determination paid off as he had an 'awfully jolly evening of it, really far and away the best we had had'. His sweetheart Mary had arrived earlier to stay a few days so he was able to dance with her as many times as they could both arrange. He felt by now that he could also dance with other 'certain' partners as his confidence grew. The group that evening was a large one – 24 young people enlarged by a fairly large number brought by Mrs Goodman. Mrs Barley did not come down to where the dancing was being held, as the numbers were too overwhelming for her, but her daughter, Miss Barley and a Miss Parkhurst came and 'helped us splendidly'.

His last dancing lesson of the holiday was the following week and he 'had a very successful evening'; he was clearly getting the hang of dancing the waltz at least, and after starting at 5.00pm the dancers kept going until 9.00. Despite his initial fears he enthused that 'instead of disliking dancing I now enjoy it very much'. He hoped that his mother would arrange more classes next year during the Christmas holidays. It was snowing when they finished, but as it was only a few steps to his house it was no hardship. Escorting his sister Mabel and also Mary back to Slepe House as the snowflakes fell silently was rather romantic.

The final dance of the holidays came the next evening when the Warren family held a soirée and he, Mabel, Mary and his mother went round to their grand house a short walk away. His father came along soon after. The Warrens' dining room made an excellent place to dance. The guests were given pretty dance programmes to use to arrange dances with partners. He chose those who could not dance very well and stayed with the waltzes, rather than other dances he did not know the steps to. He danced twice with Mary, which was a delight for them both, and he thought he only sat out five dances. The last dance of the evening he danced with his sister Mabel. Although he wrote in his diary that Mary had promised it to him, it did not seem to upset him. He got to bed about 1 in the morning. It was the end of the holidays.

CHRISTMAS TIME

During his years at King's College Choir School, Christmas was spent at school as the choristers had to sing on Christmas Day itself. For the boys it was a sad time being separated from their families. Besides being a Christian festival of joy, it was a time for family get-togethers, the more so as the century progressed and the 'Victorian Christmas' became more established. However, the Headmaster and other staff made stalwart efforts to compensate for being away from home.

Reginald described going skating in the morning and then decking out the Christmas tree on Christmas Eve at school in 1881 when was 12. On Christmas morning the choir sang in the chapel, that year the anthem being 'Hear O Thou Shepherd' by Handel. His Christmas cards arrived on Christmas Day itself, so deliveries were made then, unlike today. On Boxing Day the boys had their Christmas dinner in the evening at 7.00. The Christmas tree was up and each boy received some presents from it. The boys were allowed home on 28 December after Chapel. The festivities at home had been sadly missed.

The next year, some of the boys went out carol-singing to a few houses nearby and Reginald got 3s 3d (£37.86), which was a large sum for their efforts. His diary is not clear whether this was the total received and split among the boys, or Reginald's share. His parents sent him a Christmas hamper which must have been very welcome, and the other boys received them from home, too.

Christmas Eve fell on a Sunday and the choir practised both before and after the morning service; some Christmas cards were delivered to him afterwards. On Christmas Day there was another practice before the morning service, and Reginald sang a solo as well as a verse from the Creed. Another practice was held after the afternoon service. This year there did not seem to be a Christmas dinner, although in the evening the boys all went to Austen Leigh's, the Vice Provost, for tea and they then played parlour games, 'post' and 'charades'. Reginald received a 'splendid' book from Leigh. The boys went home on Boxing Day.

Once Reginald went to Uppingham he was always at home for Christmas. From other descriptions of Christmas, like in Molly Hughes' account mentioned earlier, the Christmas excitement built up in a similar way to today. The main difference was that no preparations were made until a week before Christmas Day itself, apart from buying cards. Reginald described going into Cambridge ten days before Christmas Day in 1882 to buy them. The excitement, especially for the children, was packed into a short space of time. There was lots of home cooking to cater for both the family itself, as well as guests, and a variety of puddings were prepared. Preparation in the week before also involved an annual play, with the plot often written by a family member.

On Christmas Eve there were last-minute rehearsals in the morning, posting cards and dashing to the shops to buy presents. Christmas Eve in 1885 meant decorating the house, and in the evening playing games; one of his cousins, Hansie Gosling, had come to stay and they played a game called 'laps'. Reginald lost 6d (£3.12) of his father's money.

In other families, the head of the family generally came home early, although Dr Grove was always on duty for emergency calls to visit patients. For the rest of the family, sweet biscuits, sweets and surprise cakes with icing on the top and threepenny bits inside began the festivities. In the evening the family play was performed with two rows of chairs in the front, acting as the stalls where mother and father sat, together with any aunt who might be staying, or family friends. According to Molly Hughes, at the back sat the servants 'who attended with much gigglement'. After the play had finished, the family progressed to the parlour where Mother had arranged all the presents – 'a little pile for each and we all fell upon them with delight', remembered Hughes. In her family there were no Christmas trees, stockings or Santa Claus, but this was unusual. At Slepe House in 1886 Reginald received a variety of gifts which he listed in his diary: a silk handkerchief from his mother, and a diamond pin belonging to his Grandfather Grove who had died in 1841. His grandmother had died a few months earlier so the pin must have been left to him in her will. He also received a terracotta ornament from his sweetheart, Mary, and a bracelet from his Uncle Frank. This was a rather strange gift and he gave no explanation – perhaps it belonged to his grandmother. This was the only occasion that Reginald listed what he received as Christmas presents. Birthdays seemed to be more important, as he always wrote down what he had been given.

Before opening their presents, the family went to church for Holy Communion at the 8.00am service. Christmas cards were opened on their return – on this occasion he had three cards, one of which was from his friend George Lloyd who was studying medicine, Miss Eliot from Redgate, and Dr Guillemard, one of his father's previous Medical Assistants. He mentioned that this year he seemed to be the only one in the family who had sent out any cards, so this practice must have been rather sporadic.

With ice on the flooded meadows by the river, the younger ones in the family went off for some skating, although the ice was in a poor condition.

For most middle-class families, Christmas dinner was turkey and plum pudding. On Christmas Day 1886 there were 13 at dinner, including three single gentlemen, Revd Paget, Mr Whitins and Mr Pollock. They sat down for their meal at 5.00pm but many families ate earlier; in fact, the year before they ate an hour earlier. After eating, most of the adults dozed off while the children played with their new toys. Later chestnuts were often roasted on the bars of the grate. In the evening punch was made by the head of the household with loaf sugar, lemons, and a large jug of water boiled in a kettle on the fire. A tumbler full of brandy and rum was then added to make a hot drink for all the adults.[654]

Parlour games then followed for the rest of the evening. On Christmas Day 1886 they 'had very good games till 12.00'. The following day, Boxing Day, a few more Christmas cards came and he had a letter from his friend Bensly from Algiers. It was a Sunday so Reginald went to both morning and evening services.

---

[654] Hughes, Molly, *A Victorian Family: 1870–1900* (Guild Publishing, 1990), p. 31.

CHAPTER 13

Hobbies and Interests

'It is too much to expect too many fellows in the School to become collectors, but I hope that some few, who do not play cricket for some reason or other may, this term, and others in the holidays, at least try to rub one brass.'[655]

Reginald Grove, 'Monumental Brasses', Uppingham School Magazine, 1887

STAMP COLLECTING

Like many boys, Reginald enjoyed collecting stamps which had become widespread as a hobby in the period before he was born. The postal service had been improved and standardised in the 1840s and became widely used as the railway network enabled mail to be delivered quickly across the country. In 1854 stamps became perforated; before this, they had had to be cut individually from the sheet with scissors. These two factors resulted in used stamps being collected, growing as a popular pastime among the middle classes. In April 1882, when he was 13, he mentioned that a new stamp book had arrived; this meant that he must have begun his hobby some time before this. Friends of the family and his Uncle Frank helped build up his collection. He mentioned that a Mrs Wright had brought him some stamps at home in a break from school in June 1882. There was someone who lived in the village of Holywell with whom he exchanged stamps – he mentioned riding over in the June holiday of 1882 with 'Mr Thorpe', who was probably another of his father's Medical Assistants. He also swopped stamps by post with boys from school during the holidays.

It was a hobby that he could lose himself in at King's when, with no lessons, the weather stopped playing outside; he did this one Tuesday afternoon in July 1882. Or if all the boys had detention for some misdemeanour where they all had to stay in, then working on his stamp collection was a good way to spend the time. On another rainy afternoon later in the year when he looked through his albums he mentioned that his stamp collection now numbered 1,078. Two months later he wrote in his

[655] Uppingham School Magazine 06.06.87.

diary about another stamp book arriving. It was a hobby that continued when he went to Uppingham and his collection grew. He subscribed to *Stamp News* regularly, which was posted to him from home, and when he was 15 he wrote to a stamp dealer about buying some for his collection. He had used a stamp dealer before when he was at King's. Whether he received any at Uppingham is not recorded, but he received sheets of stamps from his mother, sometimes, when she forwarded *Stamp News* to him from home. His interest in collecting continued until his last year at school, encouraged by his Uncle Frank. In the Christmas holidays of 1886, his uncle gave Reginald a 'lot of stamps' that he had not got. What happened to his collection after he left school is not known.

AUTOGRAPH COLLECTING

Uncle Frank encouraged him to collect autographs, and when Reginald had just turned 16 sent him some at Uppingham – how many and of whom was not recorded. In his letter his uncle thought 'some were quite interesting'. The letter survived but the autographs, sadly, did not. Collecting the signatures of well-known personalities dated back to antiquity, but in the mid-19th century the hobby was so popular that auction houses held sales of them. Reginald's diaries made no further mention, so to what extent he pursued this hobby is unclear.

CARTOON COLLECTING

One other collecting hobby he had was obtaining cartoon illustrations by an artist called John Leech from the magazine *Punch*.[656] This was a humorous magazine aimed at the middle classes which combined pieces of political satire on topical matters with drawings and pictures. Before Reginald had been born, Leech had become well known for his cartoons on the Crimean War, and he helped shape public attitudes to the conflict. We only know that Reginald had a collection of Leech's cartoons because just after his 18th birthday before he left to travel back to school, he found eight had somehow gone missing at home. He had brought them down from his bedroom to show his sweetheart Mary at the weekend, but despite hunting everywhere for them, they were nowhere to be found.

The following day he said goodbye to his family before catching the

[656] *Punch* or *The London Charivari* was first published in 1841 on a weekly basis, and reached its peak readership in the 1940s. It ceased publication in 2002.

train back to school. He put the loss out of his mind but was delighted to hear from his mother a few weeks later that the pictures had been found – in the cabinet in the drawing room where they had looked before. He found it strange but felt there was 'no use making a row about them'. Maybe he felt someone in the house, a servant or a sibling, had stolen them and then put them back. They had been found with some 'lucky farthings I [had] lost' … 'carefully wrapped up in paper'. The two finds were clearly linked, but Reginald was just glad to know that he had got them back.

BRASS RUBBINGS

During his last two terms at Uppingham Reginald became very enthused about brass rubbings. He did his first brass rubbing when he was 15 in a church in Westley Waterless[657] near Cambridge in January 1884, but his interest was awakened by the new curate at All Saints Parish Church, St Ives, who was appointed in 1886.[658] In a passing conversation he learnt that Revd Leonard Pollock had 'used to go for rubbing brasses', and showed him some 'splendid ones he had done'. Pollock had been at St John's College, Cambridge, from 1880 to 1884. One of his friends there was Revd Herbert Macklin,[659] who also shared an interest in this hobby.[660] The conversation prompted Reginald to think about 'going in for it again'. He must have been interested previously, although his diaries do not show this. He had a further chat with Pollock about brass rubbing just before going back to school. Pollock promised to contact his friend Macklin to help Reginald.

The work involved reproducing onto rolls of paper impressions of monumental brasses found in old churches, usually on the floor but sometimes on a wall. These had been made originally to commemorate a well-off knight or wealthy merchant, and sometimes their wives between the 13th and 16th centuries.[661] The image of each brass was transferred

---

657 The church contains a brass from 1324 commemorating Sir John de Creke and his first wife Alyne Clopton.

658 Pollock remained curate until 1892.

659 Macklin joined St John's in Pollock's final year, but the age difference was no barrier to their friendship and shared interest in brass rubbing. Macklin became rector of Houghton Conquest in Bedfordshire from 1897 until his early death from TB in 1917, aged 51.

660 Venn, J., *Alumni Cantabrigienses: a biographical list of all known students* Volume 2 Part 5 (1953 edition).

661 Because the rubbing process wears the brass image down gradually over time, in many churches rubbings are not allowed today.

onto large pieces of paper using black wax or graphite, like a pencil. He described this process in greater detail in the article he wrote for the School Magazine in June 1887 (see Appendix 4).

For the next seven months brass rubbing was a hobby that he entered into with great enthusiasm.

Back at school in January Reginald walked with Berry the two miles to the village of Lyddington to rub some brasses in the church – St Andrew's. The oldest parts of the church are 15th-century, but as the church underwent alterations in 1890 it is different now from when Reginald and Berry went there. He took copies of a woman, and then of a man, woman and their children. He said that the brasses were very old. The next month he described going on his own to the small village church at Stockerston a few miles outside Uppingham. This was St Peter's Church which dated from the 13th century. He took two rubbings. His interest was also stimulated during the many walks he took with his friend Berry with whom he walked to Huntingdon at the end of the Easter Term. Passing through villages during their training, they often stopped to look at the local church. This was not the first visit to St Peter's, as he noticed the old pews had been replaced with ones made from deal, and the interior looked 'very much less than a stable although still very damp and in some corners very dirty'. On this occasion he had 'an awful business to get at the brasses', as he had to move an old chest with some other things in order to get at them and then use his duster to get a clean image. The brasses were of a knight in armour and his lady. Sadly, the knight's head had gone, as had one of her hands. There were two other brasses but these were half-hidden under a more modern tomb. He thought the brasses were from the late-15th century and was correct.[662]

After their chat in the school holidays Pollock was as good as his word and Macklin wrote to Reginald at the beginning of March about the brasses that could be found around Uppingham. He wrote again to Reginald to

[662] The brasses were those of Sir John de Boyville and his wife Isabella Cheiney. De Boyville built the tower and south chantry chapel. He also founded a hospital with an income of £10.00 a year for a chaplain to care for those in poverty. He died in 1467. The other brass depicts part of a man in praying position, together with the skirt of a woman. These figures are of John Southill and his wife Elizabeth Plompton. Southill died in 1493. (http://www.sixsaintscircaholt.org/HTML/Stockerston_History.htm 20.08.2019.)

encourage him in their shared interest. Macklin[663] was a great enthusiast, became an expert on antiquities, and was a founding member and later the Honorary Secretary and President of the Monumental Brass Society.[664] Reginald was later to meet up with him in Cambridge and in 1890 went on a day trip by cycle to take brass rubbings described in Volume 3. Reginald also became a founding member of Cambridge University Association of Brass Collectors. Macklin published *Brasses of England*, which became the standard reference of its time. Virtually all those churches which he told Reginald about were ones that Reginald had visited. There were only two he had not taken rubbings of – in villages eight and 15 miles away.

Reginald and Berry showed their brass rubbings to their Housemaster's wife. She was 'charmed' with them and immediately wrote to Headmaster Thring to invite him to tea the following day to see them. Thring was due to go to Cambridge to give a lecture so was not able to see them until his return. Before this was arranged, Reginald went to see Thring in the School Room and asked him, if it was fine, if he could in two days' time miss dinner (lunch) and at noon go to Braunston to take brass rubbings. Thring was apparently 'awfully jolly about it' and said that 'it was against his rule and custom but I was in the Upper Sixth so he himself would ask me out to go and take a brass at Braunston'. It was a clever way of justifying his request. Maybe Thring was impressed by Macklin's encouragement of Reginald, or Mrs Christian's letter had impressed him, but the result was that Thring gave him special leave.

His friend Berry got permission, too, and two days later they took an hour and a half for the five and half-mile journey. They took two rubbings at All Saints Church at Braunston, with one having an inscription and the man's coat of arms. Hoping to speak to the vicar, they knocked on his door but found he was out. Not deterred from looking for more brasses, they went into St Peter's Brook on the way back ('the nicest little village church I have seen round here')[665] and then across the fields to Manton

[663] https://familytreemacklin.wordpress.com/2017/07/23/rev-herbert-walter-macklin-1866-1917/ (20.08.19).

[664] The society was founded in 1887 by a group of Cambridge undergraduates, including Reginald, who were keen to preserve and record monumental brasses. Initially it was known as the Cambridge University Association of Brass Collectors. Later it was renamed the Monumental Brass Society. (https://www.mbs-brasses.co.uk/ (20.08.19).)

[665] The church is a quintessential English one and was used in the film adaptation of *Pride and Prejudice* in 2005.

where they found three brass inscriptions at St Mary's Church. Because the 13th-century church was being restored they were not able to take any rubbings.

On returning, they shared what they had taken with Revd Christian and his wife who were very pleased with them. Afterwards word spread to the boys in the house and they 'had to show them ever so many times to different knots of fellows in the house who were really interested in them and there wasn't the slightest bit of hustle'. A few days later at teatime he and Berry went into his Housemaster's drawing room where Thring, Skrine and Howson had assembled to see the brasses. They had clearly caused a stir. This was a creative hobby, new to the school, and Thring was interested, as it aligned with his educational beliefs of encouraging boys to explore the world around them. 'They were all, especially Thring, very pleased with the brasses'. As a result, Thring gave Reginald permission to go with the Archaeological Society to Stamford to visit Little Casterton to brass rub at the beginning of April. He thought they would have elected him a full member, but the society was already full.

Word spread to another master, Charles Rossiter (Art Master 1873–97), who was also interested from an artistic viewpoint. Thring suggested that Reginald borrow a book on foreign brasses from him, which Reginald did soon after. He enjoyed the book, as the brasses illustrated were of very good quality, although he was disappointed that no English ones were included. Rossiter invited Reginald round to show him some rubbings. Rossiter was aware of the technique and showed him some old rubbings which were in very bad condition in the small museum in the Old School Room. His interest in Reginald's was because of the quality of their reproduction and because they came from villages around Uppingham.

His trip to Stamford and Little Casterton took place at the beginning of April on a Saturday, with Thring having given him permission to leave after first school. Leaving at 11.15am he took the bus to Seaton then caught a train to Stamford. Although he did not mention it, he walked the two miles north to Little Casterton and got there just before 1.30pm. Little Casterton was then, and still is, a small hamlet.[666] All Saints Church has some beautiful carved roof bosses, but Reginald had his eyes on the

[666] The hamlet is very near to the county border of Lincolnshire. Most of the church dates from the 13th century and consists of a nave, north and south aisles (1250 and 1280, respectively), chancel, south porch and an unusual tower which was added later by building it within the nave, but more on that later.

brasses only and was delighted by the 'splendid' one that he took, making two copies. He walked back to Stamford before 4.00 and went to the parish church there, also dedicated to All Saints, to take more rubbings. He tried to take a rubbing from one on a wall which was not a particularly good specimen; when a better one was seen, he did not have time to take a rubbing, as a service was about to start. It was not a saint's day, but the eve of Palm Sunday, so there may have been a special service as a result.

At Stamford railway station he came across some members of the Archaeological Society and he travelled back with them. Haslam, one of the masters, gave him a lift back in his trap. Getting back to Redgate, Mrs Christian asked him to join her and her husband so she could hear all about his visit. He gave her one of the extra copies of the Little Casterton brass to give to the Archaeological Society which delighted her.[667] The following day, Palm Sunday, he was excited to hear that Thring had accepted his brass from Little Casterton. It was something to chat to the boys in the house in the evening, and to show them the copy he had kept. He mounted the brass later on canvas, and took it to Thring a couple of days later for the Archaeological Society.

He and Berry walked eight miles before the end of term, to visit St Peter's Church at Deene, just over the border in Northamptonshire; the church was in the estate of the Brudenell family who owned Deene Park House. He was interested that there was a monument to the Earl of Cardigan, who led the Charge of the Light Brigade, and his wife. He was buried in the family vault in the church. Cardigan had died in 1868 but his widow, his second wife, who was much younger than him, was still alive and the Vicar told him 'very much flattered' by the depiction of her which 'lies in a most tremendously affected attitude'! He managed only to take one brass – a mural one – as a service interrupted his work. They walked home at a 'tremendous pace' as they had misjudged the time, but got back a quarter of an hour late for call-over.

This meant reporting to Thring the next day. Thring was cross with them and refused them any more special leave that term. As there were only a few days before the end of term it was no great hardship. At the beginning of the Summer Term he returned to Deene, this time with another friend, Evans. They were grateful that they took two umbrellas as it poured with rain on their way there and they would have been drenched

[667] https://en.wikipedia.org/wiki/St_Peter 27s_Church,_Deene (02.04.87).

without them. This was a more fruitful visit as the brass he took was, in his view, 'the best rubbing I have ever taken'. He did it very carefully, and made a difference in the shades of black. Evans took another rubbing and drew two sketches of the church which he gave Reginald later. Two hours after they arrived, the Vicar, Revd Sylvester, invited them into his home and gave them sherry and biscuits. He 'sent us on our way rejoicing'! He got back on this occasion for call-over and that evening showed Mrs Christian his rubbing. She was 'tremendously pleased'.

During the Easter holidays his enthusiasm for his new hobby continued. He met up with Revd Pollock and they talked further about taking brasses and made plans to go together on a trip locally; he also bought a book about brasses on a visit to Cambridge, probably the one he used when writing his article the next term for the School Magazine. A paper that he wrote on the brass at Casterton for the Archaeological Society was finalised, and he mounted some of his rubbings. The next day he received a fine copy of a brass from the church in Trumpington. This was given to him by a gentleman called Streeten with whom he had got into a conversation at the end of returning by train from a visit to Cambridge. Pollock continued to offer him advice and generously gave him a special case for carrying his paper for rubbings on expeditions to churches. This proved invaluable on a three-day visit to his Uncle Dan and Aunt Sarah soon after.

He took the train from St Ives to Cambridge and then continued a further eight miles to the village of Linton. Getting off at this station, be began his brass rubbing expedition by walking a couple of miles to Hildersham, a small hamlet on the River Granta. He met the vicar who said all the brasses were covered up, due to renovations, and so he walked east along country tracks for five more miles to another hamlet called Horseheath. He was more fortunate there as he found two brasses, one of them 'a good knight in armour' of which he took two good copies. The vicar took pity on him and suggested giving him a lift in his trap back to Linton, but Reginald did not think he could finish anything there in time. But he was delighted with the offer of a glass of beer and some biscuits and he 'sent me on my way rejoicing'.

It was not the first time he had gone on his way rejoicing!

By a strange chance on the way back to Linton he met up with a boy from Rugby School called Lowe who was 'on the tramp round the place alone'. They walked together for a while chatting until Lowe turned off to Baldock. Despite what he'd said to the vicar he arrived in time to take another rubbing of a small knight. But by this time, he'd walked 12 miles and with his boots being rather tight, found that the skin had been taken off the top of one foot. He limped along slowly another seven miles to the town of Haverhill, as he'd planned to meet up with his relatives, getting there at 2.30pm. It was a welcome relief to rest his blistered foot and travel by trap to his Uncle Dan's farm at The Hall, Great Bradley.

He had a break from his hobby for a few days and then carried on with two of his cousins, Bessie and Ida Long, to a nearby village called Cowling to the medieval church of St Mary of Antioch, but 'it was not up to much', so they returned without further ado for lunch, having walked four miles there and four back. His feet were still painful so he did some 'doctoring', and after they had eaten they went out again in the farm trap to Little Bradley with another cousin, Lorrie, to the small parish church, one of a few in Suffolk which had a round tower. He found five brasses and took a copy of one of the easiest to rub, which was on the floor. They got back in time for dinner and then another drive to Carleton to visit more Long relatives and family friends and play parlour games afterwards.

The next day his uncle lent him a pony and trap, gave him a 'splendid' packed lunch, and he drove to Balsham which was eight miles away. Holy Trinity Church had two brasses, one a 'very fine' one that he rubbed. The church had a number of 15th-century brasses, two of which were former Rectors, John Sleford (d.1401) and John Blodwell (d.1462), The third, that of an unidentified knight (c.1480s), was described by Reginald as 'a small battered knight'. Having spent four and a half hours at the church, he got back to his uncle after another four-hour journey at 6.00pm.

On the morning of his last day, he walked with his aunt to Little Bradley Church, All Saints.[668] It was another round-towered Suffolk church, with no less than five brasses. Reginald took the one that was well known, mounted

[668] This church became notorious as the vicar, in the 1851 National Census of Religious Worship grossly falsified the returns. Some Anglican ministers wanted nothing to do with the Census, fearing comparisons being made with local non-conformist chapels. The vicar at Little Bradley was one of them and it was the parish clerk who gave the return to the registrar who appeared to have filled in the return himself, putting the congregation down as 200 on average each Sunday over a three-month period. As there were only 35 people in the whole parish the Census figures were completely bogus.

on the wall in memory of John Daye, a printer.[669] That afternoon he went home by train via Cambridge, again having had an 'awfully jolly week', and promising his Aunt Dan and Aunt Lawsell that he would be back at his next holiday in the summer. As he stopped writing his diary at the end of the Summer Term, there is no way of knowing whether he did or not.

Reginald was finally elected a member of the Archaeological Society towards the end of May. There was a Leicestershire Archaeological Society which had been formed in 1855, and later in May it met at the house of Skrine and Reginald attended his first meeting, when a paper on Crowland Abbey, by a boy called Fisher, was read. He was a little disappointed that his article was not read, but he was able to show those who came some of his brasses and 'everybody seemed very pleased with them'.

More expeditions were carried out to take more rubbings further afield. He was given permission to travel by train to Coventry to take copies at the Church of St John the Baptist in the little village of Babington which was four miles south of the city centre. There was a party of 13 that met at Seaton station to go to Coventry, but Reginald had been tipped off by his mentor Macklin that the brasses at Coventry were not very good and so he got permission from 'the Old Man' (Thring) to travel to Babington.

The rail journey took just under four hours and he walked to the village. The brass he wanted was on a wall eight to ten feet from the ground so he borrowed two ladders from the rectory to get up there! He was rather frustrated as once he got close he found that the lines had 'comparatively recently been filled in with some black substance and part coloured red'. This did not allow him to show the lines clearly but, that said, he felt that he had 'managed to get a fair rubbing of a splendid brass'. As he finished, the curate turned up and showed him around the church which was rather unusual in design – 'old oak and other things' with a yew tree which was growing out of one of the buttresses in the chancel. The curate then showed him the ruins of an old castle nearby – Babington Castle, which was actually a 14th-century manor house. Getting back to the station by 4.00pm he was early for the train so wasted some time in the town before

---

[669] This was John Daye (Reginald spelt the name incorrectly) who was a Puritan printer who lived in Great Bradley in the 16th century. He was renowned for printing *Foxe's Book of Martyrs* in 1563. Compiled by John Foxe, this rather grisly account of those who had been put to death as Protestants during the reign of Mary I (1553–58) was placed in every Church of England church alongside the Bible during Elizabeth I's reign. The inscription on the brass reads: 'heere lies the Daye that darkness could not blynd when popish fogges had over cast the sunne'.

catching a train to Rugby where he bought a cup of tea and a bun, as he had not eaten since breakfast and was 'awfully hungry'. He got back by 6.30 and discovered the others who had gone had enjoyed themselves. Mrs Christian, who seemed to have taken a shine to Reginald and his hobby, was duly impressed with his rubbing when he showed her.

The following months saw him go on more trips to collect brasses encouraged by Mrs Christian. She invited him to travel with her to Stamford one Saturday in July to carry out some more rubbings which he thought was 'very kind and thoughtful' and he jumped at the chance. Accordingly, two days after her invitation, they went to Stamford from Seaton station after lunch accompanied by his friend Evans, a Miss Wilkinson, a 'German school fellow of hers' and Mrs Christian of course. The station was crowded with masters and boys going to a tennis match. The others in his party went off to Burleigh House[670] for a visit, leaving him at All Saints Church. He took two brasses, a large one of a man and a woman, and another small one of a girl – both he reckoned about 1480. The others met him in the church at 6.00pm and they all got back safely by 7.30 and enjoyed dinner together.

His last trip was near the end of term when he made another visit to St Peter's Church, Stockerston, with Evans and Compton. A brass had been uncovered recently – a knight dated 1467 – which Reginald described as 'fairly good and curious'. This was because the knight depicted was headless. He was John de Boyville, the Lord of Stockerston, and was shown in armour who died, having possibly fought in the Wars of the Roses. His wife, Isabella Cheiney, was by his side. It was the last time that Reginald recorded taking a brass in his schoolboy diaries.

What could have resulted in others at school being enthused by his hobby turned out to be rather a flop. An article about brasses which he wrote in the June 1887 edition of the School Magazine was not a success. There was a scare before publication as he and Berry found they had 28 pages too many for the edition, as there were more articles submitted than could be printed. Reginald wrote that he 'nearly had to leave my brasses out as we are so crowded: it is as I am afraid, we shall mortally offend one of the masters by leaving a thing out which really he ought to have given us last term'.

---

[670] This stately home one mile outside Stamford was built in the reign of Elizabeth I and was the home of the Cecil family. It has been owned within the same family for 16 generations. While it is open to the public now, it appears that it was also open on occasion for visitors in the 1880s.

Additionally, the printer, Hawthorn's, had lost some of the copy before going to print. Thankfully, the lost copy was found and it was agreed that this issue should be a bumper Jubilee issue for The Queen's Jubilee celebration that month. It was also the last edition that he helped edit and produce. He had hoped it would be a success, and Berry, in reading the draft, thought it was very good; Reginald 'rather doubted its success with masters and fellows, from the latter I am trying to get recruits for rubbing'. He was the first to admit that the readers did not think much of it: 'I am afraid my paper has not taken, most of the fellows seem to think it awful rot'.

While the contents were factual, it was ponderous and academic in style (see Appendix 4). Quite possibly it was based on an article for the Archaeological Society which the rather dry content was more suited to; in any event, it is probable that much of it was copied from another publication as this excerpt betrays:

> They are most useful and interesting to us for the costumes of ladies, the vestments of ecclesiastics, and the various parts of the armour and dress of the men during the four centuries of a most exciting part of English History. In addition to the great variety of costume, many curious customs and usages of those times are directly or indirectly very often illustrated.

His mentor, Macklin, wrote a book called *Monumental Brasses* three years later in 1890.[671] The style of the book was similar to that used by Reginald, so it is highly likely that he used notes sent by Macklin to help his young protégé. Sadly, Reginald's article lacked the personal touch that his earlier article in the February edition displayed, and its reception by the school readership was unenthusiastic.

PETS

Besides the family dog called Charlie, the only pet that Reginald had was a jackdaw that he bought at Uppingham the day before the end of the Summer Term when he was 17. It cost him 2s 15 (£17.80), which included the cage to take it back on the train to St Ives. Travelling back with him was his father and his old Headmaster, Reynell, from King's who had come up for the prize-giving. With his trunk, the cage was put in the guard's van. The bird must have been trapped by a local farmhand and then sold in one

---

[671] https://archive.org/stream/macklinmonumenta00mack/macklinmonumenta00mack_djvu.txt (21.08.19).

of the town shops. Reginald made no further mention of it in his diaries. Keeping caged birds was quite popular at the time; Thring built an aviary at School House. He described it in a letter to his brother Godfrey:

> You would be immensely pleased with our aviary in the school gardens, a bank enclosed for thirty feet by twenty in fine wire...with plants and grass and bushes and a large aquarium in it. The birds are so tame and interesting: the siskins run up and down...and curious to relate, I believe, we are the only people in the world who know the habits of the common blackbird and one of its notes. We have linnets, redpoles, greenfinches, a robin, sparrows, hedge sparrows, bullfinch, goldfinch, two Australian parquets, blackbirds, thrushes, siskins, and a plover, and it is very interesting watching them, especially now they are beginning to sing.[672]

At the horticultural shows held in the summer holidays in St Ives, birds were exhibited besides fruit and vegetables. The 1883 show had over 500 exhibits, including singing birds such as canaries, goldfinches, bullfinches, linnets, blackbirds and thrushes.

Reginald's jackdaw was not, of course, a songbird. But jackdaws were often kept as pets, responding to humans and recognising human faces and making eye contact with them.

PHOTOGRAPHY

Apart from mentioning portrait photographs that he had taken of himself to send his sweetheart Mary previously mentioned, as well as some photographs taken by a friend his study at Uppingham, photography was not one of his hobbies as a boy. However, in later life Reginald became an enthusiastic photographer with a special interest in stereoscopics which were an early version of 3D images. He became a leading figure in the Stereoscopic Society. This hobby is explored in Volume 3.

[672] Richardson, Nigel, *Thring of Uppingham* (2014), p. 243.

CHAPTER 14

Reginald's Reading

'So, Frederick had to go to bed; His leg was very sore and red! The Doctor came and shook his head, and made a very great to-do, and gave him nasty physic too.'[673]

From the poem 'The Story of Cruel Frederick' by Dr Heinrich Hoffmann

EARLY YEARS

Handed down within the Grove family is a magazine dating from 1872 when Reginald was four, which was read by his parents. This was the *British Workman* publication which is described later in the chapter. On the back cover it gives a good idea of what books were read to Reginald as a child.

The magazine advertised a list of storybooks available for parents which all had a moral purpose for the child. There was *The Tiny Library,* for instance, a series of books printed in large type with 'numerous' illustrations with titles like *The Golden Rule, Grandpapa's Walking Stick* and *Richard Barton; or, The Wounded Bird.* For 1d (52p) a month there was *The Infants' Magazine* which was 'intended for the very Little Ones. Each No contains a Piece of Music for the Nursery.' The Children's Friend Series, which boasted coloured covers and many engravings, were priced at 1d (52p) and had titles such as *The Church Mouse, Dick and his Donkey* and *Ronald's Response, or the Little Cripple.* There were other stories with a moral flavour such as the *Illustrated Temperance Anecdotes Volume 1 and 2,* priced at 1s 6d, or *The Babes in the Basket (or Daph and Her Charges)* with 13 engravings selling at 2s 6d (£15.72). These were the sort of stories that Reginald was brought up on by his Christian parents.

Stories for children and young adults were shorter than those for adults earlier in the century. Initially, the cost of books was four or five shillings which meant that those from poorer homes could not afford them. Cheaper editions at 6d (£3.12) a copy[674] began to be printed that

[673] From *'Struwwelpeter'* or 'Shock-Headed Peter', 1845.

[674] For instance, W. H. G. Kingston's books were printed at this price (£3.12), as opposed to editions at 5s (£31.50).

broadened the readership.[675] There were other differences, too, with adult books, which were that children's stories began to have magic or fantasy as a basis. The most well-known of these are *Alice's Adventures in Wonderland* and its sequel, *Through the Looking-Glass* (1871), which were written by the clergyman, Revd Charles Dodgson, under the pseudonym of Lewis Carroll.[676] While he never mentioned reading it in his diaries, it was so popular after its publication in 1865, just four years before Reginald's birth, that it is inconceivable he did not read it or that it was not read to him.

An interesting new aspect about these books was that Alice, the heroine, was motivated by curiosity, which was not a quality necessarily encouraged by all parents.[677] Reginald's father, in drawing Reginald into the world of medicine and science in his medical practice when he was older, bucked this trend, as did Thring, his Headmaster at Uppingham.

Of course, fairy tales and the magic they portrayed had existed for some centuries, but these grew in popularity in the mid-19th century largely due to the stories written by Hans Christian Andersen which were translated into English in 1846, and the Brothers Grimm whose books were translated in 1823. Books were translated from all the major European languages and Victorian children heard Norse and Scandinavian tales as well as stories about Cossacks and pirates. Revd Charles Kingsley's *The Water Babies* (1863) was a popular book which would have formed part of Reginald's reading; with a Christian background, mixed with some science, it reinforced the values of corrective punishment to bring up a child.

George MacDonald, a Scottish Congregational Minister, and mentor to Dodgson,[678] wrote a number of fairy tales while Reginald was a child, like *At the Back of the North Wind* (1870), *The Princess and the Goblin* (1871)

---

[675] Musgrave, P. W., *From Brown to Bunter* (Routledge & Kegan Paul, 1985), p. 150.

[676] Charles Dodgson wrote under the pseudonym Lewis Carroll. The heroine called Alice falls through a rabbit hole into a fantasy world populated by strange creatures. *Alice's Adventures in Wonderland* (generally shortened to *Alice in Wonderland*) was written in 1865, four years before Reginald was born.

[677] Musgrave, p. 89.

[678] George MacDonald is considered by many to be the founding father of modern fantasy writing and was a strong influence in the 20th century on the Christian writers C. S. Lewis (*The Chronicle of Narnia*) and J. R. R Tolkien (*The Hobbit* and *The Lord of the Rings*). He also wrote a number of theological works. The Christian author Oswald Chambers wrote in his *Christian Disciplines* that 'it is a striking indication of the trend and shallowness of the modern reading public that George MacDonald's books have been so neglected', cited by Hein, Rolland, *George MacDonald: Victorian Mythmaker* (2014).

and its sequel, *The Princess and the Curdie* (1872), with the intention of showing children how to grow up to be good. The Groves' close friends, the Ulphs, who lived next door to Slepe House, were Congregationalists, so it is very likely that MacDonald's books were introduced by them.

Many of these fairy tales were rooted in the reality of Victorian life: in *The Water Babies*, the hero Tom is a chimney sweep, and *At the Back of the North Wind* takes place in working-class London. Other authors, like Hesba Stretton, in writing their novels for children, portrayed slum life in *Little Meg's Children* (1868), for instance. *In Prison and Out*, written by her in 1879, she told the story about two boys who were sent to prison for stealing food. Her publisher was the Religious Tract Society,[679] whose aim was to evangelise its readers.

Like other children of his generation, Reginald learnt about foreign countries and customs. James Fenimore Cooper's tales from North America, such as *The Last of the Mohicans* (1826), and *Uncle Tom's Cabin* by Harriet Beecher Stowe (1852) gave boys looking for adventure an insight into life in America.[680]

BOOKS FOR BOYS

Young people's literature generally was designed to inspire heroism, especially for boys. The story of *Jackanapes* (1884) by Mrs Julia (Juliana) Ewing,[681] a close friend of Edward Thring's, is a good example. First published in *Aunt Judy's Magazine*, it was later issued as a slim book priced at 1/- (£6.30) in its own right, illustrated by the well-known artist Randolph Caldecott. Apparently based on the account of the death of the young French Prince Imperial during the Zulu War of 1879, the story portrays the death of the hero, nicknamed Jackanapes, as a result of his self-sacrifice in saving his friend's life in battle. Both were Cavalry officers.

'*Leave you?* To save my skin? No, Tony, not to save my soul!' cried brave

[679] The Religious Tract Society was founded 1799 with the aim of publishing the Christian message through literature aimed particularly at children, women and the poor.

[680] Walvin, James, *A Child's World: A Social History of English Childhood 1800–1914* (Penguin, 1962), p. 126.

[681] Julia Ewing wrote for *Aunt Judy's Magazine* (1866–82), a popular family publication which Thring loved for his children. He was enthralled by her portrayal of happy family life and her idealisation of rural life. Thring wrote to her frequently as he appreciated her books for young readers, as they displayed a strong Christian faith and her stories inspired heroism. He visited her for the first time in May 1885 shortly before her untimely death aged 43. (Thring's diary, 7 May 1885.)

Jackanapes, who brought his wounded friend and their horses back to headquarters but was himself mortally wounded in the process. Asked by his commanding officer if he could do anything for him, Jackanapes's final wish was for him to 'Say a prayer by me. Out loud, please':

> Pressed by the conviction that what little he could do it was his duty to do it, the Major—kneeling—bared his head, and spoke loudly, clearly and very reverently—
> 'The Grace of our Lord Jesus Christ—'
> Jackanapes moved his left hand to his right one, which still held the Major's—
> '—The love of GOD.'
> And with that—Jackanapes died.[682]

Thring was so taken by the story that he insisted that 50 copies were ordered and displayed prominently in Hawthorn's, the printer and bookseller in the High Street. In writing to Ewing, he told the whole school that if he 'had the power I would make every man jack of them buy Jackanapes a copy'![683] Thring would have been pleased to know that Reginald had bought one of the copies, which he passed on to his daughter Jane.[684]

Reginald's Grandmother Grove gave him a copy of *Tom Brown's School Days* by Thomas Hughes (1857) for his 14th birthday and this, no doubt, was a preparation for him going to Uppingham nine months later. This was the first boys' school story written, and others followed later as more boys began to be sent to boarding schools by middle-class parents.

W. H. G. Kingston became well known as an adventure story writer. He published two books in 1860 one of which – *Digby Heathcote or the Early Days of a Country Gentleman's Son and Heir* – was partly about Digby's time at an 'academy for young gentlemen'. His other book, *Ernest Bracebridge; or, Schoolboy Days,* was wholly about school life at Grafton Hall, a small private school. Written a few years before Reginald was born, these popular books were part of schoolboy reading at King's.

---

682 Ewins, Juliana, *Jackanapes* (SPCK, London, 1884) pp. 38 and 42. The Major's parting words were taken from 2 Corinthians 13 vs 14 'May the grace of the Lord Jesus Christ, and the love of God, and the fellowship of the Holy Spirirt, be with you all.

683 Parkin, George, *Life and Letters of Edward Thring (*Macmillan & Co Ltd, 1910), p. 468.

684 It is now in the Grove Family Archive. It is the 1884 edition. Reginald's name is inscribed in it, with the later addition of Jane Grove's signature.

Another well-known author was Dean F. W. Farrar[685] who wrote *Eric, or Little By Little* in 1858, a year after Hughes' story set at Rugby. Two other novels about school life followed – *Julian Home: A Tale of College Life* in 1859, and *St Winifred's, or the World of School* in 1862. These books had a strong moral message behind them. In his preface to *Eric*, in a new illustrated edition in 1889, Farrar wrote:

> The story of Eric was written with but one single objective – the vivid inculcation of inward purity and moral purpose, by the history of a boy, who, in spite of the inherent nobleness of his disposition falls into all folly and wickedness, until he has learnt to seek help from above.

At King's, *Eric* was a book which the boys read with enthusiasm. Such was its popularity that *Eric* went through 36 editions before Farrar's death.

On the same birthday that he was given *Tom Brown's School Days*, his parents gave him a copy of *Robinson Crusoe* by Daniel Defoe (1719). Together with *The Swiss Family Robinson* by Johann Wyss (1812), these two books were very popular with their tales of adventure and daring. R. M. Ballantyne's *The Coral Island* and *Martin Rattler* (both published in 1858) also told tales of adventure on the high seas. Robert Louis Stevenson's *Treasure Island* (1883) continued this type of adventure story. Reginald read this when he was 17.

G. A. Henty's stories were also extremely widely read by children. He wrote his first book for his own children and later children's historical novels generally featured a boy or young man. He wrote 122 novels in all, and his heroes, always modest, were intelligent, courageous, honest and resourceful with plenty of 'pluck'. These and other adventure stories were seen to portray the essence of Great Britain's greatness and its contribution to civilisation.[686] Many of these stories are now considered xenophobic and racist, promoting colonialism, exploitation and 'cultural appropriation'. The values that one generation holds dear, a later generation may well despise.

---

[685] Frederic William Farrar studied at King's College, London, and then at Trinity College Cambridge. He joined The Apostles, a famous intellectual group in the university. He was ordained into the Church of England and was a strong Christian. Besides becoming an author, he was also a schoolteacher. He was Headmaster at Marlborough College, and then at Harrow School, and was a contemporary of Thring's in educational circles. He became Archdeacon of Westminster and later Dean of Canterbury Cathedral from 1895 until his death in 1903. Interestingly, he was a pall-bearer at the funeral of Charles Darwin in 1882.

[686] Walvin, James, *A Child's World: A Social History of English Childhood 1800–1914*, p. 128.

Besides writing *The Water Babies*, Charles Kingsley wrote two historical novels – *Westward Ho!* (1855) and *Hereward the Wake* (1865). Reginald read the latter when he was 16. It had a special interest for him as it was set in the Fens on the Isle of Ely, which was not far from St Ives. As Kingsley described the Fens: 'a howling wilderness of meres, eas [sic], reed-ronds [sic] and floating alder-beds, through which only the fen-men wandered, with leaping-pole and log canoe'.[687] Chapter 28, which begins, 'When William heard the Danes were gone, he marched on Ely, as on an easy prey', continued to recount how William the Conqueror's army then crossed the impenetrable fens at Aldreth,[688] near Willingham, a village three and a half miles east of Earith. where his father's furthest patients lived. Reginald thought that it was 'a good historical novel with a quaint style'.

Interestingly, two years later in February 1887 he complained about the book. He had to reread it because it was set for the English exam at Easter. 'Why will they always chose 'miserable' books for this exam? Last year it was Harold – Harold is much more my idea of a hero than Hereward.' Reginald's personal copy, in which he wrote his name and which has an Uppingham School stamp in the inside front cover, is held in the Grove Family Archive.

The following year, in 1886, Reginald listed for the first time the 29 books that he read during the year with some comments against most of them. It was an eclectic list, shown at the end of this chapter, but it gives a good idea of the novels to which he was drawn, from Thomas Macaulay to Wilkie Collins. He particularly enjoyed *Dr Jekyll and Mr Hyde*, *The Vicar of Wakefield*, *The Moonstone* and *A Fallen Idol.*

ADULT READING

In his last but one term at school, he read with great enjoyment *The Angel in the House* (1854) by the American author, Coventry Patmore. This described Patmore's courtship with Emily, later to become his wife. Probably because Reginald was courting his sweetheart Mary when he read this, it struck a chord in his heart; he called it a 'jolly work which was simply splendid'.

---

[687] Kingsley, Charles, *Hereward the Wake*, T. Nelson & Sons, p. 382.

[688] *Hereward the Wake*, p. 383: 'So all his host camped themselves in Willingham Field, by the old earthwork which men now call Belsar's Hill; and down the bridleway poured countless men, bearing timber and faggots, cut from all the hills, that they might bridge the black half mile.' As a child I used to play at being Hereward the Wake at Belsar's Camp, as the site had come to be known.

Another adult work that he enjoyed reading that term was *The Professor at the Breakfast-Table* (1859) by Oliver Wendell Holmes senior, a well-known American who wrote essays on topical subjects. Reginald

> read every word of it, a thing which I do not think I have ever done in the case of any other book. There is an indiscernible charm in the Professor's ideas on subjects and every now and then you burst into a laugh over some witty saying: the little gentleman is perhaps the secret that makes me like the book so much.

Praise indeed.

NONSENSE POEMS

Nonsense verse, as exemplified by Edward Lear's *Book of Nonsense*, published in 1846, became popular with both children and adults.[689] In 1871 he published *Nonsense Songs, Stories, Botany, and Alphabets*, which included his most famous nonsense song, 'The Owl and the Pussy-cat', written for the children of his patron Edward Smith-Stanley, 13th Earl of Derby. Children and adults alike were enthralled by his charmingly eccentric verse, the last few lines of this poem being a good example:

> They dined on mince, and slices of quince
> Which they ate with a runcible spoon;
> And hand in hand, on the edge of the sand,
> They danced by the light of the moon,
> The moon,
> The moon,
> They danced by the light of the moon.

With the river flowing at the bottom of their garden in their first house it is not difficult to imagine Reginald's father reading a verse like

> There was an Old Man in a boat, who said,
> I'm afloat, I'm afloat!
> When they said 'No you ain't,' he was ready to faint,
> That unhappy Old Man in a boat.[690]

---

[689] As an author, Edward Lear (1812–88) is best known for his popular nonsense collections of poems, songs and short stories. He was an accomplished illustrator and drew botanical sketches as well as pictures for his books and stories. Less well known is the fact that he composed and published 12 musical settings of Tennyson's poetry.

[690] Lear, Edward, *The Book of Nonsense*, Frederick Warne & Co. Date of publication unknown.

and pointing to the illustration, drawn by Lear himself, showing the man in a skiff just like those used on the Ouse.

Or perhaps when he set sail on the Ouse from the bottom of their garden with his cousins, they and Reginald might have sung out the poem about the strange creatures called The Jumblies:

> They sailed away in a Sieve, they did, In a Sieve they sailed so fast,
> With only a beautiful pea-green veil Tied with a ribbon by way of a sail,
> To a small tobacco-pipe mast; And every one said, who saw them go,
> 'O won't they be soon upset, you know! For the sky is dark, and the voyage is long,
> And happen what may, it's extremely wrong In a Sieve to sail so fast!'
> Far and few, far and few,
> Are the lands where the Jumblies live;
> Their heads are green, and their hands are blue,
> And they went to sea in a Sieve.[691]

Verses like this, it has been argued, met a need for Victorians to laugh at themselves and poke fun at their stiff conventions and formalities.

MORAL INSTRUCTION

As has already been said, some children's stories were written to be morally instructive, and was a genre which told the tale in verse for amusement as well. They show the attitudes and values of the parents towards their children. *Struwwelpeter* (or *Shock-Headed Peter*) by the German author Dr Heinrich Hoffmann, first published in 1845, is a good example. It was popular with Reginald's own children before the First World War, and so there is every reason to believe it was popular, too, in the Grove household when he was growing up. The book has ten rhymed stories, mostly about children, illustrated with graphic illustrations. Each has a clear moral tale to tell, with the consequences of bad behaviour made abundantly clear. One story[692] was of a little boy called Frederick – 'cruel Frederick' who hurt small creatures. It was called *The Story of Cruel Frederick.*[693] He got his just deserts when his 'faithful Tray' whom he had hit with a whip, bit him. No doubt Dr Grove smiled as he read to young Reginald the last two verses

---

691 Lear, Edward, *The Book of Nonsense*, Frederick Warne & Co.

692 In German, '*Die Geschichte vom bösen Friederich*'.

693 Hoffmann, Dr Heinrich, *Struwwelpeter*, Routledge and Kegan Paul, p. 5.

and pointed to the delightful illustration of the doctor in his tailcoat with the bottle of medicine being dispensed to Frederick lying in bed, looking sorry for himself:

> So Frederick had to go to bed;
> His leg was very sore and red!
> The Doctor came and shook his head,
> And made a very great to-do,
> And gave him nasty physic too'
>
> But good dog Tray is happy now;
> He has no time to say 'bow-wow'!
> He seats himself in Frederick's chair,
> And laughs to see the nice things there:
> The soup he swallows, sup by sup,
> And eats the pies and puddings up.[694]

It would have made them think of Charlie, their family dog.

MAGAZINES

Besides books, Reginald read a number of magazines and periodicals. One in particular was a favourite at King's and Uppingham which he had sent from home, often with local newspapers. The *St. Nicholas Magazine for Boys and Girls* was an American children's magazine, popular in England and first published in 1873. It was aimed at children aged five to 18,[695] and its articles, all illustrated with finely executed line drawings, included poems, stories and educational information on science, geography, and so on. It was a publication of which his parents approved. The first time he mentioned it being sent to him was in February 1882 when he was 13 at King's. Throughout his schooldays until he was 17 he enjoyed reading it, and regularly mentioned its arrival in the post.

During the 1860s and 1870s there was a growth in the publication of cheap periodicals, but there was huge concern from many educationalists and parents about them, and the term 'penny dreadfuls' became used early

[694] 'Struwwelpeter' was popular with my children, too!

[695] Many well-known authors wrote for the *St Nicholas*, such as Mark Twain. A special department called the St. Nicholas League offered awards and cash prizes to the best work submitted by its juvenile readers. F. Scott Fitzgerald was a St Nicholas League winner in the 20th century. The magazine stopped publishing in the 1940s.

on. The cheap periodicals often included a school story (embracing a range of schools from 'charity' schools to public schools) to attract their readers, which were mostly boys.

In some ways they were modelled on *Tom Brown's School Days*, but they were often stories of bullying, floggings and cruelty, and lacked the moral purpose of Hughes and other authors who wanted their readers to learn lessons of life within a moral framework.

A reviewer in the *Quarterly Review* in 1890 termed these publications 'the literature of rascaldom' and 'the best that can be said of them is, that they are comparatively harmless; the worst, that no boy is likely to be the better for reading them'.[696] However, there was a real fear that the influence on young boys was harmful. The *Quarterly Review* made the point that 'this foul and filthy trash that circulates by thousands and tens of thousands amongst lads who are the most impressionable period of their lives, and whom the modern system of purely secular education has left without ballast or guidance'.[697] Reginald did not mention reading any of the penny dreadfuls, although it is likely that he did, as copies were circulated undercover by schoolboys.

The educationalist E. Salmon, in his book *Juvenile Literature As It Is*, published in 1888, gave examples of the 'disastrous effects of the dreadfuls on the minds of our boys and girls'.[698] He thought that 'the only real antidote for these poisonous sheets … is the *Boy's Own Paper*, because the *Boy's Own Paper* is the only first class journal of its kind which has found its way into the slums as well as into the best homes'.

The Religious Tract Society stepped in to offset the impact of these publications by issuing 'a monthly shilling volume for the younger members of Christian families' which was the prototype for the *Boy's Own Paper*. Success was limited mainly because of the cost each month, and a weekly paper for boys was suggested. The Society realised that 'Leisure Hour' as a title might be off-putting, so a new publication was published called the *Boy's Own Paper*. The first issue appeared when Reginald had just celebrated his 10th birthday. Priced at 1d (52p), with around 16 pages and illustrated with line drawings, it was published every Saturday.

[696] *Quarterly Review* 1890 p. 156.

[697] Musgrave, p. 113.

[698] Ibid.

It was designed to instil Christian morals during boys' formative years,[699] and its Latin motto was '*Quicquidagunt pueri nostri farrago libelli*', or 'Whatever boys do makes up the mixture of our little book'.[700] After the first volume had come out, Andrew Hutchinson, the assistant editor, was appointed editor, and under his direction the *BOP* grew in popularity. A Baptist, he adhered to the Society's policy that religious dogma should not be pushed. The *BOP* remained a weekly publication until 1914 when it became monthly. Hutchinson was adept at getting well-known authors to write stories: Jules Verne, R. M. Ballantyne, G. A. Henty, Conan Doyle and W. H. G. Kingston all contributed at one time or another what could be termed 'healthy adventure stories'.[701]

The first reference to the *BOP* in his diaries was when he was 12. Readers were encouraged to write in and he wrote to the 'Boys Newspaper [sic]'. He said nothing about the content of his correspondence or if he received a reply. The correspondence section of the magazine always contained a number of comments by readers about articles published previously; questions were also raised by readers which other readers then answered in the next edition. Correspondence came from English readers as well as those from New Zealand and Australia, for example. Initials, rather than names, were used.

Those whose letters were published gave an insight into the readership of the *BOP*. In 1879, for instance, a letter from a branch of the Technical Department of the Post Office in Scotland stated that out of 84 boys on the staff, 63 took the *BOP* each week and five monthly. A letter from a boy at Wellington College showed that readers came from public schools as well as working-class lads.[702] The 1881 edition[703] did not carry Reginald's initials so his letter never made publication. In October the following year he went into town to order the *Boy's Own Paper*, but never mentioned reading it while he was at Uppingham so he must have outgrown it.

As already mentioned, the Grove family subscribed to *British Workman*

---

699 The first issue was published on 18 January 1879.

700 Musgrave, p. 115.

701 Ibid.

702 Ibid, p. 142.

703 https://archive.org/details/boysownpaper79unse/page/750.

magazine.[704] It contained poems, short articles and stories with a strong moral message. For instance, there were a number of articles 'against smoking' with titles such as 'What Put my pipe out?' and 'How Sam Adam's Pipe became a Pig' (both these were illustrated by Cruikshank).[705] The back page of the magazine advertised a wide range of books; some were for the nursery, such as *The Mother's Picture Alphabet* and *Rhymes worth remember* (sic). Others were books for girls, such as *The Church Mouse* or *Mind Whom You Marry*, suitable for Mabel, Reginald's sister. Many pages contained Scriptural texts in highlighted boxes such as 'Love not sleep, lest thou come to poverty' (Proverbs 10:13) or 'Let us not be weary in well doing' (Galatians 6 vs9).[706]

One story which would have appealed to Reginald having visited his cousins on their farms was called 'The Farmer's Lad'.

***

> A shepherd boy once went into a bookseller's shop in Edinburgh and inquired for a second-hand Greek New Testament. The bookseller having presented one, the boy asked him the price. 'For whom do you want it?' inquired the bookseller. 'For myself,' answered the boy. 'Then,' said the bookseller, 'if you will read a few verses and translate them, you shall have it for nothing.' With much apparent satisfaction, the poor boy complied with the condition and carried off the Testament in triumph.'
>
> Many years afterwards, the late Revd John Brown of Haddington, then in the midst of his fame as an author and commentator on the Scriptures, went into the same shop and entered into conversation with the bookseller. The latter, who was no stranger to either his person or his character, received him with marked respect. In the course of conversation, Mr Brown inquired if he remembered the circumstances above detailed. 'I remember it well,' replied the bookseller, 'and I would give a good deal to know what became of the boy; for I am sure that he has risen to eminence in some line or other'. 'Sir,' said Mr Brown, 'you see him before you.' It is

---

[704] This was published monthly by Partridge and Co between 1855 and 1892. It aimed to 'promote the health, wealth and happiness of the working classes'. It was illustrated with well-executed engravings. There was a bias in favour of socialism, temperance and Christian faith. While it was dedicated to the 'industrial classes', it clearly was read by middle-class families like the Groves.

[705] George Cruikshank (1792–1878) was a well-known caricaturist who illustrated his friend Charles Dickens' novels.

[706] *British Workman,* August 1872 No 212, p. 128.

needless to add that they were both well pleased to meet each other again.

We hope that by means of the new Educational Act[707] many farmers lads who are now 'tenting'[708] all day will have the advantage of attending school under the 'half time' system and thereby have opportunity of gaining useful knowledge which will fit them, like John Brown, for positions of honour and usefulness in the world.[709]

***

This story[710] and many others printed in this magazine echoed the view put forward by the author Samuel Smiles in his classic *Self-Help,*[711] published in 1859, the same year as Charles Darwin's *On the Origin of Species* and John Stuart Mill's essay 'On Liberty'. Each had a significant impact[712] on mid-Victorian attitudes and thinking, but certainly *Self-Help* was staple reading for a middle-class family like the Groves.

Reginald was given another of Smiles' works on *Duty,*[713] published two years previously, as a school prize[714] at King's when he was 13. Curiously, Smiles was born in the same village of which Revd Brown was the minister, although Brown had died by the time Smiles was born. In *Self-Help*, his most popular book, Smiles promoted the virtue of hard work and thrift,

[707] This was the Education Act 1872, also known as Forster's Education Act, which made primary education a right for children and mandatory in Scotland. However, it was not until a further Act of 1880 that schooling became compulsory for children from 5 to 10, and became organised through the new School Boards and paid for by local rates and grants. That said, children could be withdrawn over the summer months whenever harvesting was carried out locally.

[708] A drawing on the next page of the magazine shows a young boy in a smock, sitting on a five-barred gate leading to a cornfield with a large rattle in his hand. This is presumably to scare birds away from the crop. The caption of the picture states 'Farmer's Boy "tenting" in the corn field'.

[709] Revd John Brown (1722–87) was a Scottish minister at Haddington, East Lothian (United Secession Church) who knew Greek, Latin and Hebrew, and was able to read and speak French, Italian, German, Arabic, Persian, Syriac and Ethiopic. (https://en.wikipedia.org/wiki/John_Brown_of_Haddington 02.09.19.)

[710] *British Workman*, August 1872 No 212, p. 127.

[711] *Self-Help* sold 25,000 copies in its first year and 250,000 copies by the end of the century.

[712] The eminent historian of Victorian England, Professor Asa Briggs, wrote in the centenary edition of *Self-Help* that 'there are few books in history which have reflected the spirit of their age more faithfully and successfully than Samuel Smiles' *"Self Help"*'.

[713] Smiles, Samuel, *Duty; With Illustrations of Courage, Patience, & Endurance* (John Murray, 1880).

[714] Diary 1882 note.

and claimed that poverty was caused largely by irresponsible habits, while he also attacked materialism.[715]

Self-Help has been called 'the bible of mid-Victorian liberalism'.[716] Smiles wrote that 'the spirit of self-help is the root of all genuine growth in the individual and exhibited in the lives of many it constitutes the true source of national vigour and strength'.[717] What appealed to readers from different backgrounds was his encouragement for everyone to use education and their energy and personal drive to better themselves and society. His message in a word was 'perseverance':

> Great men of science, literature and art – apostles of great thoughts and lords of great hearts – have belonged to no exclusive class or rank in life. They have come alike from colleges, workshops and farmhouses – from the huts of poor men and the mansions of the rich.

And in his book he told the story of a range of individuals whose lives demonstrated their perseverance – statesmen like Disraeli, soldiers like Wellington, and painters like Hogarth.

Of interest no doubt to Reginald were the lives of men like Charles Bell[718] who researched into the nervous system, Charles Jenner[719] who discovered the merits of vaccination against smallpox, and Ambroise Paré,[720] the French surgeon who pioneered the treatment of wounds in war. All rose from humble beginnings. Smiles' idea that 'the crown and glory of life is Character' was echoed by Reginald's Headmaster, Thring. As Smiles said, 'it is the noblest possession of a man, constituting a rank

---

[715] Smiles' father died while he was a child and his mother ran, single-handedly, the family village store to support her ten children. A firm Christian, she believed that the 'Lord will provide'. Her tireless example was a strong influence on Smiles' life.

[716] Cohen, M. J., and Major, John, editors, *History in Quotations,* (Cassell, 2004), p. 611.

[717] Smiles, Samuel, *Self-Help*, first published by John Murray (1859), p. 11, Sphere Books, 1968.

[718] The Scottish surgeon Charles Bell (1774–1842) discovered the difference between sensory nerves and motor nerves in the spinal cord. He research into another area was awarded the title Bell's palsy.

[719] Edward Jenner (1748–1823), an English surgeon, is often called 'the father of immunology'. It has been said that he 'saved more lives than the work of any other human' in history.

[720] Ambroise Paré (1510–90), a Frenchman served who Henry II, Francis II, Charles IX and Henry III. He was a surgeon/barber and is considered one of the fathers of surgery and modern forensic pathology, and a pioneer in surgical techniques and battlefield medicine, especially in the treatment of wounds.

in itself and an estate in the general goodwill, dignifying every station and exalting every position in society'.[721]

Later, as Reginald grew up, he enjoyed a magazine called *Tit Bits.*[722] During 1885 he bought it regularly priced 1d (52p). It was a British, rather than an American publication, which first came on the market in 1871 when Reginald was a baby. It was a mass-circulation magazine which, rather like a mini-encyclopaedia, printed a range of 'titbits' of factual information in an easy-to-read format. It had lots of human-interest stories as well as short fictional stories, but also well-known authors like Rider Haggard and in 1900, P. G. Wodehouse, who had his first humorous article published.[723]

When he was 17 he bought a copy of *The English Illustrated Magazine.* Priced at 6d (£3) it was a monthly publication with features that included travel, topography and a large section on fiction.[724] As he was editing the Uppingham School Magazine at this time, Reginald must have felt it could give him some new ideas; he certainly liked it and thought he might well 'get it for a year'. The following month his accounts showed that he spent 2/6d (£15.72) on a subscription and a Leech print, and then in December another 2/- (£12.60).

A publication which Reginald bought only once, when he was 12 years old at King's, was *Sports and Pastimes.* He ordered it in March 1881 by making a special trip into Cambridge town centre. *Baily's Magazine of Sports and Pastimes* (to give it its correct title) was a British sport and recreation magazine first published in 1860. Articles ranged from those about blood sports such as stag hunting, fox hunting, angling, and hare coursing to horse racing and other country sports. In addition, it gave the dates of horse races, hunt meetings and horse livestock sales. Reginald was no stranger to blood sports, as his farming uncles and aunts had a pragmatic view of killing foxes, hares, rabbits, rats and mice as vermin which threatened their livelihood.

---

[721] Smiles, Samuel, *Self-Help*, p. 246.

[722] Officially it was *Tit-Bits from all the Interesting Books, Periodicals and Newspapers in the World*, but was abbreviated to *Tit-Bits.*

[723] During the First World War Ivor Novello won a *Tit-Bits* competition to write a song soldiers could sing at the front: he penned 'Keep the Home Fires Burning'. Pin-ups of girls, which I remember, began in 1939. The magazine ceased publication in 1984.

[724] The magazine ran for 359 issues between October 1883 and August 1913.

The March edition had an article on hunting around Cambridge by the university undergraduates, so this was perhaps why Reginald bought it. Besides a drag hunting club, the hunts mentioned were the Cambridgeshire, the Fitzwilliam, the Oakley and the Trinity Foot Beagles.[725] The latter hunted hares on foot within an eight-mile radius of the town.[726] Some of their 'runs' were five miles long, and two or three hares were killed during an afternoon's sport.[727] It's interesting to compare this with the hare hunting at Shippea Hill farm described earlier. All the hunts described in the article survive to this day, although undergraduate participation is now rare.

A few years before Reginald left school, a national survey[728] was carried out by a Charles Welsh for children when he sent out a 'circular containing several questions such as: what is your favourite book and why do you like it best?' It went to 'numerous schools for boys and girls and he had 2,000 replies, including from schoolmasters and schoolmistresses. Whether it was sent to Uppingham is not known, but 790 replies were returned from boys. Their first favourite authors were:

1. Charles Dickens
2. W. H. G. Kingston
3. Sir Walter Scott
4. Jules Verne
5. Captain Marryat.

The top individual books were:

1. *Robinson Crusoe*
2. *The Swiss Family Robinson*
3. *The Pickwick Papers*
4. *Ivanhoe*
5. *Boy's Own Paper.*

The Bible was sixth, and seventh was *Tom Brown's School Days.*

---

725 There was a public house on the Cambridge to Huntingdon Road called 'The Trinity Foot' which I remember well. It was demolished in 2017, having been derelict since 2008.

726 *Bailey's Sports and Pastimes* Vol 37 (A. H. Bailey, Nicholas Lane, King William Street, EC, 1881), pp. 31–32 https://archive.org/details/bailysmagazineof37gilbuoft/page/32

727 The Trinity Foot amalgamated with the South Herts Beagles in 2003.

728 Salmon, Edward, *Juvenile Literature As It Is* (Drane, London, 1888). Charles Welsh's survey is mentioned.

In 1886, Reginald's reading encompassed some, but not all, of these authors and books:

Title	Author	Date read	Comment by Reginald
Guy Mannering	Walter Scott	5 January	*Good*
Comic Dramatists of the Restoration	Thomas Macaulay	21 January	
Essay on Lord Byron	Thomas Macaulay	24 January	
Yeast	Charles Kingsley	27 January	*Too much logic which I can't understand*
The School for Scandal	Richard Sheridan	1 February	*Good*
Kenilworth	Walter Scott	21 February	
Treasure Island	Robert Louis Stevenson	7 February	*Splendid*
Dr Jekyll and Mr Hyde	Robert Louis Stevenson	7 February	*Good*
Henrietta Temple	Benjamin Disraeli	27 February	*Interesting*
The Vicar of Wakefield	Oliver Goldsmith	8 March	*Enjoyed it!*
Silas Marner	George Eliot	14 March	
Princess	Alfred Tennyson	26 March	
Pride and Prejudice	Jane Austen	26 March	
Hard Lines	Hawley Smart	22 April	
Scenes of Clerical Life	George Eliot	30 May	
Martin Chuzzlewit	Charles Dickens		
The Castle of Otranto	Horace Walpole	6 June	
The Man of Feeling	Henry Mackenzie		
The Coming Race	Edward Lytton	25 June	
The Dilemma	Unknown	25 July	
The Moonstone	Wilkie Collins	16 September	*Very good*
King Solomon's Mines	Rider Haggard	18 September	
Kidnapped	Robert Louis Stevenson	6 October	
A Fallen Idol	F. Anstey	10 October	*Very amusing*
The Gladiators	George Whyte-Melville	17 October	
Madame d'Arblay	Thomas Macaulay	20 October	
Mansfield Park	Jane Austen	27 November	
Three Brass Balls	George Robert Sims	27 November	
The Holy Rose	Walter Besant	27 December	

CHAPTER 15

Entertainment

'In the evening we all went to Drury Lane and saw a splendid ballet and then a 'Run of Luck' which was a splendid piece, nine race horse races on stage at once; enjoyed ourselves very much.'
Reginald Grove, 11 September 1886

THE SEASIDE AND HOLIDAYS

The coast in Norfolk was within easy day reach by train via Cambridge, and Hunstanton was a favourite seaside resort that the family visited during the school holidays. When he was 12 Reginald noted in his diary going off to Hunstanton one Thursday by train in the summer holidays,[729] leaving at 9.00am, having his photograph taken on the beachfront, swimming in the sea and taking a train back at 7.00pm. They arrived home at about 10.00, exhausted but pleased with a pleasant day out.

During the period before Reginald was born, the growth of the railway network, the prosperity enjoyed by the growing middle classes and the desire to have a break in the healthy environment of the sea meant that seaside towns promoted themselves as elegant holiday resorts.

Families would stay at guest houses or rent a house for a few weeks in the summer. After Reginald caught scarlet fever in the autumn of 1883, he convalesced in Hunstanton after the worst was over, lodging with a Miss Marsters who lived at No 2 Greeve Gate Terrace. He stayed there for a fortnight and in his diary wrote that he 'enjoyed myself very much at the seaside', getting better and regaining his strength. The sea itself was seen to be healthy, as were the fresh air and gentle walks along the seafront. Promenades, gardens and seating areas were built in the new resorts like Hunstanton, and local businesses catered for food and drink. Theatres, concert halls and bandstands were built to attract visitors.

Hunstanton was very much a 19th-century resort town, initially known as New Hunstanton to distinguish it from the adjacent village

[729] When he was at King's Choir School, the summer holidays were held in September, rather than in July–August.

from which it took its name. The new town soon exceeded the village in scale and population. Well before the Grove family visits, the first main building was erected in 1848. This was the Royal Hotel (now the Golden Lion), which was the work of the renowned Victorian architect, William Butterfield, a friend of Le Strange's. Overlooking a sloping green and the sea, and for several years standing alone, it earned the nickname 'Le Strange's Folly'. In 1850 Le Strange, an amateur architect and painter, appointed a land agent to survey the site and prepare a plan. Le Strange drew and painted a map and a perspective of the scheme, showing shops, a station and a church. He consulted William Butterfield on the design. Their shared passion was for an 'Old English' style of architecture for domestic buildings, owing much to medieval precedents and the earnestness of the Victorian Gothic Revival. Hunstanton became an exemplar of a 19th-century seaside town. Most of the fabric and character of the original development survive.

Like many Victorian seaside resorts, Hunstanton had a pier[730] stretching out to sea with fine attractions which included a pavilion and miniature steam railway running up and down it. Interestingly, piers were built using a system of screw piles – wrought-iron pillars with a screw thread at the end screwed through the shingle/sand to the bedrock.[731]

Bathing was seen as a medical tonic to stimulate and invigorate the circulation.[732] In the early days, sea bathing meant standing waist-deep and dipping oneself under the surface a few times. By the 1850s bathing huts became popular, which were sheds on wheels fitted with steps at the front which Queen Victoria used at Osborne House on the Isle of Wight. Their

---

730 Sadly, the pier pavilion was destroyed by fire in 1939; the pier was damaged by fire again in the 1950s, before almost the entire structure was washed away by a storm in 1978.

731 The method of pier construction was invented by Eugenius Birch. He built 14 piers all over the country such as West Pier Brighton and North Pier Blackpool. By 1900 there were 80 piers offering bands, Punch and Judy shows, steam excursions and arcade amusements. (Hart-Davis, Adam, *What the Victorians Did for Us*, 2001, p. 109.)

732 Besides the sea itself, the air at the seaside was deemed to have beneficial qualities (similar approach to taking spa water). The gas ozone had been discovered in 1839 and had been found to be a good disinfectant. It had a distinctive smell, associated with electrical discharges, and so was believed to be healthy. The smell of decomposing seaweed has a similar smell and so sea air was thought to be beneficial. Dr T. Herbert Baker wrote in *The Times* in 1865 that 'There can be little doubt that ozone is Nature's grand atmospecific [sic] disinfectant. All the facts which have hitherto been developed tend to prove this.' He noted that no ozone was found near cesspools or in crowded churches. (Hart-Davis, p. 107.)

use declined by the 1890s by the time Reginald was at Cambridge, and they were replaced by lines of changing huts or tents along the promenade edge.

In 1872 Francis Kilvert, who was a Welsh curate,[733] described the pleasure from stripping off and swimming naked on holiday at Weston-super-Mare: 'there was a delicious feeling of freedom in stripping in the open air and running down naked to the sea where the waves were curling white foam and the red morning sunshine glowing upon the naked limbs of the bathers'.[734] Soon, however, prudery took over and men were forced to cover up. Nude bathing did occur, as described in Volume 2 about swimming in the Cam at Cambridge, but it was confined to town urchins rather than middle-class curates! With the prevalence of swimming wear, mixed bathing slowly became common and this is what Reginald experienced on family outings to the seaside.

Most beaches were segregated by sex, and women wore bathing suits which were woollen stacks with a drawstring neck and simple slits at the side for arms. As the century drew to a close, women wore knee-length tunics and below-the knee-drawers made out of serge, not flannel (absorbed less water and not so heavy), with a belt. This was the type of swimming costume that Reginald's sister Mabel would have worn.

Almost everything about the seaside that is common today stems from Victorian times – buckets and spades, donkey rides, slot machines, ice cream, Punch and Judy shows and piers; the only entertainment not seen today was the travelling groups of 'pierrot' entertainers who were dressed as white-faced clowns.

A day trip in mid-August 1886 is a good example of the Groves enjoying the seaside. His diary describes a family day trip by train with his mother, his brothers and sisters and a 'Miss Schiralm', who was probably the younger ones' governess. The day before his father had travelled to Hunstanton himself for a holiday, as his rheumatism had been painful and a break from work on the coast would do him good. When they arrived they found he was a little better for his stay, even after just one day

Starting off at 8.15am, Reginald and his mother had intended to meet

---

733 Robert Francis Kilvert (1840–79), known as Francis, was an English clergyman whose diaries reflected rural life in the 1870s and were published over 50 years after his death.

734 http://www.thekilvertsociety.org.uk/assets/downloads/archive/kilvert-society-newsletter-1979-march.pdf (13.04.19).

up at Ely with their Long cousins from Shippea Hill Farm, but they sent his cousin Dick Long to Ely in the trap to tell them they thought it was going to rain, so they had decided not to go. In fact, the weather was fine and the Groves had 'a splendid day' bathing in the sea, with the Borissow family[735] who joined them when the train stopped at Cambridge. Whether it was a chance meeting or both families had planned it is not clear, but meeting up with the Borissows filled the gap of the Longs not coming. The Borissows were a large family of nine who lived in Trumpington, just outside Cambridge. The boys were a similar age to Reginald and his brothers and they knew each other from King's College Choir School. Their eldest sister, Edith was the same age as Mabel and the children all got on well.

The Borissows travelled back on the same train to Cambridge but at Ely Reginald left his family to take the train to Shippea Hill to stay the night there before he returned early next day to Cambridge to stay a few days at King's with the Vice Provost.

FAIRS AND CIRCUSES

In Reginald's late-teens, home-grown entertainment and dramatics were the main entertainment that he enjoyed, whether at home or at school. And at school there were the occasional concerts that he attended, which frequently featured well-known musicians and singers.

But to add to other entertainment there were also travelling circuses, fairs, theatres and events that came to St Ives, Cambridge and Uppingham. Reginald also visited theatres in Cambridge and London when he was older during the school holidays.

While legal restrictions on these entertainments in the 21st century

---

[735] The Groves knew the family well. Revd Louis Borissow was the Chaplain and Precentor at Trinity College, Cambridge and he and his wife, Harriet lived in Trumpington, just outside Cambridge. They had 10 children with the first three being boys who all started at Kings College Choir School in August 1881 as detailed in Volume 2 Chapter 1. Ernest was 13, Clement 12 and Henry 10. Ernest became an architect in later life and the borough surveyor for Huntingdon. Tragically, he died in 1915 aged 47 while serving with the Royal Army Medical Corps in Greece. Clement became a solicitor. (http://slatters.org.uk/ 09.10.20.) In 1888/9 Borissow became the tutor at Trinity College for Sir Ranjitsinhji Vibhaji Jadeja (often known as Ranji), who was the ruler of Nawanagar from 1907 to 1933, as Maharaja Jam Saheb. He was a famous Test cricketer who played for England, Cambridge University, and county cricket for Sussex. Ranji lodged with the Borissows until 1892 when he moved in to his own lodgings in Cambridge. Sadly, the loss of family life contributed to his loneliness. He left Cambridge in 1894 without graduating. He remained close to the family after leaving Cambridge. (https://en.wikipedia.org/wiki/Ranjitsinhji 09.10.20.)

appear minimal, legislation introduced before Reginald was born endeavoured to bring in some constraints to define what was acceptable on the streets. The 1834 Poor Law Act meant that travelling entertainers could be arrested for vagrancy. The 1835 Highway Act allowed street entertainments and sports to be classified as nuisances, and the 1835 Cruelty to Animals Act banned dog fighting, bull-baiting and cock fighting. The Victorians loved sensational exploits, such as high-wire acts like Blondin's,[736] with the ever-present possibility of a horrific accident occurring.[737] The last public hanging took place in 1868.[738] Perhaps the melodramatic circus and high-wire acts replaced the thrill of these cruel spectacles?

The two annual fairs were held in St Ives in the Bullock Market and Market Hill, and one in Uppingham, held in Market Place in March which lasted three days. The boys from the school were banned from visiting the fair – a 'tawdry encampment and its boorish revels'.[739] No doubt a few boys sneaked out to join the fun – Hornung described how two boys sneaked out of one of the Hill Houses at night 'disguised in bowlers and false beards'.[740] They were expelled as a result.

These fairs featured rides with a central steam engine. Their eventer was a Norfolk man, Frederick Savage, who had a workshop in King's Lynn making fairground rides. An early one, made in 1860, was called the Velocipede which comprised six bicycles welded together in a circle. Savage progressed to the Galloper later, which was a roundabout, often still seen today, with rising and falling horses (or cockerels or geese) on twisted brass poles. He also made Gondolas – a string of half a dozen 'boats' decorated with brass and gilt carvings which chased one another round and round on

---

[736] Blondin (whose real name was Jean Gravelet[t]), having performed his spectacular stunts crossing the Niagara Falls in 1859–60, visited England in 1861 and travelled all over the country, including Crystal Palace, wowing huge crowds with his exploits. He died aged 73 in 1895 after a career performing stunts over a 65-year period.

[737] Some of Blondin's rivals were killed or badly injured: Mme Genevieve, styled as 'The Female Blondin', was killed at a fete in Ashton Park, Birmingham, in 1863 when the ropes broke as she was carrying out a high-wire crossing blindfolded. She was eight months pregnant at the time which made the accident all the more dreadful.

[738] This was in May 1868 and was of the Irish terrorist Michael Barrett who was executed at Newgate Prison for mass murder. He was involved in the 'Clerkenwell explosion' in London which had killed 12 people.

[739] Hornung, *Fathers of Men*, p. 196.

[740] Ibid, p. 200.

rails on a steep switchback course, each carrying four couples. Music was supplied by a steam-powered organ that played popular tunes loudly and created 'the fun of the fair' atmosphere loved to this day. For those living nearby, 'the incessant strains of the steam merry go round became part of the place for the time being and made night especially hideous in the town houses nearest the scene'.[741] The Uppingham schoolboys described by Hornung bemoaned the fact that 'Over the Garden Wall' and 'Lardy-dah'[742] were played incessantly.

As the two annual fairs held at St Ives were held in the school holidays, Reginald missed these once he went to boarding school.

Travelling circuses were a popular feature of Victorian life and small ones often came to St Ives. By the mid-19th century there were hundreds of circuses operating in Britain offering a wide range of entertainment. Jugglers, clowns, acrobats and trick horse riding were essential for performances.

Such was their popularity that theatres also presented circus acts such as jugglers and aerial acts on stage. Even the Drury Lane Theatre in London had a circus ring so it could present equestrian acts. Reginald went to a performance there in September 1886 when he was in London taking his Apothecary examinations, described in Volume 3. On the Saturday evening he went with his cousins Hansie Long and Wilfred Long to see 'Run of Luck',[743] 'which was a splendid piece, nine race horse races on stage at once; enjoyed ourselves very much'.

One of the factors that made the circus so popular was that fairground entertainers travelled to their audiences, and even the smallest towns like St Ives and Uppingham were visited. The use of tents,[744] especially for small circuses, enabled shows to be put on for the local inhabitants in fields near the town centre; St Ives had plenty of meadows and fields within a

---

741 Hornung, *Fathers of Men*, p. 196.

742 'Over the Garden Wall' was a polka composed by Warwick Williams in c.1870. 'La-di-da' or 'City Toff' was written by V. Page with music composed by Vincent Davies in c.1865. It was sung by Miss Nelly Power, a well-known music hall, burlesque and pantomime artiste. Sadly, she was only 32 when she died of pleurisy in 1887, the year Reginald left Uppingham.

743 This was a production put on by the Drury Lane Company with leading actors E. W. Gardiner, William Rignold, Harry Nicolls, Sophie Eyre, Alma Murray and J. G. Grahame.

744 The large tents associated today with circuses ('Big Tops') began to be used from the 1820s in the United States. The Powell and Clarke's Circus in the 1880s had a tent which could seat 7,000 spectators (The Victorian Circus – Victoria and Albert Museum website www.vam.ac.uk/content/articles/v/victorian-circus, 29.09.19).

few minutes of the centre, and Reginald saw a number of shows when they came to town. The performances held in the evenings used candles put on the wooden barriers that were erected to separate the audience from the performers.

The development of the railways enabled large circuses to travel all over the country, and indeed across Europe and the United States. In April 1887 'Buffalo Bill' Cody and his Wild West Show landed at the Albert Dock in the Thames 14 days after sailing from the United States. 100 Native Americans were part of the troupe, as were 160 horses. The show was spectacular and took London by storm when it opened the next month at the American Exhibition in Earls Court. Admission was one guinea (£132.81) which was beyond most people. Besides Cody's show the exhibition displayed American products and technical innovations, but it was the show that was the big attraction, with members of the royal family including The Queen visiting. Reginald was at school at the time so was not one of the estimated one million visitors that went. The show returned in 1892 and 1903/04.

Another show from the United States that stunned audiences was Barnum and Bailey's circus which was billed as the 'Greatest Show on Earth'.[745] The circus parade was another way in which publicity for the entertainment was generated and a natural advertisement for the circus, always drawing large crowds. The Barnum and Bailey circus arrived by train to Norwich in 1899 and the parade from the station to their site, included a military band, a wagon pulled by 40 horses, a menagerie of wild animals, 70 horses and a collection of 'living human curiosities'; this was a freak show of those with deformities which, sadly, were a popular attraction of the time.[746]

A circus came to St Ives during the summer holidays in 1885 when

---

[745] Barnum and Bailey's Circus from the United States (The Greatest Show on Earth) visited Europe from 1897 to 1902. When it was at London's Olympia it had at least ten displays, including aquatic acts, aerialists, elephants and an act with 70 horses in the ring at once. A military band played before each performance and there were also races and ballets, a menagerie and a spectacular re-enactment of a well-known American sea battle with the Spanish fleet at Santiago.

[746] One such unfortunate who became very well known was Julia Pastrana, known as 'The Nondescript'. She suffered from hypertrichosis which caused her to be covered in long, thick hair and to have exaggerated facial features. She toured England in the 1840s and 50s, and her mummified body continued to attract an audience after her death. https://the-line-up.com/freak-show-peculiar-attraction-victorian-era 29.09.19.

he was 16. Circus performers generally included clowns, trapeze artists, magicians, horse riders, and often a small menagerie of exotic animals. Reginald did not note the programme, but he enjoyed himself and thought it was 'not all bad'. The following month, the day before he was due to travel back to Uppingham, he watched a circus procession or 'parade', as he called it; it must have been another one visiting town.

The next summer another circus came to St Ives, possibly the same one that had come 11 months previously. This time the whole family went, apart from his mother, and it 'was great fun' and they 'enjoyed it very much'. The next month a travelling theatre came to St Ives and Reginald went with his friend, Arnie Ulph. They found it amusing, not least because the actors could not act very well and the 'letter h' was pronounced wrongly – but perhaps that was part of the play!

Circuses were out of bounds at Uppingham if they stopped in the town, but watching a circus convoy of horse-drawn carts was the next best thing. In March 1887 the boys watched a circus caravan pass through the town and this provided great free entertainment. Reginald was in his house reading and found out later that he had missed a 'grand sight', as the circus passed through the town. It was a long procession he heard and he observed in his diary that 'they had great difficulty in getting up the hill'. As it had rained earlier in the day, it must have been even more difficult on the slippery cobbles through the town. As Reginald would have seen and heard the convey when he was at Redgate on Red Hill, the circus must have passed from Stamford to Leicester or vice versa.

PLAYS, PANTOMIMES AND THEATRES

Reginald occasionally went to Cambridge to the theatre to see both pantomimes and more serious plays. Plays were put on at the Theatre Royal in St Andrew's Street. When he was at King's he occasionally was taken to the theatre when he was in the 'first division', which was what the older boys were called. They saw the Greek play *Ajax*[747] and he thought it was 'awfully jolly'. The play ended just after 10.30pm so they got back to school late. As the boys only had an hour's lesson the following morning, they managed to get through the rest of the day despite their late night.

He made a visit in the Easter holidays 1885 to stay at King's with the Vice Provost Austen Leigh for a couple of days when he played cricket.

[747] The play was by Sophocles.

On his first evening he went to the Cambridge Theatre[748] to watch a performance of a play called *The Member for Hocum.* Unfortunately, he thought it was 'not very good'.

Just before Christmas 1886 he was staying with his cousins Dick and Mary Long at Shippea Hill, and the two boys drove in the trap in the evening to Ely to meet up with his parents to see a production of *The Sorcerer* put on at his brother's school. His brother Ted played the prima donna ('looked an awful good girl'!) and Ernest was in the chorus. Dr and Mrs Grove stayed at the Lamb Inn and his sister Mabel with a friend of the family. After the play had finished they went to dinner together joined by his uncle and his sweetheart Mary, whom he sat next to all evening. After this, the others retired but he and his Uncle Hanslip went to see another family friend, Dr Francis Beckett, and they did not get back to the farm and to bed until 2.00am. It had been an enjoyable evening.

Pantomimes had the same level of slapstick and double entendre as today; one pantomime he visited in Cambridge during the Christmas holidays, when he was nearly 18, he found 'some parts very vulgar'.

When Reginald was 12 he 'went to see some Zulus in the afternoon'. Whether they were actual Zulus from the British province of Natal in South Africa or not is not known. It is possible that they were; the recent Anglo-Zulu War of 1879 was very much at the forefront of the public imagination. The annihilation of the English expeditionary force at Isandlwana and the heroic stand of the small contingent at the mission station at Rorke's Drift (where 11 Victoria Crosses were awarded) had been widely reported in the press.[749] The Zulu warriors were held in respect.

More probably they were a troupe of black and white minstrels. On another occasion, just after his 15th birthday, Reginald went to the St Ives Corn Exchange one evening in the Christmas holidays, and saw what he termed a '****** [750] entertainment'. He enjoyed it very much. This is

[748] Which theatre this was is not clear but it was not the well-known Cambridge Arts Theatre which was only founded in 1936.

[749] On January 22 1879 the Zulu army of King Cetshwayo destroyed a British column at the Battle of Isandlwana – arguably the greatest military disaster in colonial history. The South Wales 24th Foot lost 602 men in the attack by 20,000 Zulus. At Rorke's Drift, the following day, B Company of the 24th – all that was left of the regiment – fought off 4,000 Zulus for the loss of only 17 men.

[750] Pejorative racial term used interchangeable with 'negro'.

likely to have been a black and white minstrel troupe.[751] These originated in the United States in the early 19th century when white people put on blacking as an entertainment. It has been argued that white, working-class audiences in North America, who were squeezed politically, economically and socially, invented 'minstrelsy' as a way of earning a living.[752] It became a distinctly American art form with its own songs, costumes and shows, grew commercially and crossed the Atlantic with ease. Whether Reginald saw the show as simple entertainment or racial mimicry is not known; but it was probably the former.

At the end of that year on New Year's Eve 1885 when he was 16, Reginald noted in his diary that everyone in the family apart from him and his father went to see 'some local negro minstrels'. He did not 'care to go' and sat the old year out smoking and reading with Mr Snell, his father's assistant.

The golliwog, or minstrel doll, grew out of the same tradition and was invented by an English woman, Florence Upton, who had grown up in the United States. In 1895, when Reginald had returned to run his father's practice, she wrote *The Adventures of two Dutch Dolls and a "Golliwogg"*[753]. In the book, the black doll was an object of fear.[754] But in contrast, ten years later, she wrote another children's book, *The Golliwogg's Fox-Hunt.*[755] This was given to Reginald's eldest son by his Uncle Fred and Aunt Ethel in 1905. The book was a Christmas present and featured a number of wooden peg dolls as well as a 'golliwog' who went fox hunting. The fox is the villain of the story, not the golliwog:

---

[751] White performers in New York first put on blackface to mock slaves on the Southern plantations depicting them as lazy, sexually avaricious and larcenous. By the mid-19th century it was a major form of entertainment. The first blackface character to become well known was 'Jim Crow' played by Thomas Dartmouth Rice who, from the 1820s performed a song called 'Jump Jim Crow', which had the lines 'First on de heel tap, den on the toes, Every time I wheel about I jump Jim Crow'. Often the performances re-enforced racial prejudice and the laws brought in by southern states after the Civil War to enforce segregation were known as Jim Crow laws. ('Blacking up was never just innocent fun' by Ben Macintyre, *The Times* 20.09.19.)

[752] Cockrell, Dale, *Demons of Disorder: Early Blackface Minstrels and their Work* (New York, Cambridge University Press, 1997).

[753] This word was sometimes spelt with three 'g's. The word nowadays is a pejorative one.

[754] The book contained the lines: 'They all looked round, as well they may, to see a horrid sight! The blackest gnome stands there alone; they scatter in their fright'.

[755] *The Golliwogg's Fox-Hunt,* Longmans, Green and Co, London.

> At night, the Golliwogg set forth, with lantern, pick and spade, to fill with faggots, stones and earth, the holes he had made.
> Said he, 'that knave is now abroad, killing the farmers' chicks, by stopping up his every door, we'll put him in a fox.'

The book is held in the Grove Family Archive.

EXHIBITIONS

There were occasional visits to exhibitions held in London. On the visit described earlier when he sat for his examinations for the Apothecaries qualification, he stayed with his Uncle James and Aunt Louise Gosling who now lived in Walthamstow, north of the East End, a stone's throw from the railway station. After their Saturday evening out in Drury Lane, first thing on Sunday morning they took a horse-drawn omnibus to London and visited the tourist sites: Horse Guards Parade and the Changing of the Guard, as well as a boat trip on the Thames. Often a journey on a London omnibus took longer than walking. Molly Hughes remembered as a child in the 1870s stopping everywhere, as there were no set stops and the driver and conductor's earnings were based on the fares generated:[756] '…the plenty for passengers rather than rapid progress was the main idea. I reckon that a journey from Islington to the West End took over an hour for a journey of about two miles.'[757]

In the afternoon Reginald and his relatives went to a service at St Paul's Cathedral, and then in the evening to another service at the large, well-known church of St Mary's Stoke Newington, five miles from where they were staying. They heard 'some good singing but did not care for the sermon'.[758]

On the Monday, Reginald, Ernest (who had joined them) and Dick walked the five and a half miles to 'the Exhibition' in Olympia from Willesden station where they had left their luggage. They spent the rest of

[756] Initially there was no set fare on omnibuses and the conductor charged what he thought the passenger would pay, passing on as little as he could to the company and sharing his gains with the driver, hence the more passengers, the better! (Flanders p. 364.)

[757] Hughes, Molly, *A London Child of the 1870s* (Papamoa Press, 2018), p. 39.

[758] St Mary's was a large church built in 1858 in the Gothic style with the renowned Sir George Gilbert Scott as the architect ; at the end of the century, besides the rector and four curates, it had 120 Sunday school teachers, 1,000 children who attended, 100 choristers and 140 mission visitors. (https://www.stmaryn16.org/history.html)

the day seeing the exhibition, and 'enjoyed it very much indeed'.

The Exhibition was spectacular. A visitor who was there the same month wrote that she

> ...also saw the riderless race of thirty-two horses, and the furious Jehu [sic] race of chariots, driven by young women in flowing robes of brilliant colours. Then the race of lady jooks [sic], a dashing pace, splendidly ridden. A grand rare show, in which the chief actors are animals ... the performing elephants are wonderful, and when at the close of their performance you felt there was literally nothing more for an elephant to do!
>
> Had the little one sat down and played on the piano, the big one singing, 'By the twilight, O my darling,' I should have taken it as a matter of course, though a little critical as to its 'method'!

The report concluded:

> There is sitting accommodation for 9,000 people, and the night I was there there were few vacancies. On Saturday, hundreds were unsuccessful in gaining entrance. Such a show has never been seen in London![759]

Such was his enthusiasm that Reginald persuaded his parents to visit in March the following year while he was still at school. The Victorians knew how to put on a good show!

Three months later another exhibition was put on – the American Exhibition featuring Buffalo Bill Cody's spectacular Wild West Show, as already described.

The forerunner of these exhibitions was staged 30 years before, called the 'Great Exhibition' which was Prince Albert's brainchild. It opened in 1851 in Hyde Park to show to the world Great Britain's technical and industrial process in goods for sale. It was later moved to a permanent location in South London on top of Penge Peak next to Sydenham Hill, an affluent suburb of large villas. Made out of cast iron and plate glass, it became known as the 'Crystal Palace'. It continued to showcase British inventions and goods until it burnt down in 1936.

In 1899, when Reginald was studying medicine at Guy's Hospital, the Greater Britain Exhibition was held at Earls Court London and opened in great style by Prince George, Duke of Cambridge. A colonial exhibition, it had a twice-daily equestrian show called 'Savage South Africa'. The

---

[759] *Western Mail* (Perth, Australia), Ladies London Gossip, 5 March 1887.

exhibition also had four mud hut villages in which 174 native men, women and children lived for the duration of the exhibition. Besides the Swazi, Zulus, Basuto and Matabele from Southern Africa, this human zoo also had Amazons from the Dinka country.[760] Again, the Victorians knew how to put on a good show!

MUSICAL CONCERTS

Reginald was taken to concerts in the town when he was at King's. It is not surprising, given that the school was a choir school steeped in classical choral music. In May 1881 he went to a 'promenade concert' in the Fellows Garden of King's College, having been given tickets by a 'Mr Poole'. In the Summer Term of 1882, he went with Reynell and older boys from the school (called 'the first division')[761] to what he described as 'a People's Concert' in the grounds of Emmanuel College which is the centre of the town. Given the magnificent grounds of the college, it must have been an impressive occasion.

Reginald went to a number of concerts at Uppingham which are described in Volume 2, as well in the school holidays when he attended smoking concerts. These were popular in this period and were men-only gatherings, which introduced new musical forms to the public. At these functions men would smoke, listen to live music and talk politics. The concert Reginald attended was put on by the Primrose League, described earlier, and held in the Corn Exchange at St Ives.

---

[760] Jackson, Lee, *Palaces of Pleasure* (Yale, 2019).

[761] They were older boys aged 12–14.

CHAPTER 16

Country Pursuits – Blood Sports, Cycling and Skating

'And you, good fenmen,[762]
Whose limbs were made in England, show us here
The mettle of your pasture; let us swear,
That you are worth your breeding: which I doubt not:
For there is none of you so mean and base,
That hath not noble lustre in your eyes,
I see you stand, like greyhounds in the slips,
Straining upon the start.'

Neville and Albert Goodman, *The Handbook of Fen Skating*, 1882

Sports and games were perhaps the biggest pastime for men as the 19th century progressed. The development of organised games is dealt with in Volume 2, but this chapter deals with Reginald's participation in popular country pursuits like blood sports, cycling and skating.

BLOOD SPORTS

The sport of aristocrats and gentry in the 18th century was game sports: hunting, fox hunting, hare coursing and horse racing. Shooting seasons were an accepted part of the annual calendar, and diaries[763] gave the dates of open and closed seasons:

> February: the pheasant, partridge shooting ended; as did hare hunting.
> March: the fox hunting ended.
> April: the oyster season began; the buck (deer) hunting season ended.
> August: the grouse and blackcock season began.
> September: the buck hunting began.
> October: the partridge shooting season began; hare and fox hunting began.
> December: the grouse and blackcock season ended.

[762] An adaptation of Shakespeare's *Henry V* Act 3, changing 'good yeomen' to 'good fenmen'.

[763] Reginald's diaries highlight most of these dates.

Living in the country, and with uncles, aunts and cousins who were farmers, shooting was a necessity to protect crops and keep vermin down; Reginald shot rooks with his uncles and cousins. Shooting game, such as pheasants, was a gentleman's sport and was part of Reginald's upbringing, especially when he stayed on holiday with his Long relatives. The game they hunted was standard fare for farmers and their families – pheasants, partridges, pigeons, snipe, hares and rabbits.

He was taught to shoot by his Uncle George when he stayed at his farm in Carleton Grange in the Christmas holidays when he 12. His diary note made no mention of what they shot but it is probable that hares were their quarry; the next day he went to a haystack to catch mice, so his hunting encompassed a range of prey! He returned again in the summer holidays in 1883 when he was 14½ years old and shot at rooks in the fields with his uncle's shotgun. At home in St Ives in the Christmas holiday when he was 15, he spent a day out with a local family, the Battcocks, mentioned previously, who farmed in the Hemingfords. He did not say what they were shooting or how the day went, but probably the quarry was snipe. Snipe was certainly in their sights when his uncles, George and Lawsell, went with some of their friends for a few days' snipe shooting in Welney[764] in the Fens in the summer holidays in 1886. That Christmas, during the holidays, he stayed with his sweetheart Mary at Shippea Hill, and went out with his cousin Hansie to shoot on the farm, but only got one shot at a pheasant and missed!

The year before on a visit to his Aunt Martha in Harpenden he went out shooting with his cousins, Henry and Frank Mardall, but the day was rather unsuccessful with only three birds winged, and of these, one was not recovered. No doubt the two were taken back to his aunts and were served up on the dining table after they had hung for a few days.

Reginald only went shooting when staying with his farming relatives.

HUNTING

Fox hunting was widespread in England but, despite living in the country, none of the Groves or Longs rode with a hunt. The main fox hunts in Cambridgeshire were the Fitzwilliam and the Oakley, while hares were

[764] Welney is a village about ten miles south-west of Downham Market and 20 miles south of King's Lynn. The group must have taken a train from St Ives via Ely to Downham Market and a trap from there to the village.

hunted by the Trinity Foot Beagles. Around Uppingham the main hunt was the Cottesmore, which was one of the earliest formed in England.[765] Cottesmore is ten miles from Uppingham to the north of Oakham. The other pack that hunted near Uppingham was the Quorn, named after the village of the same name. Quorn is 22 miles from Uppingham, so it was rare for them to come near Uppingham.

While not a fox hunting man, what Reginald was keen on at school was running with the hounds. Stoke Dry was one village where the hunt met, which was only three miles from Uppingham, and another was Ayston, even less of a distance. Sometimes, Reginald just went to watch the huntsmen and hounds, but more often it was to run behind them after the hounds gave chase to a fox. It was good training for cross-country running, of course, as well as being an exhilarating experience hearing the huntsmen's cries, the baying of the hounds and the unique sound of the hunting horn. In the Easter Term in 1886, when he was 17, he went for a ramble with his friend Berry, and near Wardley Wood, two and a half miles from Uppingham, they came across the pack and 'had a good run after them til they stopped for the day'. He went for another walk with Berry four weeks later, and this time at Ayston they encountered the hunt and 'a short run after them, but soon lost them'.

HORSE RACING

Horse racing was very popular in 19th-century England and drew large crowds from across society – especially at Ascot and Newmarket, and at the Grand National at Aintree. Observer sporting activities, like today, had a great following amongst all classes, and newspaper coverage enabled those not able to attend to be kept informed.

When he was 17 Reginald enjoyed a visit to Newmarket with his uncle and cousins to see the 2,000 Guineas Race in April 1887 as described in an earlier chapter. At Newmarket, there was flat racing but nearer home, at the Huntingdon Racecourse near the village of Brampton, steeplechasing was held. Reginald went on a couple of occasions when he was older during his holidays in September 1885. In August the following year he went with his father where they watched three races. Gambling was very

[765] It was named after the village of Cottesmore but the hunt's kennels were moved just after Reginald left Uppingham to Langham where the buildings housed 100 couples of hounds, 50 horses, and most of the 40 grooms and kennelmen of the hunt.

popular at racecourses, although Reginald never mentioned placing any bets himself.[766]

BOXING

Boxing was popular, too, during the 19th century with working men, aristocrats and gentlemen – for the latter more as a sport to be viewed, rather than to be played. For those drawn to the blood and gore there was a similarity with watching animal fights where betting intensified the excitement of the sawdust ring. While cock fighting, bull-baiting, bear and dog fighting had been outlawed in 1835 in England,[767] bare-knuckle boxing continued to be permitted.

Some measure of respectability was given by the formation of the Amateur Boxing Association in 1880, with the Queensberry Rules[768] being adopted across the country. Bare-knuckle boxing began to be replaced by the use of boxing gloves. Surprisingly, bare-knuckle fighting is still legal in Britain; the last major heavyweight bare-knuckle fight in the USA took place in 1889.

Boxing was not a sport played at Uppingham, although Reginald did have a couple of friendly bouts in his last year of school, as described in Volume 2. He boxed with his brother Ernest and was rather proud that he drew first blood. A few weeks later he had another bout with his friend Heald at Redgate but was pommelled. Heald was his own age, and his brother Ernest was two years younger and smaller, so this might explain the results of his two fights. He did not mention boxing again.

CYCLING

The development and improved design of the bicycle in the second half of the 19th century changed the lives of thousands in Victorian England; as a revolution in transport it was a close second to the railway. Before its use

---

766 The Betting Act of 1853 restricted gambling to on-course race meetings, one of which was the 2,000 Guineas meeting at Newmarket.

767 The Cruelty to Animals Act 1835 outlawed these activities in England and Wales, but they continued to be lawful in Scotland until 1895.

768 The four principles of the Queensberry Rules, named after the Marquis of Queensberry, were that contestants wore padded gloves; a round consisted of three minutes of fighting followed by a minute of rest; wrestling was not permitted; and any fighter who went down had to get up unaided within 10 seconds – if a fighter was unable to get up, he was declared knocked out, and the fight was over.

became widespread, the only transport on roads was by horse, and the cost of upkeep was far less, as was the ease of maintenance. The bicycle became affordable to many who previously could only walk.

The breakthrough in design came in 1863 with the invention of pedals by Kirkpatrick Macmillan, as propulsion of the early designs, called 'velocipedes' by the original French designer, was carried out by the rider striding along with his feet touching the ground and with no breaks. The new pedal machine was first demonstrated in London in 1869, the year of Reginald's birth, and sales immediately took off. They had solid, rubber-rimmed wheels. It could be said that he grew up in the age of the bicycle.[769]

The new craze for riding was rapid and Reginald became caught up in it in the summer holidays of 1881 when he was 12. At the beginning of the holiday he went over to the village of Earith with his father to visit Ellen Jewson,[770] a family friend and a patient, for tea. Her husband, John, died in April the next year, so it is possible that Dr Grove may have gone to see him professionally. Her husband's father, George, had started a timber business in 1836 at Earith. This expanded to include coal and building supplies when her son, also called George, moved the business to Norwich in 1868.[771]

Reginald was shown one of the new bicycling machines. He had great fun all afternoon trying to learn to balance on the two-wheeler 'boneshaker' (so called because of their solid tyres) which made for a bumpy ride. It was only after 1888 that John Dunlop invented the pneumatic tyre and riding became more comfortable. But Reginald was so delighted with it that he and his father did not get back home in the trap until 8.00pm. A few days later the family were invited to Mrs Jewson's for dinner, but it does not appear he had another try on the bicycle.

He was lent a tricycle ten days later by a 'Miss Wright' for an hour as she had heard of his interest, and he found it much easier to ride of course. He was confident enough to hire one soon after for the day from

[769] The word 'bicycle' comes from the Latin 'bi' (two) and the Greek 'kuklos' (circles, i.e. wheels) and is attributed to a Cambridge undergraduate, G. Herbert, who bought a machine and learnt to ride it around the town (Paterson, Michael, *Life in Victorian Britain* (2008), p. 144.)

[770] Mrs Ellen Jewson (1825–1904). Her husband John died in 1882 aged 66.

[771] Jewson is one of the country's biggest builders' merchants today.

'Hill's',[772] and rode to the village of Holywell to visit another family friend, Mrs Spencer, where he had dinner and then rode back. He hired it again the following morning. He was really taken by this new sport, but had to borrow another tricycle the next day from a Mr Herbert as 'somebody had broken Hill's'. He was back at King's at the end of the month, and on his second day the craze had reached the school and he was out riding again. As the weather turned colder, and the evenings drew in, football took over for the rest of term; but his appetite for riding had been whetted.

Reginald was too young to have ridden the first type of bicycle that was popular – the 'penny-farthing' – which began being manufactured in 1871. Using a larger front wheel that was thought to increase the potential speed of the bicycle, its exaggerated-sized front wheel (four-foot diameter) and much smaller rear wheel (one-foot diameter) led to its nickname. It was an apt name, as the bronze Victorian penny was perhaps four times the size of the much smaller farthing coin.

The handlebar and seat of the penny-farthing were positioned right at the top of the front wheel, so mounting the bicycle needed skill and nerve, as well as when getting off; unless a reasonable speed was achieved, the penalty was a series of wobbles ending in falling off – from a height! These difficulties led to the design of the 'safety' bicycle which Reginald rode. These look similar to those ridden today. Some versions had two seats, the tandem, where a lady might take the front seat with a gentleman, taking the rear one 'under masculine convoy and protection'.[773]

At the same time the tricycle was manufactured which did not require riders to balance and were more stable. Initially tricycles were driven by a double-cranked axle, and they might have a small steering wheel. A sales flyer from the Surrey Machinists' Company, based in Great Suffolk Street, Borough, South London,[774] of 1888 in the Grove Family Archive advertises at this late date two types of penny-farthings: the 'Invincible' Roadster No 40 and the 'Invincible' Racing Bicycle No 38. Also advertised in the Invincible range were two models of two-wheel safety bicycles, two models of tricycle, and two models of tricycle for two riders. The testimony of E. S.

---

[772] The only business person in St Ives with this surname was John Arthur Hill in Bridge Street who was a 'hairdresser and perfumer'. It seems unlikely he would hire out a tricycle.

[773] Paterson, Michael, *Life in Victorian Britain*, p. 148.

[774] The business was run by a Mr J. S. Smith with his wife; she never raced on a single tricycle or bicycle, and never on a tandem, except with her husband. (https://gracesguide.co.uk/Surrey Machinist Co)

Cheel, Esq, who was captain of the London Wheelers cycle club, enthused about the Roadster Safety Bicycle No 44 that 'it combines absolute safety, comfort and great speed over any surface, being certainly faster all round than the ordinary bicycle, and last, but by no means least, there is next to none vibration'. The flyer said that one of the tricycles for two riders was the type of machine that 'Mr and Mrs J. Smith broke the tandem records from 20 to 25 miles on 8 October 1887 (20 miles one hour 3 minutes and 44 seconds) and 25 miles (one hour 20 minutes and 6 seconds)'. A Major T. Know Helms said that 'for a resident in London, I consider this the best and safest Machine I was ever on'.

Women (or rather ladies, as cycling was a gentlewoman's activity) took up riding with enthusiasm, as for the first time it was possible to go out in public unchaperoned or without a male escort. They could only ride tricycles to begin with because the penny-farthings were unsuitable. But with the design and production of the 'safety' cycle it was possible for women to ride them in skirts by the late-1880s by which Reginald's sister was in her late-teens and likely to have taken up the activity with other young women in St Ives. Gwen Raverat describes riding at night with just a candle or oil bicycle lamps which were blown out by any gust of wind. As a young girl, being out alone was very unusual.

Riding was not without its mishaps, as the roads in towns and particularly in the country were in a poor state. Potholes, wheel ruts, cart tracks and gravel surfaces made the new craze hazardous; it was only in 1888 that borough and county councils were made responsible for maintaining the major roads.[775] This improved towards the end of the century with the growth in popularity, as well as the first tentative production of motor cars.[776]

Once the skill of riding a bicycle had been learnt (never to be forgotten!) the sense of personal freedom and mobility for this generation is difficult to imagine today. Reginald rode when he came home in the holidays, sometimes on his own and sometimes with friends like Bert Mence and Dick Naish.[777] He never owned a machine himself, but borrowed one from brother Ernest and from his friend Arnie Ulph who owned his own. As Ulph's father ran

---

[775] Under the Local Government Act.

[776] The first four-wheeled, petrol-driven car in Britain was made in 1892.

[777] Mence was the son of a local doctor who lived in Fenstanton, and Naish's father was a 'provision merchant' in Bridge Street.

an ironmongery business, he had probably begun to sell this new product to meet the growing local demand. Sometimes his rides were just for fun, like when he and Arnie rode to Earith and then Somersham.

On another occasion he rode to Cambridge but then it rained all day, and he returned by train, having arranged for Ernest's bicycle to be sent on by train. 'Ernest's bicycle came down by morning train and all was safe; he was going to ride over to Ely to see Ernest [where he was at school] but it was very dull and there was some wind', and so he dropped the idea. As the round trip to Ely was about 36 miles, this was probably best. When staying at King's College in the summer holidays with the Vice Provost Austen Leigh, he borrowed a tricycle and went for a ride to Shelford, Sawston and Babraham with Austen Leigh and two other fellows, a round trip of 16 miles 'where we saw the park but the wind was rather strong'. The park was part of Babraham Hall.[778]

At other times he ran errands for his father, like taking some medicine to Earith for a patient when he hired a tricycle for the visit in September 1885 when he was 16.

Cycling as a sport took off and cycling clubs were formed to encourage groups to ride cross-country. A club was formed in St Ives in 1877 and it carried on until 1884 when interest waned. But in May 1889, when Reginald was at Sidney Sussex College, Cambridge, a meeting was held in the Corn Exchange of 20 gentlemen to revive the club. This was agreed and the new St Ives Cycling Club was formed with Mr B. Brown of Hemingford as President, the Captain Mr H. H. Hankin as Secretary, and Treasurer Mr H. Wadsworth. It was typical of other cycling clubs. The annual subscription was fixed at 2s 6d; no uniform was required; members could wear what they wished and simply have a badge on their cap. Meetings were on Thursday evenings for a 'ride out' and occasionally there were day-long excursions. The first run was arranged for the following Thursday at 6.00pm, starting from Market Hill.[779] Reginald was not involved, but he was a keen cyclist at Cambridge and later in London, too, when he was training at Guy's Hospital and living in lodgings in south London (see Volume 3).

Cycling became a very popular pastime as the century drew to a close. In a guidebook for both visitors as well as residents, four routes from St

---

778 The Hall now houses the Babraham Institute which carries out medical research.

779 *Cambridge Independent Press* 03.05.89.

Ives were suggested, ranging from 13 to 32 miles. The shortest was from St Ives to Huntingdon via the Hemingfords and Godmanchester, returning via Hartford, Wyton and Houghton (13 miles). The longest was to Ely via Earith and Sutton, returning by Stretham, Haddenham and Earith (32 miles).[780] The countryside being flat, these routes were not arduous.

SKATING

Reginald, like his brothers and sisters, as well as his cousins, were keen Fen skaters. The origins of skating on the frozen Fenlands waters of the Isle of Ely and Cambridgeshire date back to the 17th century when Dutch engineers came to the area to build the drainage dykes and brought this sport over from Holland. The landscape today reflects their accomplishments; and they left another mark – that of the gabled roofs of the houses built in the Dutch style in the villages like Earith where some of the engineers lived.

The Fens are an area in East Anglia of deep, dark dykes (or drains, as they are called locally), intense light, willow-arched fen droves (tracks) and magnificent cloudscapes where today green and golden crops contrast sharply with the jet black, fertile soil, the fruit of the draining 200 years ago.

The two massive 21-mile drainage cuts that were dug made what became the 'Old Bedford' and the 'New Bedford',[781] half a mile parallel to each other from Earith to Denver Sluice on the coast; the 'Wash' between them flooded in winter. The fields either side of the Ouse, Cam and Lark flooded, too, creating ideal expanses for skating. The flooded meadows on the banks of the Ouse around St Ives as well as around the villages of Bluntisham, Earith and Swavesey were popular, as were the dykes and flooded meadows of the River Lark near to Prickwillow when Reginald visited his Long cousins. The best skating was to be had on the man-made drainage cuts and flooded meadows, rather than the rivers themselves, which were wide and fast-flowing with winter rain. Besides the local locations near St Ives, there were a few occasions when he skated at Uppingham, although the nearest river, the Welland, was some miles away.

Skating matches were held from the beginning of the 19th century; but the golden age of fen skating was the second half of the 19th century when the railways enabled spectators, often in their thousands, and some from as far away as London, to travel easily to the skating locations to watch

780 *Huntingdon and the Great Ouse: A handbook for visitors and residents* (1905) p. 96.

781 Sometimes called the 'Hundred Foot'.

championship matches.[782] Seven years before Reginald's father started at Huntingdon Hospital, the *Cambridge Chronicle*[783] gave this evocative description of an event in 1855 when there was an exceptionally hard winter:

> The clergy and 'squires', gentry and tradesmen – hale ploughboys and rosy milkmaids – ladies parties in carriages, gigs and carts, made their way to the bank near the bridge, and took their respective positions, where the view was excellent, and all that could be wished, for the 'St Ledger [sic] day on the ice'. A brass band of music from Chatteris was placed on the bridge, and played the most lively tunes: at the starting of a race, 'Cheer boys, cheer', and at the winning, 'See the conquering hero comes'. The number of persons present was stated at from five to eight thousand, and some said ten thousand. Punctually at the time appointed, half-past one, the racing commenced. The bold Fen-men soon appeared, whose iron frames, lion sinews, elasticity of action and body, astonished all beholders. They were a fine specimen of the bold peasantry of England. The fenmen were a hardy breed, called Fen Tigers because of the opposition their ancestors had put up to the draining of the fens two hundred years before. They addressed each other then, as they did when I was a boy as 'Bor'[784] meaning 'man'.[785]

As with sporting heroes today, Fen skating had its local champions, men like William 'Turkey' Smart (1830–1919) and 'Gutta Percha' See (1832–98). There were a number of well-known skater families – the Smart family of Welney, the Drakes of Chatteris, and the Porters of Southery.[786] The National Skating Association was set up in Cambridge in 1879, and St Ives had its

---

[782] Skating matches were held in towns and villages all over the Fens when men, and sometimes women and children, would race for prizes; sometimes cash, sometimes food (like joints of meat) and even clothing. The course was usually about a mile and a half long (660 yards twice up and down) with a barrel with a flag on it at each end. Local winners, men and women, were often invited to take part in larger championship matches. These matches attracted skaters from across the Fens. Cash prizes were put up by local landowners. These championships attracted huge crowds. Often there were up to 30 competitors paired off in heats against each other, with the winner of each heat going through to the next round. Virtually all those competing were agricultural labourers. Challenges were often made; one made in 1821 was for the fastest man to skate a mile in under 3 minutes for £100 guineas (£1,898). At Prickwillow, where Reginald was later to skate himself, a John Gittam of Nordelph skated one mile in 2 minutes 53 seconds and won the bet. The typical wage of a farm labourer was about 11 shillings a week (£69.30), so the prize money was monumental.

[783] *Cambridge Chronicle*, 17 February 1855, p. 7.

[784] Barrett, W. H., *Tales from the Fens* (Routledge & Kegan Paul, 1969), p. 64.

[785] This form of address was also used in Norfolk as well as Cambridgeshire.

[786] Dring, W. E., *The Fenland Story*, p. 32.

own branch whose Honorary Secretary was a Mr James G. Hankin,[787] whom the Grove family knew; there is no evidence, despite his enthusiasm, that Reginald joined. This branch worked hard at formulating the championship rules which were published in great detail.[788] The rules covered the heats, suggested amounts for prizes, entrance fees, the number of runners, the course length, starters, time-keeping ('the man with a bell') and the use of a blackboard to write on the name of the winners of each heat.

Up until the 1890s when a new, lightweight design made from steel was introduced from Norway, the skates used in the Fens were metal runners ('patterns') fitted onto a wooden base made of beech wood, called 'Fen Runners'. This base was then screwed into the sole of a boot[789] with three small spikes at the front which kept the skate steady. There were holes in the base for leather straps to tie it to the foot to give greater stability. The metal blades were slightly higher at the back than the front. This was the type of skate that Reginald used. His best friend's father, John Birt Ulph, besides being an ironmonger, sold 'standard' skates which were approved by the St Ives branch.[790] The price of such skates was 13–14s (£82–88).[791]

Fen skaters stooped low as they skated with a rolling gait and an extravagant, sidelong stroke of the leg. This gave an easy stride and maximum speed. There were two skating styles to achieve the poise and grace of the long, swinging, easy stride with which the fenmen covered miles of ice at lightning speed. The first was the low sweeps of the legs with the hands locked behind the skater's back,[792] and secondly, using the arms like windmills to propel the skater, much like a runner uses their arms to increase speed.[793] This was the style probably used by Reginald. Those who have skated using either style will know the thrill of hearing the ice ring to

787 Hankin ran a stationery and bookshop, and was also a printer. His business was located at The Pavement in St Ives.

788 Goodman, Neville, and Goodman, Albert, *Handbook of Fen Skating*, pp. 65–66.

789 Stout walking boots with broad, thick soles were best with the hole in the heel made with a gimlet. The advice given by the Graham brothers in their book on fen skating was that the hole should be filled with lard or soap when not in use to preserve the twist of the screw and prevent small stones getting in.

790 Goodman and Goodman, p. 250.

791 Goodman and Goodman, p. 74.

792 A method pioneered by 'Turkey' Smart who got his nickname because with his chest pushed forward he looked like a turkey.

793 The method was for both arms to be swung from side to side, keeping time with the stroke of the legs.

the swish and crackle of the skates.

For the skilled skater, considerable speed could be achieved. The average skater could cover a mile in three and a half to four minutes. A timed test of George Smart's speed over a mile course, without the advantage of any wind, resulted in a time of three minutes, which is 20mph. One champion skater, a man who went by the unusual name of Larman Register, accepted a challenge to race against a steam train in 1870.[794] The Ouse ran alongside the railway track from Littleport to Ely, a distance of 4–5 miles.[795] Racing alongside the rail track, he beat the train by about half a minute, despite the train driver apparently throwing cinders onto the ice at Adelaide Bridge from his boiler.[796] The Graham brothers reckoned that a first-class skater could achieve 16–17mph,[797] and an average one could travel at 12mph with little trouble.[798]

A game called 'bandy' was developed on Bury Fen, near Bluntisham, where Reginald skated. It was similar to ice hockey, with 11 players on each side, played with sticks and a ball, rather than a puck. The pitch was the same size as for football. Bluntisham became the home of the Bury Fen Bandy Club when it was formed in 1882 after the harsh winter of the previous year. The club laid down the rules for play; the game spread to Holland and then other northern European countries, but after the First World War it died out in the Fens. However, it is still played in Scandinavian countries.

There were three very cold winters in 1878–81, and every year there were opportunities to skate somewhere in the Fens.[799] This enabled the sport to be enjoyed during the Christmas holidays when Reginald came home; as already mentioned, there were occasionally opportunities to skate at school.

Reginald learnt to skate when he was eight or nine, which was the recommended age because by then the ankles became sufficiently strong to

---

794 *Chasing Ice: The Story of Fen Skating.* https://www.youtube.com/watch?v=mg8cpEE3pQo (12.11.19).

795 During World War II the Oxford vs Cambridge Annual Boat Race was held on this stretch of river due to the danger of aerial attack when rowing on the Thames.

796 Today the train journey takes nine minutes from Ely to Littleport.

797 Goodman and Goodman, p. 60.

798 Goodman and Goodman, p. 59.

799 The Graham brothers said that over the 40 years that preceded the writing of their book on skating in 1882 there was only one year when it had not been possible to skate somewhere in the Fens for at least one day due to the mild weather.

take the exertion and balance needed. He probably used the tested method of a wooden, high-backed chair to learn to balance. Having mastered this, the next step was to practise the leg movements needed to propel forward. The first mention made in his diary was when he skated on his 12th birthday on the flooded fields besides the Ouse from St Ives to the Old Ferry Boat Inn[800] at Holywell– a round trip of six miles.

It was here that *Hereward the Wake* was rumoured to have crossed the Ouse using the ferry at this spot when he was fleeing the troops of William the Conqueror after the Battle of Hastings in 1066.[801] As mentioned earlier, Charles Kingsley's tale in his novel *Hereward the Wake* was on Reginald's reading list of books, so no doubt his daring exploits were on Reginald's mind as he turned back towards St Ives. The following day he went skating on the nearby meadows before going back to school in the afternoon. The meadows between Hemingford and St Ives often flooded but because there were no embankments, once the ice had been formed the water underneath often drained away which left a hollow called 'cat's ice' which was very brittle and less suitable for skating. However, above the bridge at St Ives there was often 'a good piece of ice for skating'.[802]

Back at King's, the freezing weather continued as first thing in the morning the Assistant Master, Kelly, took the boys skating in Cambridge for a couple of hours. When the weather permitted, skating definitely came before school work! After the weekend, once lessons had finished at 11.00am, the boys went skating again.

Reginald went skating again the next day but wrote that it was so windy that he and other boys were blown along. That night and the following day, it snowed very hard. This was when the 'Blizzard of January 1881' struck. More heavy snow then fell which put paid to further sport, as did a head cold that landed Reginald in the sickbay for a few days. There was no further skating after this, as it thawed and the weather changed.

The weather for the next couple of years was not cold enough for skating, although on Christmas Eve 1881 when he was at King's, the boys

---

800 The inn claims to be oldest in England, with the foundations dating back to c.660 AD. The present building dates from the 17th century. The artist, William Fraser Garden, lived in the inn for 17 years until his death in 1921.

801 Another pathway was used by Hereward, known only to the Fenmen, to get to the safety of the Isle of Ely through the fen swamp and reeds of Aldreth Causeway north-east of the village of Willingham. See note in Chapter 14.

802 Goodman and Goodman, p 168.

were able to skate on some 'bad ice'. The next December snow fell and the temperature dropped: the boys at King's were able to do some skating in a field which had flooded and frozen over – perhaps on the Backs opposite King's Chapel, although Reginald was not specific.[803] Reginald chaffed that he had not brought his skates so he wrote for them to be sent to him. Sadly, they arrived after the thaw set in. The rest of December was mild and wet.

The weather in the winters of 1883 and 1884 was also mild, but while he was at Uppingham in December 1885 the temperature fell and Reginald heard that there was some skating on the Welland River. The Welland was one of the many rivers which drained into The Wash.[804] The nearest spot from Uppingham was the little village of Caldecott which was four miles from the school. A 'good many fellows went skating', Reginald noted, but not him. The next day some boys managed some skating at a spot about 2½ miles from Uppingham on an area of about an acre, but as he did not have any skates this time either, he was not able to skate. The ice and snow began to melt then, but there was still some skating before the ice vanished.

But during this Christmas holiday the weather was colder than in previous years, and in January 1886 it snowed for a couple of days and the temperature fell dramatically. On the Saturday, Reginald managed to skate for half an hour on some ice not far from his home on the side of the railway line. Word had spread that the fields at Bury Fen[805] between Bluntisham and Earith were flooded and frozen over. This area flooded easily and the ice was a mile long and a quarter of a mile wide from Bluntisham church to Earith village. By Reginald's time, the new railway from St Ives (by which he got to the skating spot) had cut the original area of fen in half, but it was still considered 'one of the best skating grounds in the Eastern Counties'.[806]

Taking the train at 11.30am from St Ives, he travelled with many others to a place where there was 'a splendid big piece of ice', although it was 'a bit rough in some places' due to the wind rippling the ice when it thawed slightly.

---

[803] A meadow was flooded for skating at Grantchester called Lingay Fen where the River Granta and the Bourne Brook met. It was three miles from the city centre. There are still lamp-posts standing in the fields where skating took place which lit the area for evening skating.

[804] Besides the Welland, the other rivers which drained into The Wash were the Withy, Nene and Great Ouse.

[805] On Ordnance Survey maps of the period this is called Bluntisham Fen, but all other references call it Bury Fen.

[806] Goodman and Goodman, p 169.

His cousin, Ted Long, and a friend, Will Langhorne, were there, and they travelled back together on the train and all had tea at Slepe House. After the weekend the thaw set in as he travelled to Shippea Hill Farm, Prickwillow, to stay with his uncle and aunt and sweetheart Mary. The weather turned cold again and his cousins went skating on the 'drains' (dykes) nearby, leaving Reginald learning his lines for the play they were putting on. After his stay was over, Reginald went home and then travelled to Cambridge to stay with Austen Leigh, King's Vice Provost. The weather was below freezing and he tried 'all morning to find skating, but they would not let anyone on'. The nervousness of the civic authorities was understandable, even before the constraints of health and safety of the 21st century.

The reason was the memory of a horrific accident that had occurred 19 years before in London Regent's Park which, coincidentally, had involved a boy from Uppingham among many others. Both Reginald's parents would have remembered the accident and been glad that the Cambridge authorities took precautions against something similar happening again.

Edward Thring, Reginald's Headmaster, wrote in his diary then that

> A fearful ice accident yesterday in the Regent's Park. Some thirty or forty people drowned; the numbers not known yet. Among them poor Woodhouse, one of our boys – a good fellow.[807] It is a great regard for true work, or trying to work truly, the not being afraid to think of those who have departed from us, but being comforted rather…[808]

The accident was widely reported with some gruesomeness in the national and provincial press[809] as the death toll was established as 41, while those

[807] Henry·Woodhouse was in Thring's house and lived in Bedford House, Tavistock Square, in Bloomsbury, London. He was 17 at the time of his death.

[808] Parkin, George *Life and Letters of Edward Thring* (Macmillan & Co Ltd, 1910), p. 13,6 Thring Diary 17.01.67.

[809] The newspapers of the time also highlight the extraordinary impact of the accident. In a society divided very much into the 'have and have nots', with the rich often being very rich and the poor being very poor. The tragedy did not discriminate between the classes. The *Glasgow Evening Post* stated that: 'Every grade of society was represented by the mourners for the lost ones. Ladies of station were sorrowfully looking after sons who had not returned last night to the homes they had left yesterday morning full of life…Poor Irish women who earn an honest penny by the sale of oranges were 'keening' at the gate, and wildly calling upon the name of the husband who brought his hot chestnuts yesterday among the skaters at the park, and ventured his life and lost it in selling them.' The same sentiment has been expressed at modern, natural disasters in 21st century.

involved were over 150. It is best described by those who experienced it themselves. One of the survivors was a Mr Dunton whose story was printed in his local paper.[810] He was on the lake with his two children, when 'without a second's warning the ice seemed to glide from under us, leaving us in water quite five feet deep'. He went on to describe his harrowing experience:

> Such a sight I hope never to see again. Quite 150 persons were struggling for life. Heads and arms were to be seen all around amongst the broken masses of ice. Two yards from me a little boy was drowning…I stood in this position for nearly half an hour, sinking down in the mud deeper every minute, until the water reached my chin. I held my children as high as possible above water until I felt my legs being cramped with the cold. I said to the eldest, 'Is there any help coming, Fred? Wave my walking-stick, for I am sinking down in the mud.' Presently the boy said, 'Father, a man is swimming to us, and we shall be saved.' On looking round, I saw a brave young fellow plunging through the ice towards me.

The frozen water was no respecter of class or age. The list of victims, printed in *The Waterford Mirror and Tramore Visitor*, showed the varying classes of people on the lake that day. Listed among the dead was 'H Woodhouse Esquire, of Tavistock Square [Thring's pupil], and an officer, Lieutenant R Edwin Scott'. Besides them there were many working men, just trying to earn a living from the skaters at the park – like James Griffin who was selling oranges to the skaters or John Bryan who was selling roast chestnuts when the ice broke up. It was reported that his portable stove later surfaced with his body. Thames fishermen from Kew were drawn in to drag their nets along the bottom of the lake to retrieve bodies, as were divers using the latest equipment of the day.[811] It was an accident that remained at the forefront of people's minds for long afterwards.

But other, less publicised tragedies occurred. The waters of the Ouse were dangerous once a thaw set in, as the flow of the river, under the ice, could wear it away from beneath so that it became treacherous. In 1881 two young men from Cambridge were drowned near Bottisham almost

[810] *Oxford Chronicle & Reading Gazette* 26.01.67.

[811] https://blog.britishnewspaperarchive.co.uk/2019/01/14/the-regents-park-skating-tragedy/ (12.11.19).

before the thaw began.[812] Another incident, which could have proved fatal, occurred upstream from St Ives below Huntingdon Bridge: a large sheet of ice on which 50 or so people were skating broke away and floated downstream. 'All those unwilling voyagers escaped, some dry and some wet, but the fright was so great that some of them have never returned on the ice since'.[813]

By the time Reginald returned to school the weather had turned milder. Sometime during the annual closure of the swimming baths and early in 1886, the south side of the baths at the school was covered in asphalt with an outer rim a few inches high to allow it to be flooded in winter to give the boys an ice rink for skating.[814] In December, Reginald's last at school, it snowed and froze for a few days but the weather then became milder, although it snowed again on the day that school broke up and on his return the weather was too mild to skate.

However, during the Christmas holidays of 1886 the conditions were ideal for skating. He managed a trip with his 15-year-old sister Mabel on some ice in Meadow Lane,[815] but they had to stop due to a snowstorm. That day he went to stay with his uncle and aunt on their farm at Shippea Hill primarily to see Mary. The next day he and his cousin Dick found a spot in 'splendid condition about a mile along the side of the river' and spent an hour and a half gliding over the ice. The next day a thaw started but he went to the same spot nevertheless, this time with cousins Hansie, Mary and Dick. The ice had a covering of water on it and the three of them fell over together. One of Reginald's legs got thoroughly wet but the others seemed all right. They decided to get back to the farm and the rain then started to come down.

In the New Year the weather turned very cold again and it remained like this for a couple of weeks. Others at Slepe House went skating on St Ives' meadow the day after New Year, but the next day there was great excitement as Uncle Hansie Long arrived to go to the skating championships being held at Swavesey on Middle Fen. The National Skating Association originated from the championships held there in January 1879.[816] Taking

---

812 Goodman and Goodman, p 164.

813 Goodman and Goodman, p 166.

814 Tozer, Malcolm, *Edward Thring's Theory, Practice and Legacy* (2019), citing a letter from Grace Thring to Parkin 06.02.86, p. 200.

815 Meadow Lane was a stone's throw from where they lived at Slepe House.

816 Goodman and Goodman, p 169.

the train from St Ives, his uncle was able to get off at the village station and, together with 6,000 to 15,000 spectators, watched 'Fish' Smart win 'again easily'.[817] The salute to such fenmen, written by the Goodman brothers whose *Handbook of Fen Skating* written in 1882 was the 'manual' on skating, could have been written for him and the others who stood, ready for the start of each heat that cold January day:

> and you, good fenmen,
> Whose limbs were made in England, show us here
> The mettle of your pasture; let us swear
> That you are worth your breeding: which I doubt not:
> For there is none of you so mean and base,
> That hath not noble lustre in your eyes,
> I see you stand, like greyhounds in the slips,
> Straining upon the start.[818]

Reginald was not able to go with his uncle as that afternoon he had to go to Cambridge to sit for a scholarship at Sidney Sussex. However, he caught the atmosphere of the event on the train. In the next carriage there were a lot of skaters who got on at Swavesey, making a lot of noise 'singing comic songs'.

But there was further skating for him after he got back home and before going back to school. Reginald skated near the 'low road' which went from St Ives to Fenstanton: 'was very grand; getting on very well with the outside edge', and then the next day his brothers and a cousin Wilfred went off to Bury Fen again by train to skate and 'seemed to have had a good day' while he stayed at home as Mary 'of course could not go', but he, Mary and cousin Ethel took to the ice by the side of the St Ives to Huntingdon railway line about 120 yards long, and he and Mary skated up and down together, enjoying themselves very much.

In the afternoon, a heavy mist came down and it seemed to wet everything through, so they stayed at home in front of a blazing fire. The last skating before going back to school was a few days later when all the younger members of the family walked to a large, flooded, frozen area between the Woolpack Inn[819] and the St Ives Workhouse, and enjoyed

---

817 Fish Smart won his third and final championship in January 1887 at Swavesey, beating his cousin Isaac See, who was the younger son of Gutta Percha. See earlier mention.

818 Goodman and Goodman, p 72.

819 There was a Woolpack Public House on the Bullock Market (now number 32, The Broadway) but this one must have been on the London Road across St Ives Bridge.

themselves for a couple of hours before walking back. That evening the thaw set in.

While he did not take part himself, at the beginning of the Easter Term there was some skating at Uppingham by boys on the Leicester Sports Ground. It was not what Reginald was used to in the Fens, as the ice formed in the water between the furrows after the ground had been ploughed.[820]

[820] Walker, Henry, *Memoirs 1886–1889* (1957), Uppingham School Archives.

CHAPTER 17

Country Pursuits – Walks and Rambles

'He was interested in every wayside flower, every bird's note, every striking bit of scenery, every shifting cloud which changed the appearance of the sky.'
George Parkin, writing of Edward Thring

The entry on New Year's Day that Reginald made in his first diary of 1881 said: 'Had three walkers to tea from Mrs Honeybourne'. Walking in the countryside was popular in Victorian middle-class society as a social activity, enabling the opportunity to chat with walking companions, and enjoy fresh air and nature; and it cost nothing apart from shoe leather. Both at his two boarding schools and at home during the school holidays, walking played an important part in his growing up.

At the time of this diary entry Reginald and his family were living in the Bullock Market in the heart of St Ives. Mrs Honeybourne was the wife of the Headmaster of the small grammar school at Manchester House which stood in front of the parish church a few minutes' walk from where the Groves lived in the Bullock Market. Manchester House had been built in the 18th century and the blue plaque at the front of the house today states that it was used as a grammar school from 1858 to 1939. Dr and Mrs Grove were extremely sociable as a couple, and in a small town like St Ives knew socially or professionally all the other residents, including the Honeybournes.

As Reginald's diaries revealed, guests, relatives as well as local friends and acquaintances frequently were invited for tea or dinner, or stayed for a few days in their home. While a walking holiday was more popular in warmer weather, St Ives was on the edge of the bleak Fen country which had a beauty of its own in winter. This may have been the attraction for the three walkers who stayed with the Honeybournes.

Walking had become a leisure activity for the middle classes by the mid-19th century, rather than a means of travelling from one location to another as it still was for agricultural and industrial workers. Horse transport was used for travel about town and trains for longer trips, for the middle classes, and walking as a means of transport was only for those from the lower-middle class in impoverished circumstances. For instance, while the painter Vincent van Gogh was living in England in the 1880s[821] and earning a modest salary as a schoolmaster, he described in his letters to his brother, Theo, the many journeys that he made on foot. After the school that he was teaching in moved from Ramsgate on the Kent cost to the village of Isleworth near Richmond, he walked the 90 miles on foot to continue in his job. Living in Isleworth, he then spent some of his free time walking to London and back, a distance of 11 miles.[822] While there was relatively cheap public transport in London and the growing suburbs for him to use, he walked instead, partly to save money but also because he enjoyed, with the eye of an artist, everything around him.

Fifty years before, when travel by train was not available, walking both short and longer distances for the less well-off was customary. The diary of a boy living in London begun in 1826 at the same age as Reginald made this clear. John Pocock's family lived in rural Kilburn on modest means, as his father was in prison for debt and died when John was 15. While there was money for clothes, presents and food on the table, John described walking everywhere, sometimes as much as 30 miles a day visiting friends in Fulham, Edgware and Battersea, or visiting the British Museum and the Royal Academy exhibitions.[823] Before he sailed as an assistant to a ship's surgeon aged 16 to Cape Town in the Cape Colony, he was a clerk to a solicitor, a house agent and a timber merchant.

What happened to the three walkers after their teatime visit to the Groves in 1881 is not known. Reginald went off by train a few days later to visit his aunt and Uncle George at their farm not far from Newmarket where he stayed a few days shooting game. After a week he returned home and took the train back to school. But ten days later, on 18 and 19 January, England was struck by a massive snowstorm, subsequently known as the 'Blizzard of January 1881'.[824] If the three walkers were still on their holiday they were confronted with nearly seven inches of snow which fell across

[821] Young van Gogh taught at three schools in England between 1876 and 1877: one in Ramsgate, and two in Isleworth, South-West London.

[822] Van Gogh, letter No 92 dated 03.10.76 (2007 edition) Van Gogh Museum, Amsterdam.

[823] Pocock, John Thomas, *The Diary of a London Schoolboy 1826–1830* (Camden History Society, 1980), edited by Marjorie Holder and Christina Gee.

[824] https://en.wikipedia.org/wiki/Blizzard_of_January_1881 (11.10.2019).

Southern England. Transport and communication links were paralysed and three-foot snowdrifts were reported in London. It was recorded in the press that about 100 people had died. By the time of the blizzard, Reginald had gone back to boarding school on 13 January where it was cold enough for him to go skating.

AT KING'S

At King's Choir School, walks to the surrounding villages around Cambridge were encouraged by the staff for the boys. Dr Reynell, as Headmaster, often went strolling with boys like Reginald, as did the Vice Provost Austen Leigh on Sunday afternoons. Playing games like tennis or football on a Sunday was not permitted, nor was boating on the river, so afternoon walks passed the time. These walks were opportunities to take in fresh air, see the countryside and chat with companions on the journey. Sometimes they were long, five- to ten-mile hikes along country roads or field tracks; or often they were more like short rambles. On Whitsun Sunday 28th May 1882, for example, Reginald walked with Reynell to Madingley church in the evening. The relationship between the boys and the Headmaster, the Vice Provost and College Fellows was relaxed, innocent and social. Walking was part of this friendly, adult-child relationship.

Reginald sometimes went to the Provost's college room for breakfast, or to pick flowers in the Fellows Gardens. This was a few hundred yards from the school on the corner of West Road and The Backs.

Walks on Sunday afternoons generally tended to take place during the winter months, rather than in the summer when he was at King's and at home for the holidays. After chapel one Sunday in the month soon after the blizzard described earlier, Reginald went for a brisk six-mile walk in the afternoon with his Headmaster, Reynell. This was the first of many such walks with Reynell; for instance, he went out walking with him in August that year, too, this time on a Saturday afternoon. While he does not mention being on any of these walks with other boys, it is likely that there were. Taking advantage of the light evenings in the summer, he went for a walk on another Sunday later that year. This walk appeared less of a hike and more of a ramble. Austen Leigh frequently played football with the Choirboys and was friendly with them all but especially with Reginald, as their letter-writing at Uppingham as well as visits in the holidays to see Leigh demonstrated.

But there were a number of adults who invited Reginald and the boys out for Sunday afternoon walks. Just before Easter that same year, Miss Reynell, the Headmaster's sister, took him for a walk on Good Friday afternoon, after chapel; in the evening on Easter Day itself, the Assistant Master, Mr Kelly, went for a walk with him, too. Kelly went with him again a year later in May 1882 on a Sunday afternoon walk to the villages of Grantchester and Trumpington.

Sometimes Reginald gave details of the walking routes taken at King's. For instance, Austen Leigh went for a 6-mile walk with him to Coton Hill and back via the Madingley Road in May 1881; they repeated the same walk a couple of months later. The same route was taken in April 1882 with Reynell. And he mentioned that in another walk taken with Austen Leigh later in the summer, the village of Madingley was their destination. Then again they did an eight-mile walk two months later on a Sunday afternoon with a Mr Briscoe, nearly reaching Haslingfield which is six miles south-west of Cambridge. In May the next year he did a ten-mile walk to the other side of Coton with a Mr Nixon, and then with a Mr Biscoe another similar walk two weeks later; both were Fellows at King's.

ST IVES

During the school holidays, a gentle walk into the countryside around St Ives or along the riverbank was a family affair, which including guests staying for the weekend or perhaps for the day. One Sunday afternoon in June 1882, when he was 13, before going to the evening service at church was one such time. Reginald, his cousins Dick and Hansie Long (who had come for tea), and Mr Ewart, his father's Medical Assistant, all went for a walk. In 1882 Reginald got home for the Christmas holidays on Boxing Day, and the next day he and Mr Ewart walked to the village of Needingworth – a round trip of just under four miles. Another example was in January 1885 when he walked with cousin Edith Gosling after church to see their Uncle George in Hemingford and had tea.

At home, Reginald described numerous Sunday afternoon walks with his family and visiting guests.

UPPINGHAM

When he went to Uppingham he enjoyed walking with other boys, and it was an activity encouraged by Edward Thring. John Skrine, a boy at Uppingham and later a master, commented that

> the Rutland pasturelands are excellent for walker. The views are pleasant, if not remarkable, and you may wander to see them almost where you like. The woodsides, the broad, greenrides [sic], the field paths, and their styles…[825]

Another boy who joined in 1888 described 'the peace of the rolling pastures, the wide undulating valleys, and the warmth of its rich red soil, dotted with villages and homesteads of mellow tawny stone'. He went on to say that he was

> free to explore Stoke and Wardley[826] woods, to spend afternoons failing to jump the Stockbrook or other streams, to follow the hounds with perhaps the friendly help of a stirrup leather from some kind hearted sportsman to help us back home to call-over or tea.[827]

Reginald loved the area and enjoyed wandering in this countryside.

Thring himself was a keen walker who continued to take 'really good' walks until within a few days of his death.[828] As stated at the beginning of the chapter, his friend and biographer Parkin said of him that 'he was interested in every wayside flower, every bird's note, every striking bit of scenery, every shifting cloud which changed the appearance of the sky'.[829] His favourite Latin tag was 'Solvitur Ambulando' or 'we solve it by going on' (literally 'it is loosed by walking').[830] Thring encouraged his pupils to take an interest in nature through these rambles, and Reginald loved to go out into the countryside around Uppingham. Sometimes the route taken by Reginald was the road from village to village; on occasions it was across fields, footpaths or bridleways. Edward Hornung,[831] in his novel *Fathers of Men*, based on his personal experiences at Uppingham,[832] described the sort of walk that Reginald and his friends took:

---

825 Skrine, John, *A Memory of Edward Thring*, p. 113.

826 Stoke Wood was a couple of miles to the south, and Wardley Wood a mile or so to the west of the town.

827 Graham, John, *Forty Years of Uppingham* (Macmillan & Co., 1933), p. 5.

828 Thring's diary 12.10.87 Uppingham School Archives.

829 Parkin, George, *Life and Letters of Edward Thring* (Macmillan & Co Ltd, 1910), p. 503.

830 Thring used this tag as a motto for the first meeting of the Headmasters' Conference in 1869 (Alicia Percival, *Very Superior Men* (1970) Charles Knight, p. 186).

831 Ernest Hornung was at Uppingham 1880–83 in Mr Constable's house just before Reginald joined. (Uppingham School Roll 1824–1905.)

832 Hornung, E. W., *Fathers of Men* p. 70.

> And off they went, but not with linked arms,[833] or even very close together; for Chips still seemed annoyed at something or other, and for once not in a good mood to talk about it or anything else. It was unlike him; and a small boy is not unlike himself very long. They took the road under the study windows, left the last of the little town behind them, dipped into a wooded hollow, and followed a couple far ahead over a stile and along a right-of-way through the fields; and in the fields, bathed in a mellow mist, and as yet but thinly dusted with the gold of autumn, Carpenter found his tongue.

The first friend with whom Reginald went for walks to the surrounding villages like Ridlington was a boy called Charles Blois from Redgate, Reginald's house. From January to May 1884 they went on ten walks together. Blois was the son of Sir J. R. Blois of Cockfield Hall, Yoxford, Suffolk.[834] Sadly, the Uppingham School Roll records that Blois died on a voyage to Australia in 1900 when he was 33. Another friend in his first year, with whom Reginald went walking, was Charles Evans, also from Redgate. They went walking together four times from January to April 1883. Evans died young, too, in 1892 aged 23, having become an engineer.

Reginald had other friends like Evans, and the three of them also went off for walks together – in March 1884 they walked to the Glaston Tunnel and back. There were walks in 1885 to Oakham, Stoke, Wardley and Thorpe. But the walk that capped them all was a much longer one.

THE GREAT NORTH ROAD WALK

Walking home at the end of term was Berry's idea. Early in February 1887 he put his proposal to Reginald to walk from Uppingham to Wansford, cross the River Nene to join the Great North Road, and then turned south to Huntingdon. A total distance of 36 miles.[835] At Huntingdon, Berry suggested that they parted company – he going on by train to Sandy, and Reginald to St Ives. If they got up and started very early, they believed they could do it in a day.

The plan was hatched and training commenced over the next ten weeks. They were used to walking some distance – the previous November

---

833 In fact walking arm in arm by friends was common and accepted as a token of friendship, nothing more. *Fathers of Men* p. 79: 'they were always about arm in arm together'.

834 The Hall stood in 40 acres. The house remained in the ownership of the Blois family until 1997.

835 In fact, the distance from Uppingham to Huntingdon is 46 miles according to the Uppingham School prospectus 1960.

they had walked eight miles together to the village of Belton. In fact, after second chapel on the day the plan was agreed, they both went for 'a sharp walk', Reginald noted in his diary. The next week they went for a walk to Kirby Hall,[836] a distance of six miles. Writing of Kirby Hall, Reginald commented that it must have been a fine old building in its day. But it had been 'left to go to ruin and is now little more than a shell remains'. But to Reginald and Berry, 'this itself is worth our visit'. On part of the way back to school they ran about a mile downhill and got back in an hour and a quarter. Training continued the following day with a walk around Wardley and Stockerston of about seven miles.

Taking time out of school study to train did not seem to be a problem, although they had not shared the plan with anyone else. But training was sporadic and not particularly as demanding as studying and editing the School Magazine which took up much of his time (see Volume 2). Reginald's interest in taking brass rubbings began to grow and he combined visits to local churches with training for the big walk. So, for example, they went to Braunston Church and took two brasses, then into Brook Church on the way home, then across fields to Manton for more rubbings.

Both went for a 'good grind',[837] as Reginald described their walk on 4 April to the small village of Blaston to the south of Uppingham and across the county boundary into Leicestershire; they returned through the hamlet of Horninghold, which was a round trip of 11 miles. This area was all new to them both. By now their plan had been shared with their Housemaster, and the next day after dinner, with both having been given 'call-over' leave by Revd Christian, they walked to Deene about eight miles away to visit the church there. They returned through Harrington and Seaton at 'a tremendous pace', and after Seaton were 'just about done out'. They got back to Redgate a quarter of an hour late. This was a serious matter, especially as they were praepostors; setting a good example for the rest of the boys in the house was an important part of their role. The penalty was to report themselves to Thring the following day! This was not a pleasant prospect.

However, Thring's punishment was to cancel any further times when they were excused 'call overs' that term. Given that the term ended in less

[836] Kirby Hall is now owned by English Heritage. It is deemed one of England's greatest Elizabethan and 17th-century houses. It was once owned by Sir Christopher Hatton, Lord Chancellor to Queen Elizabeth.

[837] Taken from the expression 'keeping one's nose to the grindstone'.

than a week, Reginald did not feel this was harsh.

A 'slope into the fields' with Berry in the afternoon after school the next day was a far from pleasurable experience as there was a cold north-east wind on their way home; Reginald developed a nasty cough that evening and did not feel up to any study or even reading a novel. He felt better the next day, which was Good Friday, and had a lie-in before morning chapel. Before afternoon chapel, Berry and Reginald went for a short walk at a slow pace. It was now just four days before their epic walk at the end of term. He got a letter from his father on Easter Day[838] asking, tongue in cheek, whether a stretcher should be provided next Thursday! On Bank Holiday Monday, Berry and he managed an eight-mile walk to the north-west of Uppingham, passing through Wing, Manton, where there was a small station, and back through Preston. Back at school, he had to go in for an exam at 4.30pm in Latin translation.

Two days before the end of term, on Tuesday 12 April, school work carried on as normal and Reginald was meant to write about the life of Cicero. He 'couldn't do a word nor remember a date so I hadn't the least groundwork to go on and had to show up a blank. The day was wasted and I hope that Thring will not be wild with me.' But he felt, in mitigation, that several others had done as badly. Thring's reaction is not known.

Afterwards, Reginald went for a walk with Berry to a nearby village, Ridlington, north of the town, over the fields, and went back by a different way – a six-mile round trip, and further preparation for the walk to Huntingdon. 'The weather was splendid', he commented. This was in stark contrast to what he was to face on his walk two days later.

That evening, after callover, he and Berry went for another walk east over fields to the village of Bisbrooke, and then continued further to reach the Rugby and Stamford Railway three miles from the town. Walking beside the lines along a deep cutting and before a tunnel, they turned back towards Uppingham, returning through another village called Glaston (where they had been previously to see the house where the vagrant had died) totalling a round trip of seven and a half miles. This last part of their walk was the route they were to take two days later on their walk home.

The next day, Wednesday 13 April, was the last day of term.

Reginald packed his 'play box'. There were no lessons (or 'first school'); second school was supposed to be a lesson with one of the masters, with

[838] Interestingly, there was a postal delivery service on a Sunday.

Howson,[839] but the lesson was cancelled and individual work in studies was meant to take place but 'nothing much to do', Reginald commented. He prepared for the following day by buying a stick of tobacco for the walk. Whether this was to chew or smoke is not clear.

Getting up at 4.00am when it was still dark,[840] Berry and Reginald had a quick breakfast and then got underway just after 5.00. Dawn was just breaking but it was a cloudy day. Their walk down to the village at Wansford to join the Great North Road was 14 miles from Uppingham. Reginald described this part of the trip as 'lovely' in the cool of the morning. As the modern A47 road from Uppingham to Peterborough was built years later, their route took them on narrow country lanes which were little more than tracks through the villages of Glaston and Morcott. They then went over fields to Tixover. There they joined a lane at Duddington and thence to Wansford.[841]

Arriving at 8.25am they wanted a short break at an inn, and having crossed the River Nene over the medieval bridge, they walked into what they believed was the Haycock coaching inn.[842] They found to their consternation that, only a week before, the inn sign had been taken down and it was now a private house. They were directed to the Mermaid Tavern nearby; they then had a 'splendid breakfast' of milk and eggs. They were told with pride by the staff that Dick Turpin had apparently stopped there for a drink during his famous ride.[843] The inn was demolished in the next century to improve the traffic flow from what then was the Leicester Road and the Great North Road.

It was only a 45-minute break and then they went on their way down Ermine Street (or the Great North Road, as it was also known). The modern A1 road is now a motorway and the modern route bypasses the villages

---

839 George Howson taught at Uppingham from 1886 to 1887 and then went on to be the Headmaster at Gresham's School, Norfolk. (see Volume 2). One of Reginald's sons, David Grove, went to Gresham's (see Volume 3).

840 Sunrise was at nine minutes past 5.00am.

841 Ordnance Survey Map first edition.

842 The Haycock Inn, now a hotel, was built as a coaching inn and called this, so tradition records, because a man was swept down the river in flood when he fell asleep on a haycock (bale of hay) which got stuck under the bridge there.

843 Legend has it that the highwayman Dick Turpin on his sturdy mount, Black Bess, rode the 200 miles from York to London in 1735. His route was the Great North Road. It is estimated that if he had stopped at every inn that claimed he had visited it, then his journey would have taken many months!

that they walked through – Chesterton and then through the crossroad of Norman Cross to Stilton, famous for its unique cheese.[844]

Shortly after starting this nine-mile stretch the weather changed dramatically, with heavy hail lashing down on them. Such was its ferocity that they had to walk sideways, heads bowed against the hail. The choice of inns in Stilton, despite being where the cheese was sold, was limited, and eventually they chose 'The Talbot' which still stands today in the centre of the long village street. Reginald said it was 'an awful hole'. However, they managed to wash their feet but found that Berry had a very bad 'smashed blister' on his heel. Reginald had lost a lot of skin off his toes, too, so they were not in good shape. Downstairs they had some bread and cheese (surely Stilton?!) and beer.

It was 11.15 in the morning and they had been going for six hours. An hour later they were on the road again, but being very footsore their progress was slow to start with; they soon quickened their pace as they got back into the rhythm of walking. They stopped at another wayside inn for a quick break of ten minutes. Reginald does not say where this was and they then continued for another 12 miles to Huntingdon, arriving at 3.35pm very footsore. It had taken them just over ten hours in all.

They kept their muscles from seizing up by walking around the town until Berry's train left for his home at Sandy at 4.45pm, and Reginald caught his train for St Ives 45 minutes later at 5.30pm. Before they parted they agreed that despite the blisters and tiredness they had had a very enjoyable day:

> Coming down the old North Road we had the wind behind us and hardly any sun and though there were a good many hail storms they only caught our backs so really everything was in our favour.

He was home by 6.00pm and had a bath and a 'good rub down', and he 'anointed my sore places which were really very trivial'. An early night followed and next day he only felt stiff in one foot. His family was surprised that he had walked the distance. Their reaction is interesting as walking long distances in Victorian times whether on holiday, for leisure or for work, was commonplace. So ended Reginald and Berry's epic walk.

---

[844] The particular type of blue cheese known as Stilton was first sold in c.1730 by the owner of the Bell Inn in Stilton, having discovered the distinctive cheese in a farm in Melton Mowbray in Leicestershire. Wagonloads of the cheese were sold to him and because of the inn's location on the Great North Road its popularity spread. Reginald does not mention the Bell Inn on his visit to Stilton, but it still stands today.

Part 3

Belief and Unbelief

***

CHAPTER 18

Nisi Dominus[845]

'Unless the Lord builds the house.'
Inscription above the porch at Tenterleas House,[846] St Ives,
built in 1937 by Reginald and Hilda Grove.

Seventeen-year-old Reginald had had a busy day on New Year's Eve 1886. After spending the morning with his old Headmaster from King's, Dr Reynell, who had come with his wife the day before to stay with the family, Reginald took the train to Bluntisham, spending the afternoon until 4.00 skating there. After writing some cards and letters, and seeing the Reynells off by train, Reginald, his sister Mabel and their cousin Alice Long went to All Saints Parish Church. He saw in the New Year listening to a sermon given by the young vicar, Revd Luke Paget. The service started at 11.30pm and they were home by 12.45am, and in bed at 1.15.

'Watch night' services, when Christians saw in the New Year through worship, prayer and reflection, had been a custom at All Saints for some years. A newspaper report seven years previously recorded that evensong on New Year's Eve (1878) was sung at 10.45pm: 'A very large congregation were present, the sermon preached by the Vicar[847] as the old year passed away and the bells ushered in the new year, the whole congregation knelt for some minutes in silent prayer. Holy Communion was immediately administered to a great number.'[848] The church had seating for 680, although it is doubtful whether there were that number there that night.

Reginald had previously gone to a midnight service on New Year's Eve 1882 when he was 13, but this could well have been because it was expected of him, rather than because he wanted to be there. But as he grew older, he became his own man and went to services for years on his own accord because of the personal faith he now had.

---

845 Psalm 127: Unless the Lord builds the house.

846 The original spelling used was 'Tenter Leas' (*Kelly's Directory of Huntingdonshire 1914*).

847 Revd Charles Dashwood Goldie was vicar from 1866 to 1886.

848 *All Saints Church Magazine* February 1879.

On the cross surmounting his grave is inscribed a verse from Psalm 57:8. Taken together with verse 9 it reads:

> My heart is fixed, O God, my heart is fixed. I will sing and give praise. Awake up, my glory, awake, psaltery and harp, I myself will awake early.[849]

Why it was chosen by Hilda, his wife, and their children is not known, but it is likely to have been a favourite of his. In the psalm the writer cries out to God in the midst of difficulties, and expresses that He alone can save him. It ends with a declaration of praise. If the psalm and these verses were not a favourite of his, perhaps the choice reflected how his family saw Reginald's life and faith, lived to God's glory. For there is no doubt that his lifelong faith as a Christian was nurtured both at home and at the two schools he attended as he grew into manhood. His faith, as a boy and a young man, was relational and shaped by his parents and particularly by three men in his life – Dr Vincent Reynell at King's, Revd Luke Paget at St Ives, and Revd Edward Thring at Uppingham. Thring's contribution is described in Volume 2 although Reginald did not recognize this at the time. When he was in his third year at Cambridge, his Old Uppingham friend Edward Weaver[850], who was at Trinity reading law, gave him a copy of John[851] Skrine's *A Memory of Edward Thring.*[852] He was delighted to be given it but commented in his diary:

> what a splendid man he was and how little I cared for him and why didn't I attend more to his teaching. But I'm afraid I am any common or garden person and must get all my ideas second hand.[853]

A GROWING FAITH

After his confirmation as a boy at King's aged 14, he attended church at home and chapel at Uppingham. He took Communion as often as he could. At Uppingham this took place after first chapel for those boys and

[849] From the King James Authorised Version of the Bible, which Reginald would have used.

[850] Edward Weaver went to Uppingham the year before Reginald and was at The Lodge; he left at the same time as Reginald in the summer of 1887. Both went up to Cambridge in September that year, one to Trinity and one to Sidney Sussex. Both had been School Praepostors. Weaver went on to become a barrister.

[851] He called Skrine 'Jock', a nickname that has never been identified as being used before.

[852] This 1887 first edition copy is in the Grove Family Archive, with Weaver's inscription in the fly leaf.

[853] Diary 12.02.90

masters who stayed on afterwards. Reginald took a keen interest as he grew older in what was preached on Sundays, whether at home or at school. Some sermons were commended in his diary, others less so. In the Easter holidays of 1886, when the parish church at St Ives had no vicar, prior to Paget's appointment, he went with his father to a Lenten evening service at All Saints and commented that Chamberlain[854] of Godmanchester preached 'splendidly'. In the summer holiday that year, when he was staying with his uncle and aunt at their farm, he attended the local village church at Prickwillow in the evening, and noted that 'Mr. Kingdon [the vicar] preached a splendid sermon on "our mission in life" from the text of the barren fig tree'. This parable was about a tree not producing fruit as it was designed to do.[855]

At school he noted those preachers whose sermons resonated with him; for instance, Revd Alfred Tuck, one of the masters, preached in February 1886 'rather a good sermon'. The next month, Revd Vale Bagshawe, who was the Master of the Lower School, preached with 'great effect'. In his last few weeks at school, he heard 'a splendid sermon in aid of St John's Foundation School[856] for the Sons of Clergy at Leatherhead'.

In the last two terms at Uppingham he began to go to Thring's own house, School House, for prayers on Monday evenings, which he commented was a 'new experience' for him. Clearly he was seeking something new in his spiritual life, but these evenings were not always uplifting; in June 1887 the 'prayers were awful lengthy (and) included a hymn'!

MATER AND PATER

Reginald's parents had been married at the parish church of Carlton-cum-Willingham in Cambridgeshire in February 1868, a year before he was born. He was 30 and she was 24. They arrived in St Ives as newly-weds just before the appointment of Revd Goldie as vicar. They attended the parish church all their lives in St Ives throughout Goldie's ministry and that of his successors;[857] and all their children were baptised there. Both his father

---

[854] Revd Henry Hart Chamberlain was an Oxford graduate appointed to Godmanchester St Mary's Parish Church in 1874. He was aged 44 when he preached at St Ives. He died in 1899 aged 57 and a plaque to his memory is in the chancel of the church.

[855] Luke 13:6–9.

[856] The school was founded in 1851 and is still in existence as St John's Leatherhead.

[857] The vicars during the period covered by this book were Revd Charles Dashwood Goldie 1866–86, Revd Luke Paget 1886–87, and Revd Edward Tottenham 1887–91.

and his mother played an important role within the life of the church, with Reginald's father serving as one of the two churchwardens[858] in the 1880s. As he was the Vicar's warden he must have got on with Goldie, although many others did not; Goldie was an abrasive man.

Reginald noted in his diary that Goldie died on the morning of 11 January 1886. While his father had been in attendance at the vicar's bedside, Reginald had other things on his mind as he left that afternoon to visit his sweetheart, as described in an earlier chapter. Six days later, Goldie was buried. Reginald did not attend the funeral as he was still staying with Mary, as she 'had pressed me to stay'.

The fact that his parents were married in church did not necessarily mean they were believing Christians, although registry office[859] marriages had been legal for 30 years as an alternative to a religious ceremony. Many couples continue to be married in a church purely as nominal Christians. Reginald was christened[860] as a baby on 17 February 1869 when he was one month old at St Ives Parish Church. This public ceremony was arranged by his parents with the vicar, as the christening of babies was, and still is, the custom of the Church of England. His godparents made promises at the christening service to support him in prayer and by personal example. They were his father's brother Joseph Francis Grove (Uncle Frank)[861] and his mother's brother Hanslip Long (Uncle Hanslip) and her sister Martha Mardall (née Long). Interestingly, Hanslip had signed the marriage register as a witness at Reginald's parents' wedding. Their marriage and Reginald's christening could have been merely a rite of passage conforming to the custom of their class, but other evidence points to them being professing and practising Christians.

His father left no diaries or any personal writings, so his reflections on faith have not been recorded directly. However, at his father's funeral in December 1895, as Dr Grove's coffin was interred in the drizzle of an

---

858 *Hunts County News* 01.05.86 report on the annual vestry meeting.

859 Prior to 1836, all marriages took place in Church of England churches even if the couple were not members. Civil marriages became lawful with the Marriage Act of 1836. This allowed for non-religious civil marriages to be held in registry offices set up across England and Wales in cities and towns. The act also meant Nonconformists and Catholic couples could marry in their own places of worship, according to ways of expressing the vows in their own rites.

860 All Saints Church St Ives Parish Register 1 1853–1920 Huntingdon Library Archive.

861 As noted earlier, Reginald had to wait for his christening present until he was nearly 18. At Christmas 1886 Uncle Frank gave him a christening mug with his name and the family crest engraved on it.

overcast winter's day, the mourners sang the hymn 'Now the Labourer's task is o'er'.[862] As the local newspaper reported, it was 'rendered with much effect'.[863] This hymn, plus its refrain, was chosen with care by his widow and family to reflect his Christian life of love and service. The first line was 'Now the Labourer's task is o'er; now the battle day is past; now upon the farther shore lands the voyager at last'. The refrain after each verse was: 'Father, in thy gracious keeping, Leave we now thy servant sleeping'.

Back in 1869, Reginald's parents, mindful of the instructions given in the book of Proverbs that a child should 'keep your father's commands and do not forsake your mother's teaching, bind them upon your heart for ever: fasten them around your neck',[864] brought him up to honour God and follow Christ's teachings. This was similar to many, although not all, in middle-class Victorian England. The Groves' denominational tradition was the Established Church of England. For many families, and certainly for most middle-class families, weekly church attendance was customary whether they belonged to the Anglican or Nonconformist churches or the growing number of Roman Catholic churches. Reginald was brought up to attend services each Sunday at the parish church a short distance from where the family lived in the Bullock Market. The wisdom of the proverb to 'train a child in the way he should go and when he is old, he will not turn from it'[865] was followed by Reginald's parents at an early age.

Manuals for parents were popular then, as now, and *Train Up a Child in the Way He Should Go* by John Charles Ryle, the first Anglican Bishop of Liverpool, was a popular guide which Dr and Mrs Grove were likely to have used. Originally published in 1846, it ran to a number of reprints. In another of his books, *Thoughts for Parents,*[866] he advised that 'kindness, gentleness, long suffering, forbearance, patience, sympathy,[867] a willingness to enter into childish troubles, a readiness to take part in childish joys, these are the cords by which a child may be led most easily, these are the

---

[862] This hymn was written by John Ellerton (1826–93) for *Church Hymns* (1871). Ellerton was one of the editors. It was printed in the second edition of *Hymns Ancient and Modern* (1875) which was used in the Church of England and was thus well known to the Grove family.

[863] *Hunts County News* 04.01.96.

[864] Proverbs 6:20.

[865] Proverbs 22:6.

[866] Ryle, John, *Thoughts for Parents* (William Hunt & Co, 1886), p. 8.

[867] These qualities are given in Galatians 5:22–23 as evidence of the fruit of the Holy Spirit.

clues you must follow if you would find the way to his heart'.

He continued:

> Children are weak and tender creatures and, as such, they need patient and considerate treatment. We must handle them delicately, like frail machines, lest by rough fingering we do more harm than good. They are like young plants and need gentle watering, often but little at a tim.[868]

From Reginald's diaries there is a real sense that this was his experience. In most middle-class households, family prayers were held daily with the children and servants. Reginald made no mention of family prayers in the Grove household when he was at home during the holidays; this may have been because it was so usual that it merited no mention. More likely it was because of the frequency of his father being called out to visit patients at all times of the day and night, which made it difficult to establish a morning pattern of family prayers.

DR VINCENT REYNELL AND HIS SISTER MARY

When he went to King's Choir School, choral practice in the Chapel on weekdays and attendance at services on Sundays became the regular rhythm of his week. As highlighted in Volume 2, he noted the different anthems sung each week and enjoyed Chapel. Reginald was steeped in the services and ceremonies of the Church of England. Attendance at church and at King's College Chapel was initially a duty; it later became a joy for him.[869]

Reginald's enthusiasm at King's was such that he also went to other services in Cambridge. He was encouraged by Mary Reynell, the sister of the Headmaster. She lived at the school as the housekeeper[870] before her brother was married in the summer of 1883. Reginald accompanied Miss Reynell on Sunday evenings to the 13th-century St Edward's Church[871] in the centre of the town where a new preacher was becoming well known.

---

[868] Ryle, pp. 9–10.

[869] From the Book of Common Prayer: The Communion Service; 'it is *our duty and our joy*, at all times and in all places to give you thanks and praise, Holy Father, heavenly King, almighty and eternal God, through Jesus Christ …'

[870] Reynell had two sisters, Mary and Rosa. It is not clear from any records whether Mary or Rosa helped him as his housekeeper. As Mary was the elder, I have assumed that she was his housekeeper before he got married.

[871] St Edward King and Martyr is on Peas Hill in Central Cambridge.

He was Revd John Lias[872] who had been appointed as the vicar in 1880. Word spread about him and Reginald went on four consecutive Sunday evenings in July 1881. He also went in the Autumn Term of 1882 on further occasions, once with four other boys. On another he went again with Miss Reynell and two other boys – Buck and G. Lobb. In addition to his role as a vicar, Lias was a lecturer in Literature at the university and went on to write a number of theological works later recognised for their erudition. One publication, arising out of lectures that he gave in 1883 was *The Atonement Viewed in the Light of Certain Modern Difficulties*.[873] In the view of an unknown critic, 'the evangelical theory of the Atonement may pass as a possible explanation or contribution towards an explanation of a stupendous mystery', but ought to be neither imposed nor accepted as 'a fundamental article of faith'. Those who hold it therefore 'have no right to impugn the orthodoxy of those who resort to other explanations of the Lord's proprietary work'.

Then, as now, theological arguments persisted.

But whatever his theological views, Lias must have had a powerful preaching style to draw a young boy like Reginald and Miss Reynell to hear him. Reginald went with her to services on other occasions, too, and her influence helped sow the seeds of Reginald's growing faith. How many like her have played a pivotal role in quietly nurturing faith in the young?

Reynell and Reginald joined King's Choir School more or less together. Reynell and his sister took young Reginald under their wing as a boarder and they (and then Reynell's wife) became friends of the Grove family. Some years after Reginald left King's, Reynell felt a call to ordained parish ministry, having been Headmaster for nine years. He left in 1887 and by then had carried out a number of significant reforms which had a lasting impact on the school. In the testimonial given him by the Provost at that time, Augustus Austen Leigh, it stated that:

---

872 He was rector from 1880 to 1893 and went on to become Chancellor of the Diocese of Llandaff in South Wales. He wrote for the *Encyclopaedia Britannica* 1911. He died in 1923. He was the University of Cambridge Hulsean Lecturer in 1883/84. These lectures were on divinity. One of his works was 'Are Miracles Credible?' (https://en.wikisource.org/wiki/Author:John_James_Lias (19.03.19).) A framed photograph of him is displayed at St Edward's Church which shows a bewhiskered, serious-looking man.

873 Lias, James, *The Atonement Viewed in the Light of Certain Modern Difficulties* (1888), James Nisbet.

> the boys are drawn from a higher class than formerly, and come from all parts of England, and they receive a classical education, at very small cost to their parents, until their voices break, or they are of an age to go to public school. Besides the musical gain to the College something is thus done towards restoring the advantages of a liberal education to a class which the founder meant to benefit, but which is apt to be left behind in an age of unrestricted competition.
>
> Austen Leigh also said that
>
> in his general teaching Mr. Reynell is careful and conscientious. The boys, who have left the choir school, have generally taken good places and are doing well in public schools such as Uppingham and Malvern College.

But more importantly, Austen Leigh said that

> his strongest point appears to me to be the moral and religious training of young boys. Under his eye the school has been singularly free from moral taint, and the tone of the boys has always been a high one. Indeed, the excellent character of these boys, who have passed through the school, is the best testimonial that can be given to their headmaster.[874]

Reginald was one such boy.

While Reynell was tough on moral discipline (see Volume 2) and gave out punishments of detention and caning, his personal example and encouragement were a strong influence on Reginald's life. With the formality of the age, Reginald referred to him in his diary as 'Dr Reynell', but he corresponded with him after he left King's regularly, even remembering to send Reynell birthday cards.[875]

At King's the Reynells became friends with the Grove family and they were invited to St Ives for day visits or to stay longer. Dr Grove and his wife clearly enjoyed their company. In August 1883 in the summer holidays before Reginald went to Uppingham, the newly-wed couple visited the family at St Ives for the day; in the evening they and the Goldies dined together at the Groves and then left afterwards to go back by train to Cambridge. Two weeks before Christmas 1886, Reginald got permission to leave Uppingham to take scholarship exams for Corpus Christi College in Cambridge, staying a couple of nights at the school while he did

---

874 Cited by R. J. Henderson, *A History of King's College Choir School*, p. 33.

875 Reginald's card for Reynell's birthday on 8 April 1886 cost 4d (£2.00).

this. On arrival he chatted with 'Dr and Mrs Reynell all the evening'. After Christmas that year, the Reynells came to stay with the Groves before returning home before New Year. During some of his holidays at Uppingham Reginald visited the Reynells and stayed with them.

Reynell also wrote regularly to Reginald and vice versa. Such was their friendship that gifts were regularly exchanged; Reginald bought some photographs of Uppingham to send him in March 1884. He posted Reynell a birthday card[876] again in April 1886, and Reynell sent a thankyou note a few days later. While staying at King's with Austen Leigh, the Vice Provost, he saw Reynell who gave him 'two books bound in parchment (*Vicar of Wakeford* and *English Dramatists*) for getting on so well at school'. Clearly he was very fond of Reginald and wanted to encourage him. When he resigned from his position at King's in October 1886, he wrote to Reginald to let him know. Reginald wrote in his diary that he supposed it was 'on account of frequent trouble with the College'. Reynell must have told him about these difficulties in his previous letters. Later, Reginald was asked to subscribe to a testimonial (leaving present) by Alan Guy, one of the boys from the King's Choir. He wrote that 'it was very awkward as they do not know what sort of present they want to give him and how much they want from me'. He wrote back to Guy to ask what other Old Boys were giving. Guy wrote back to ask for a sovereign[877] (£132.00) and Reginald then wrote to his father for help, as this was a large sum for a schoolboy. Thankfully his father sent him the sovereign as requested.

Reynell left no record of his own beliefs or thoughts (in either a diary or letters that have survived) but his mentoring of his old pupil was hugely influential. He encouraged Reginald to be confirmed in his faith aged 14 on 10 March 1883. Reginald was younger than most who sought confirmation. When he was at Uppingham he noted in his diary that the boys being confirmed in the school chapel for boys were generally older than he was. The fact that he wanted to be confirmed at an earlier age points to a personal decision to affirm his beliefs.

Reginald's confirmation service took place at All Saints Church[878] in Jesus Lane in central Cambridge, and was conducted by the Bishop of Ely,[879]

[876] This card cost 4d, too.

[877] A guinea was 21/- or one pound and one shilling, and was a gold coin.

[878] All Saints Church was a modern building opened in 1870.

[879] Diary 10.03.86 when details of the bishop were noted.

James Woodford.[880] His school friend Radcliffe was confirmed with him. His mother and father were in the congregation. During the service he publicly affirmed the promises made by his parents and godparents at his christening 14 years earlier. The bishop then laid hands on him to pray and confirm the gift of the Holy Spirit in him and the others being confirmed. Reginald was to remember this date on both the first anniversary[881] as well as the third anniversary[882] of the service. It meant much to him spiritually.

Unfortunately, Reginald had had a heavy cold in the days before the confirmation service. Other boys at school had German measles, with some being sent home as a result. Ten days after his confirmation and just before Palm Sunday, Reginald went down with it as well. Throughout Holy Week[883] he was in the sickroom at school covered in spots.

He wanted to take his First Communion with his mother or father, as was the custom of the time, but this had to be delayed during the holidays due to his mother being ill with a cold and his father being called to attend a patient. Eventually he took his First Communion with his mother at the St Ives Parish Church on 15 April 1883. Taking Communion on most Sundays was to become the pattern of his boyhood from then on, throughout life. He was also drawn to attend the confirmation addresses conducted by Thring each year in the spring. It acted as a refresher for him. Thring held sessions with different year groups in preparation each night. Often he compared the boys to the Israelites crossing the Red Sea into the Promised Land, exhorting them to be pure, showing true courage and manliness.

He used the sessions to warn the boys that those he termed 'secret poisoners' who practised indecency would be expelled.[884] Being manly for men meant being pure as, in the same way, purity for women was a demonstration of being womanly.[885] As Thring noted in his diary in June 1879: 'I am so thankful, though, at being able to speak to them and give to them a solemn warning against uncleanness of all kinds. They shall not sin

[880] Woodford died two years later in 1885 aged 65.

[881] Diary 10.03.84 when he received a letter from Revd Reynell.

[882] Diary 10.03.86. He wrote to Radcliffe, with whom he was confirmed, the same day 'by a strange co-incidence'.

[883] The week in the Christian calendar between Palm Sunday and Easter Day.

[884] In 1886 four boys were punished for having 'an indecent photograph' and three more left after they were found with 'an indecent note' by a master. (Richardson, p. 239.) Reginald made no mention in his diary about these incidents although it would have been widely known by the boys.

[885] Richardson, p. 215.

blindly.'[886] Candidates had a personal, confidential meeting with Thring as part of their preparation, and were encouraged to pray daily, as he did, and to read the Bible similarly. After their confirmation boys were encouraged to take Communion regularly. In his last year Reginald went one evening to the School Room 'with all the fellows who have been confirmed; had a very helpful address from Headmaster'; sadly, he did not note the details. Thring's approach to purity is covered more fully in Chapter 14 The Battle for Purity in Volume 2.

Sunday was very much a day of rest from school work and worshipping in church: both morning and evening services were the norm when Reginald was home in the holidays from school. Sometimes a third service was attended in the afternoon. During this period, Sundays were set aside for worship, and day-to-day activity was kept to a minimum in most families. A sense of this can be found in the recollections of Molly Hughes, a young girl who was a little younger than Reginald. She described Sundays where she lived in London:

> the outer world closed down. It was wrong to travel except for dire necessity and then very difficult. It was wrong to work and wrong to play. However, we did the best we could with the day and it had the advantage of my father being with us all the time.

Sunday service was at St Paul's Cathedral and the family endured long services, but she found that the music from the organ and choir was inspirational.

> It was worth all the endurance, even of the Litany. No footling sentimental hymns, but Te Deum, Psalms, Creeds, Introits and Kyries that intoxicated us. Sermons, of course, were on the endurance side, but had some alleviations. I had a nice long sit down and as I was always close to the pulpit, I enjoyed the colours of the marble pillars.

She also noted that 'sermons were seldom less than ¾ hour'.[887] Reginald never made any mention of the sermon lengths that he experienced (Thring's were generally 10–15 minutes) but on Easter Day 1887 the Communion service took 2 hours 20 minutes as there were so many who attended the school chapel.

---

[886] Parkin, George, *Life and Letters of Edward Thring* (1910), p. 387, 14.06.79.

[887] Hughes, Molly, *A Victorian Family 1870–1900* (abridged edition, Sidgwick & Jackson, 1990), p. 58.

For Reginald at both King's Choir School and at Uppingham, services were held on Sunday mornings which every boy attended. At Uppingham, 'evening prayers' on Sundays were informal times of singing and praying held in each house. At Uppingham each day began with prayers at an assembly often led by Thring himself. Each evening during the week also ended with prayers, and in his last year at Uppingham hymns were sung in the hall of his house after prayers on a Sunday evening, too, which he enjoyed.

Leisure activities on Sundays at home were limited to walks along the river; outdoor games were not played, although parlour games were allowed. At Uppingham, games like cricket were not played. In the evenings after prayers, letters were written and private work was often carried out. Towards the end of the century, the Victorian Sabbath became less stifling through the growth of Sunday recreation like cycling and train excursions to the seaside. In 1896 museums and art galleries owned by the state or municipal authorities became open to the public and encouraged a less rigid use of Sunday afternoons.

REVD LUKE PAGET

Reginald had little to say in his diaries about Goldie's ministry, but Revd Luke Paget,[888] his successor, was different. He was one of the sons of Sir James Paget, the renowned surgeon who was the President of the Royal College of Surgeons of England, a Fellow of the Royal Society, and Surgeon to Queen Victoria for 41 years. His son, Luke, was a High Churchman like Goldie, but had the personal charm and warmth that the latter lacked. Paget was to say years later that 'I had two admirable churchwardens, one a great corn factor who was one of the shrewdest men I have ever met; the other a country doctor, wise and revered, who had an immense practice in the neighbourhood'.[889] This was, of course, Reginald's father. Paget, who was a bachelor at the time, was invited by the Groves for Christmas lunch when there were 13 seated for the festive meal at Slepe House in 1886. And, as mentioned at the start of the chapter, Reginald saw in the New Year at a watch night service at the parish church listening to a sermon given by Paget. His charisma and his preaching were powerful.

Keen to pastor his flock, Paget arranged a Bible class for 'the more careful study of the Scripture' over the winter of 1886 on Tuesday evenings;

---

888 Revd Luke Paget was vicar from 1886 to 1887, and became a friend of the Grove family.

889 *Henry Luke Paget: Portrait and Frame* by Elma K. Paget (his wife) (Longmans Green 1939).

on Thursday evenings he held a Communion class on the subject of 'The Office of Holy Communion in the Book of Common Prayer'.[890] These initiatives were held during term-time when Reginald was at school, so he was not to benefit from them personally, but he heard about them in the letters he received from home. Paget's ministry at All Saints lasted only a year and Reginald was away at Uppingham for much of the time; however, such was his impact on Reginald that he mentioned Paget on a number of occasions in his diary when he was at home. Reginald heard Paget preach at St Mark's, Kennington, his church in London, when he was studying at Guy's in 1891. Paget was Prebendary of Newington in St Paul's Cathedral at the time. Reginald went to the service with his cousin Carrie Long. During the service Paget 'recognised us at once and as she said, got us near winking at him as she could'. They chatted after the evening service and Paget invited him to spend Whit Sunday with him[891]. Unfortunately, Reginald did not write in his diary for a few weeks during this period so it is not known how the visit went.

After Paget's death in 1937 aged 84, his obituary was published in *The Times*.[892] Written by Sir Samuel Hoare, his father-in-law, it said that

> he could not help making friends wherever he went. He was one of the best after-dinner speakers in the country. His taste for good stories was as sure as his taste for good wine and tobacco. For whilst strict and simple in his habits, his very humanity made him appreciate the good things of life. His Churchmanship was as human as his life. He had been trained in the school of Liddon and Church. But, unlike certain of the Tractarians, he had never let his Catholic principles harden into pedantry or archaeology. His outlook upon his fellow churchmen was the outlook of a parish priest who understood instinctively their hopes and fears.

Some years after leaving St Ives, Paget was made Bishop of Stepney in the East End of London and then Bishop of Chester. Hoare concluded that

> he had humanized the relations between episcopacy and laity, between ecclesiastical and civil life, and between one branch of the Christian faith and another. Here, indeed, was the central feature of his life – an overflowing and irresistible Christian charity. He was one of those men who make you love the Christian, and one of those Christians who make you love the Church.

[890] *Hunts County Guardian* 12.11.86.

[891] Diary 03.05.91

[892] *The Times* 28.04.37.

In July 1887 Paget was offered the parish of St Pancras Church to the north of Bloomsbury on the Euston Road in London. He was to be greatly missed at St Ives. His influence on Reginald, although for a short period, was profound.[893]

Reginald did not express his feelings a great deal in his diaries. This had much to do with the fact that his diaries could not be kept private easily. He never wrote directly about his spiritual life, but it is clear from his life after Uppingham that his Christian faith matured and was integral to his life. As Jesus said, 'by their fruit will you recognise them'.[894] As a medical student in London he was a regular church-goer, as well as being a Sunday school teacher in his twenties at St Mark's Church, Kennington. He shared his faith in letters exchanged with Hilda Stevenson,[895] whom he courted and who became his fiancée and later his wife. In their many letters written before they married, they both declared a mutual trust in Jesus as their Saviour, and frequently prayed for each other whilst apart. A letter[896] to Hilda written on Whit Sunday 1894, which happened to be her 23rd birthday, speaks clearly of their shared faith as Christians, and is reproduced in Volume 3.

Towards the end of their lives, Reginald and Hilda built a new family home at Tenterleas, St Ives, in 1937. They put the Latin inscription carved in stone above the front porch: 'Nisi Dominus' meaning 'unless the Lord', taken from Psalm 127. In full it reads:

> Unless the Lord builds the house, its builders labour in vain.[897]

Reginald and Hilda chose this as a clear and public declaration of their faith.

The child was the father of the man.

---

[893] The influence on Reginald of Sir James Paget, Luke Paget's father, as an eminent doctor, is described in Volume 3.

[894] Matthew 7:20.

[895] Hilda's father was the renowned Lecturer in Chemistry and Forensic Medicine at Guy's Hospital Medical School, London, Thomas Stevenson, who was knighted in 1904 for his public services to medicine. His faith was firm. In his obituary in the *British Medical Journal* in August 1908 it stated, inter alia, that 'he was a diligent student of the Bible; indeed, his character and life were the direct result of his constant and abiding faith in God, every act being simply and solely done for His glory'.

[896] Letter to Hilda Stevenson 12.05.94.

[897] Psalm 127:1: 'Unless the Lord builds the house, its builders labor in vain. Unless the Lord watches over the city, the watchmen stand guard in vain. In vain you rise early and stay up late, toiling for food to eat–for he grants sleep to those he loves.'

CHAPTER 19

Making Disciples of All Nations …

'Went in to breakfast with Mr Christian, there was quite a big party there. Cholmondeley, an Old Boy from this house, has come down to say goodbye before going out to be a missionary to Japan: had a very jolly breakfast.'
Reginald Grove, 14 February 1887

REACHING OUT WITH THE GOSPEL

Christians from the Established Church, as well as Nonconformists, shared a desire to reach out with the good news of salvation to those in poverty or with little education in their own country, as well as those overseas in the expanding colonies.

Back in the early 18th century, the Society for the Propagation of the Gospel in Foreign Parts, founded in 1701, was perhaps the first missionary society. In the late-18th century and early 19th centuries there was a worldwide movement of renewal and revival with considerable missionary emphasis. Numerous missionary societies were formed – the Baptist Missionary Society (1792), the Church Missionary Society[898] (1799) and the British and Foreign Bible Society[899] (1804).

Forty years later, the Young Men's Christian Association (YMCA) was founded, the Young Women's Christian Association (YWCA) in 1855, and the Evangelical Alliance, which brought together Christians across the Protestant traditions for prayer and unity, was established in 1846. Other prominent missionary societies founded just before Reginald was born were the Universities' Mission to Central Africa (1859) and the China Inland Mission (1865).

Later, in 1877, there was the Cambridge Mission to Delhi, and then in 1880 the Church of England Zenana Missionary Society, the Cape General Mission (which became the South African General Mission) in 1889, the Africa Inland Mission in 1895, and the United Free Church of Scotland Foreign Mission in 1900. Ten years later the first Conference of

[898] CMS's original name was the Society for Missions to Africa and the East.

[899] It was founded to translate the Bible into the vernacular and was interdenominational.

British Missionary Societies met in Edinburgh.[900]

Outreach into slum areas of cities across Britain through street evangelism as well as establishing mission halls and employing outreach workers was not the prerogative only of The Salvation Army, as Nonconformist[901] churches as well as the Evangelical and the Anglo-Catholic wings of the Church of England were also active. However, The Salvation Army worked in urban areas of extreme deprivation. The stories told in their weekly publication – *Darkest England* – were harrowing.[902] Home missions were set up to work in specific districts[903] or parishes in the Church of England. Some were sponsored by a university or a public school, of which Uppingham was a pioneer, as explained later in this chapter.

HOME MISSION

Through education

In what would be termed today as inner-city areas informal schools were set up by Christians to meet the needs of children from poor backgrounds who were often excluded from Sunday schools due to their challenging behaviour; because of their often smelly and dirty clothes, the schools were nicknamed 'ragged schools'. The London Ragged Schools Union was established in April 1844 to co-ordinate resources and ensured the provision of free education, food, clothing, lodging and other home missionary services for poor children. There was no need for these schools in St Ives and other similar market towns as the conditions were very different from the expanding large metropolitan areas in London, the Midlands and the North.

But providing basic education for children who could not read or write, despite the development of elementary schooling for children after the passing of the Education Act, was a priority for congregations across the denominations. Many children dutifully attended the growing number of

---

[900] Cook, Chris, *Britain in the Nineteenth Century 1815–1914* (2005), p. 173.

[901] For instance, The Home Missionary Society for Congregational Churches was formed in 1819 with the aim of evangelism, distribution of bibles, and teaching of children. In 1846 there were 139 'agents' or missionaries across the country working with local churches.

[902] This publication first came out in 1893. Priced 1d. It aimed to report on their social work and appeal to a broad audience with an illustrated mix of reports, poetry, stories and fiction.

[903] The Congregational Church in Richmond, Surrey, employed a Home Missionary called Henry Wardley for three years. At the church meeting held in October 1839 when he left, the congregation recorded that 'his labours in visiting the poor and preaching in the cottages were much prized and no doubt the last great day will declare that much good was done through his instrumentality'.

Sunday Schools if only because it gave them a greater opportunity to learn to read and write. Besides basic literacy skills, the stories in the Bible were taught and faith explained. Reginald's sister, Mabel, was a teacher in the Sunday school at All Saints Parish Church for some years, and the parish magazine recorded 'a sustained loss' to the Sunday school when she moved after her marriage in 1894.[904]

Reginald's father was involved in the running of the local 'National Schools', which were managed by the Church of England and provided free elementary education. Alternative education was provided by the British schools which were supported by the Nonconformists. Thomas Birt Ulph, who died in 1859 and was the grandfather of Reginald's friend, Arnie Ulph, was the main founder of the British School in St Ives. In his obituary it was said that 'the British Schools owed much of their prosperity to his fostering care'.[905]

Through poverty relief

In the mid- and late-19th century Christian mission and social work for the urban and rural poor developed through a growing awareness of social deprivation and its consequences. At local and national level there were philanthropic, Church-sponsored initiatives which supported the work of men like Thomas Barnardo[906] in the East End of London to alleviate poverty through the efforts of countless volunteers.

Reginald noted in his diary in May 1887, when he was home for his last school holiday, that he had driven his mother in their horse and trap to the nearby village of Holywell to support a couple who were getting married there. She had encouraged them to get married as they were living together but not married, and were on the edge of poverty. His mother bought them outfits to wear; the husband's suit was from a friend of the Grove family, and the wife's wedding dress was given by Reginald's mother. As he said, 'the people there were full of her ladylike action in coming to see them married'.

Soup kitchens were organised in St Ives by the church congregations. There was considerable poverty in the St Ives area in the 1880s as a result of the agricultural depression from poor harvests as described in Chapter

[904] *All Saints Parish Magazine* 30.04.94.

[905] Norris, p. 45.

[906] Barnardo moved from Ireland to London in 1866. Concerned at the number of young children left orphans in a cholera outbreak, he opened a school to educate children. This led to him in 1870 to found a boys' home in Stepney, and later a girls' home. He died in 1905 and it is estimated that by then Barnardo's homes cared for over 8,500 children in 96 locations.

23, as well as the decline in the river trade which affected the townspeople's livelihoods. The ladies of St Ives parish church set up a weekly soup kitchen for those in food poverty, which was supported by tradesmen supplying the ingredients 'on very liberal terms'. The congregation gave towards this work, too; in January 1892 it was reported that £1 19s 0d (£246.51) had been donated, which made 468 quarts of soup, and the cost of cooking and the discounted stock had been £1 15s 0d (£221.31).

At the same time the Town Relief Committee set up another kitchen on similar lines to serve the other end of town near the railway station. The ladies of the parish church breathed a sigh of relief at this because without this extra resource the growing welfare needs would not have been met. As the parish magazine reported, 'demand shows no sign of falling off'.[907]

And at Uppingham the wives of some of the Housemasters had extra soup made on Fridays for the poor people in the town and surrounding area who queued up with their bowls.[908]

In St Ives

The congregation of All Saints Parish Church supported both home and foreign missions; Reginald's mother was the Treasurer of the Church's Home Mission Ladies' Association.[909] In January 1887 Reginald went with his family to the Corn Exchange for what he described as a 'missionary tea fight'. Reginald did not sit with the rest of the family, as all the seats were taken, but sat at Mrs David Northrop's table. The tea was 'awfully grand', he wrote, attributing this, wrongly, to 'cattle dealing prospering'. This was a fundraising evening for missionary work in Canada which was led by the Vicar, Revd Luke Paget. Reginald was involved in a raffle 'in a most successful manner'. Before the missionary lecture there was an embarrassing episode when the Vicar, having said prayers, invited everyone to sing a hymn ('From Greenland's icy mountains')[910] which no one knew the words to apart from the Vicar, who ended singing solo.

907 *All Saints St Ives Parish Magazine* January 1892.

908 Walker, Henry, *Memoirs Book 1 & Book 2* (1957), Uppingham School Archives, p. 11.

909 Norris Museum newspaper cuttings 19.05.1888, *Hunts County Guardian.*

910 The hymn was written in 1819 when Reginald Heber, Rector of Hodnet, sitting with his father-in-law, Dean Shipley, and a few friends in the Wrexham Vicarage, was suddenly asked by the Dean to 'write something to sing at the missionary meeting tomorrow'. This he did and the words were sung in Wrexham Church on the next Sunday morning as Shipley preached in aid of the Society for the Propagation of the Gospel in Foreign Parts.

To urban areas of deprivation

At Uppingham, Thring was the first Headmaster in a public school to support urban mission in the inner city. He realised that a Gospel that did not tackle poverty and deprivation in practical terms was not a true Gospel. He expounded in his sermons Jesus' teaching that Christians should make disciples of all nations and to teach about obedience to everything Jesus taught.[911] His faithful encouragement to boys and Old Boys for following the call to ministry overseas was clear. But equally he knew the importance of putting into practice Jesus' teaching[912] of compassion for those who were hungry, thirsty, sick, in need of clothes, lonely or in prison. It gripped his heart. And Thring's teaching of the Gospel of salvation, linked to compassionate care, was propounded week after week from the pulpit of the school chapel.

He believed that 'rich boys must learn to help the poor boys', and this was the motivation for him encouraging the school's support of mission work in areas of poverty in the East End of London.[913] The idea came from a lecture given in 1869 by a Revd J. Foy who was the Travelling Secretary of the Additional Curates Society.[914] He described the dreadful conditions of the slums in the East End of London. Several boys asked what they could do, and the idea of a school mission took hold of the boys' and Thring's imagination. The masters collected £40 (£5,072) for the project, and the boys were encouraged to give small sums. Thring thought it 'a great thing to put the idea into the boys of giving personal help to the poor', and was proud to 'have started a thing likely to be imitated and to bear fruit'. In April 1869 the first Public School East End Mission was started, and for many years the school paid £150 (£19,000) annually for this ministry.[915] This was a substantial sum and the School's commitment was demonstrated in a very clear way.

The mission was established in the parish of St Marks in the Victoria

---

[911] Matthew 28:26.

[912] Matthew 25:31–46.

[913] Thring made this remark in 1864 to Mr G. W. Bell, one of the founders of The Boys' Home Industrial School which stood where the British Library, in Euston Road, London, now stands.

[914] The Society was founded by a layman, Joshua Watson, a Tractarian, in 1837 to promote Christian mission to the poor by funding assistant priests; interestingly, it was then and is now Anglo-Catholic. Watson was friends with a number of those in the Oxford Movement, including Newman.

[915] Rawnsley, *Edward Thring*, p. 51.

Docks out of which the school established a mission plant in North Woolwich, where overcrowding and poverty was rampant. One Housemaster visiting found 'plenty of dirt, plenty of children, plenty of pigs: all three to be found in the astounding ruts of the main thoroughfare'.[916] The project started with a schoolroom and a mission room; Sunday services were held twice a day, and the Sunday school attracted 240 children (soon rising to 400 in two shifts!). There were weekday activities, too, such as a clothing club, a mother and toddlers group, and men's evening classes.

The school supported the work all through Thring's headmastership,[917] and speakers from the mission came to give updates.[918] Thring took care not to equate poverty with sin, which was a tendency with some philanthropists of the period. He told the boys that their duty as adults was to 'make the life of Christ live in the miserable haunts of our great cities in pure and comforting power, wherever God calls you to work, unselfish, giving happiness'.[919] In an address that Thring gave to the Carlisle Church Congress in 1884 on 'The Best Means of Raising the Standard of Public Morality', he highlighted the difficulties of those living in slums: 'Men and women, who have no earthly pleasure save sex and beer, cannot be chaste'.

Thring was emphatic that Christians should address the needs of the poor before building grand, new church buildings in areas of deprivation, and felt there was much hypocrisy about moral issues of purity:

> Whole families pigging it in one room, cannot, in a civilised country, be chaste ... we talk of divine truths, and build churches, when we ought to be going around with a scavenger's cart and a navvy's pickaxe, carting off filth and making sewers....I hold the man who provides good amusement for the poor, and teaches them to enjoy it, to be eminently a man of God.[920]

First offer educational help, then improve the slums, and lastly evangelise was Thring's approach. Public health was a topic of much discussion

---

[916] Richardson, p. 224.

[917] The mission building was destroyed by bombing in World War II, but in 1898 the mission had transferred to the Mersey Missions to Seaman in Liverpool, and then in 1937 to a Boys' Club in the new town of Corby, not far from Uppingham.

[918] Revd Vivian Skrine and E. Hartley spoke on 2 March 1887 in the School Room about the mission which Reginald noted. There was another given a few weeks later on 31 March on the mission.

[919] Richardson, p. 227.

[920] Richardson, p. 302 footnote.

between Reginald and his father as the local Medical Officer of Health in St Ives (see Volume 3).

But it was supplying men for this ministry, rather than the financial support, which was closer to Thring's heart. Revd Wynford Alington [921] was the first Old Boy as the missionary curate of St Mark's. Thring wrote after the commissioning service that 'I'm wonderfully cheered. England has never before had this fastening of a school on to real life work in the world outside.'[922] The School transferred the mission in 1883 to St Saviour's Poplar, another deprived district where Revd Vivian Skrine, another Old Boy, was the vicar. Thring ensured that the boys at Uppingham were kept in close contact with the mission and its progress by talks given by Alington and Skrine; in March 1887 Skrine (and a Mr Hartley) came to Uppingham and 'gave the school an excellent simple, strong account of the life there and difficulties', Thring wrote in his diary, continuing that 'I feel it a great boon to have such a breath of true life sent into the school'.[923] Reginald wrote that it was a 'rather amusing lecture'. Groups of boys also visited the mission to sing in concerts which Reginald referred to in his diary.

In an address Thring gave in 1885 in London to ex-public schools under the auspices of the London Mission, in what he called his 'Charter of Life',[924] he emphasised strongly the importance of community responsibility, particularly in areas of social deprivation, and of teaching those living there 'how to be happy'. He spoke with passion of the need to 'make them human beings first. Let Mission Rooms, and attractive teaching and attractive amusements, and life [persuade] them. Music will reach everybody: reach it.'

Echoing Jesus' teaching in Matthew 25:31–46 from the parable of the sheep and goats, he said: 'Get [them] clothed and in their right mind [and only] then preach to them'. He concluded his address with the imperative of Jesus' 'do to others what you would have them do to you'[925] by mentioning Charles Kingsley's character of Mrs Doasyouwouldbedoneby in *The Water*

[921] Alington later went out to South Africa as a missionary, tragically dying of typhoid fever in 1879.

[922] Thring's Diary 24.09.72.

[923] Thring's diary 02.03.87.

[924] Vaughan, C. J. (edited), *The School Life* (1885). Seven Addresses delivered to the London Mission 1885 in St Paul's Church, Knightsbridge.

[925] Matthew 7:12.

Babies as a topical point of reference.[926]

In May 1884, not long after Reginald went to Uppingham, he wrote about the visit of about 60 boys by train, with masters and their wives, via King's Cross station to Woolwich to give a concert 'for the poor'. They stayed overnight and returned the next day in the afternoon. Reginald was not in the choir so did not attend; neither did he in his last term when another concert was given in July 1887, as he was never placed in the choir. This concert was given to celebrate Queen Victoria's Golden Jubilee. About 40 boys with several masters travelled to Poplar and Reginald wrote that 'we were the first public school, or in fact, any private body of any sort, to send out a mission of this sort. I don't suppose,' he continued, 'that the "Poplarites" will enjoy our music very much but it will show them we look after them with something besides £10 [£1,268] a year'. The school actually gave much more than this, as mentioned earlier. The works played were a violin piece by Beethoven and choruses by Handel. As one of the pieces was a popular song, 'Sally in Our Alley', sung by one of the ladies, Reginald may well have been wrong in his assessment of their reception! Thring's daughter, Grace, was amazed at the 'roads lined with troops saluting the Royalties as they drove past. The houses hung with bunting and flags, the corridors and balconies crowded with people.'[927] But as the celebration in Uppingham showed, there was an emotional outpouring of pride in The Queen and the Empire across the country.

OVERSEAS MISSION

Besides social and mission work at home, it was a period which saw the growth of missionary societies which sent people to the colonies to convert the indigenous people of the expanding British Empire in Africa, Australasia and Asia. Churches raised money through all sorts of activities to support mission. The Revd Thomas Lloyd, who was the Minister of the Free Church from 1864, had at first contemplated becoming a missionary overseas; it was not to be but he was the Secretary of the London and Baptist Missionary Society and was particularly interested in Madagascar. Naturally, under his leadership, the congregation supported this society's work.

---

[926] This character was one of the two sub-aqua spinsters who looked after the water babies in this fairy tale: she lavished unlimited love (and sweets) on those in her care.

[927] Richardson, p. 226.

To China

Two years before Reginald went up to Cambridge in 1887 there was a remarkable Christian revival in the university which stirred the hearts of many young men in public schools. This was when Charles (C. T.) Studd,[928] captain of the university cricket team, and six others volunteered as missionaries to go out to China. Three had been at Eton College, three at Repton, and one at Clifton College. The press called them the 'Cambridge Seven',[929] and public schoolboys like Reginald, keen on cricket and rowing, were caught up by this major news sensation. In fact, when he was 13 Reginald went to watch the Cambridge University Cricket Team (including C. T. Studd) play the Australian team in 1882. The university team beat the Australians by six runs. C. T. Studd left Cambridge the next year, as Reginald did when he left King's to go to Uppingham.

These sportsmen were men from middle-class backgrounds who heard the call to take the Gospel to the people of China and were accepted by the renowned missionary to China, Hudson Taylor, to join his China Inland Mission.[930] At the time, this mission had 163 missionaries in China. Due largely to the publicity generated by the Cambridge Seven, by 1890 the number had doubled, and by 1900 there were 800.

C. T. Studd's daughter, Edith Buxton, said that 'in the history of missions, no band of volunteers has caught the imagination of the public as much as these men'.[931] Besides her father, the Seven comprised the stroke of the Cambridge University boat,[932] the stroke of one of the trial eights, a dragoon guardsman, an officer of the Royal Artillery, and the son of a titled family in Norfolk.[933] Such was their fame that Queen Victoria received a booklet giving their testimonies.[934] Their sailing had to be put

---

[928] Charles Studd's father, Edward Studd, became a Christian when he was invited by a close friend to hear the American Evangelists, D. L. Moody and I. D. Sankey, who were conducting gospel meetings in a theatre in Drury Lane, London. Besides C. T. Studd, his other two sons became committed Christians. Each of them in turn were Captains of Cambridge University Cricket XI.

[929] Actually, only six of the seven were educated at Cambridge; Dixon Hoste was educated at the Royal Military Academy. He died in 1946, two years before Reginald, having survived internment by the Japanese. He was the last survivor of the Cambridge Seven.

[930] The China Inland Mission is now called OMF (Overseas Missionary Fellowship).

[931] Buxton, Edith, *Reluctant Missionary* (Lutterworth Press, 1968), p. 25.

[932] Stanley Smith who captained the University Eight in 1882.

[933] This was Sir Montagu Harry Proctor-Beauchamp, 7th Baronet.

[934] This was a description of their personal conversion to Christianity. C. T. Studd was converted at Eton when a schoolboy.

off so that they could go to Edinburgh and speak at the urgent request of the leading professors. In a hall packed with 2,000 students they were cheered again and again as they rose to speak.

Given Dr Grove's interest in rowing, and the fact that one of them, Stanley Smith, had captained the Cambridge University Eight in 1882, the Seven would have been a sure topic of conversation in the Grove family; added to this was that John Goldie, one of the sons of the Vicar of All Saints, St Ives, had been captain and Stroke of the Cambridge University Boat in 1870–72. Young Goldie was well known to the Groves and visited the family often, as did his father and mother.

What Revd Goldie's views, as an Anglo-Catholic, were of the Seven is not known.

To Africa

At Uppingham in the summer of 1886 George Pilkington, an Old Boy, visited the school. He was a missionary with the Church Missionary Society in Uganda. He was four years older than Reginald, having gone to Uppingham in 1878 when he was 13. He had been in Fir croft, on the opposite side of the road to Redgate, Reginald's house. Leaving in 1882 in Reginald's second year, he had gone up to Cambridge. Revd Skrine, writing the introduction of his biography,[935] said that

> he was much transformed. No wonder for the tide of that religious impulse which set in during his Cambridge days was running strong … a chivalrous boy from an English Public School is one of beautiful things in God's world of men; and for me, that knightly tale from Africa will be most thought of as the full blowing of a beauty of soul which first saw and shall last remember in a boy at Uppingham.[936]

A good role model for the boys.

Reginald heard a number of stirring accounts of the work of the

[935] Harford-Battersby, Charles, *Pilkington of Uganda* (Marshall Brothers, London, 1899).

[936] Pilkington was friends at Cambridge with a number of young men who became Christians as a direct result of the example of the Cambridge Seven. Two of them rowed – Sidney Swann and Cecil Tyndale-Biscoe who were both in the Cambridge University Boat in 1884. Many became missionaries for the CMS. Tyndale-Biscoe went to Srinager, Kashmir after Cambridge and briefly met Reginald's brother Ernest, when he spent time in the town while serving in the British Army in India. 'This band of brothers were stirred to become the Varsity to Christian men in seeking to win their brother undergraduates to Christ'. (*Pilkington of Uganda* by Charles Harford-Battersby, 1899, p. 24.)

Universities' Mission to Central Africa. The Mission had been founded in 1859 at the request of David Livingstone[937] with the special purpose of fighting the slave trade.

The first note in Reginald's diaries about hearing the call to take the Gospel overseas was one Sunday in the Autumn Term in 1881 when he was still at King's. This was when a 'Mr. Hutt[938] gave us a lecture on missionary life in Africa in the evening'. Hutt was a very distinguished politician with a deep concern for West Africa.

A year later the boys were told the sad news of the death of Charles York,[939] an old King's boy, who was a missionary with the same society, the Universities' Mission to Central Africa,[940] in Zanzibar in 1880. He was a man whose life was inspirational. In the history written years later of the work of the mission,

> dying amid his converts [he was] carried to the grave by catechumens, and mourned by all Umba. In those eighteen years the doctrine of 'Jesus and the Resurrection' had indeed been a light to lighten African darkness.[941]

---

[937] Livingstone died in 1873 when Reginald was four. A medical doctor by training, he was a Congregationalist, and was sent to Africa by the London Missionary Society.

[938] Sir William Hutt was a Liberal MP (for Hull and later Gateshead. During his career he was Paymaster General and Vice-President of the Board of Trade. He had a special interest in the Gold Coast, West Africa and the slave trade. He spoke on a debate in the House of Commons in 1850. *HC Deb 19 July 1850 vol 113 cc37-6937.* He was very elderly when he spoke to the boys of King's and died the following year aged 81.

[939] *The History of the Universities' Mission to Central Africa 1859–1898* (1898) p. 148 Revd Charles York was a missionary with the Universities' Mission. This is an extract from a history of the mission:

[940] Anderson-Morshead, A.E., *The History of the Universities' Mission to Central Africa 1859–1899* (1899). Gibson, Alan G.S., *Eight Years in Kaffraria 1882–1890.* http://anglicanhistory.org/africa/kaffraria_gibson/03.html.

[941] 'His work at Umba and elsewhere had been much blessed. There is a letter giving an account of Wrestling in prayer an argument for the soul of an old dying woman, turning out the charmers in the face of a council gathered against him, and finally having her baptized and buried as Christian, allowing no wailing till the first Christian funeral at Umba was over. He was much loved, and being laid up on Christmas Day at Magila, had striven to reach his people again two days later, bringing on Jan. 6 a return of fever, of which he died, and was laid to rest near the newly enlarged church of St. John Baptist, Umba, beside Maria Mapindu, his convert. He was the first of the Mission clergy to be buried in a group of graves by the Shire. At the Mission Anniversary that year, Bishop Harvey Goodwin (Carlisle), the biographer of Mackenzie, drew attention to the contrast of the desertion and loneliness of the first Bishop's death, and the Hagar-like putting his grave out of sight, with the Joy and attention surrounding Charles Yorke, dying amid his converts, carried to the grave by catechumens, and mourned by all Umba. In those 18 years the doctrine of "Jesus and the Resurrection" had indeed been a light to lighten African darkness.'

Reginald's diaries show how the call of others to overseas mission touched his heart, especially when he grew older and was at Uppingham. The first missionary he heard speak at Uppingham in his first term had been one of Thring's first pupils joining in 1858. He was 38 when he spoke at the meeting Reginald attended. He was Revd George H. Swinny[942] who served the Universities' Mission to Central Africa. Tragically, he died a few years later from fever in what is now Malawi. In June 1885 there was another talk given about UMCA, this time by Revd Percy Lisle Jones-Bateman, on missionary work in Zanzibar. Jones-Bateman worked for the UMCA in Malawi, and at the time was the Archdeacon of Zanzibar.[943] He had been active in campaigning against the slave trade.[944]

The work of this mission was also supported at St Ives when the Vicar, Revd Arthur Stapleton Barnes, held two evening meetings to promote the work of the Universities' Mission to Central Africa after Reginald had left Uppingham and was studying Medicine in London. The first meeting was held for children and 200 attended. An hour later the meeting for adults attracted 100. On both occasions pictures of the country and the work were shown through a magic lantern show. The church wanted to support a freed slave, and the congregation was encouraged to send as much money as possible to the Mission. Joining the 'Coral League' by giving 3d (£1.50) a year, and praying for the Mission was one suggestion the Vicar made

---

942 Revd George. H. Swinny joined the Universities' Mission to Central Africa and ministered from a mission in Chiesi, then Nyasaland from 1885 to 1887 when he died tragically. His wife died soon afterwards on the voyage back to England. 'He was son to the Principal of Cuddesdon, a bright, merry young Oxonian, full of reverence and humility. He had such a training as falls to the lot of few men. First in a 'holy household', but the 'home delights so keen and pure' did not beguile his heart, and when 'a sterner sound' summoned him he was not found wanting. After a curacy at Clewer, and a short time at Cowley, he sailed for the Cape, where he took charge of Newlands, a few miles from Cape Town. But his face was set towards Central Africa, and as a step, he went up to Zululand in 1882, and took charge of Kwamagwaza. It was here that he felt called to minister among the Magwangwara, whose language was still Zulu, so that he would be understood. Meantime he had married Miss McKenzie, the Bishop of Zululand's sister, and together they devoted their hearts to this work. Thus, it will be seen that the work at Likoma was to them only a preparation for carrying the kingdom of Christ to that wildest of all races in the Nyasa district'. Before he died of fever he said, 'There is the Land we have so long desired; all our loved ones are there'. He was laid in the burying ground at Bandawe, the first of the Mission to rest on the western shore of the Lake (Nyasa) in what is now Malawi. (Anderson-Morshead, A.E., *The History of the Universities' Mission to Central Africa 1859–1898* pp. 173–74, 177.)

943 Tengatenga, James, *The UMCA in Malawi: A History of the Anglican Church 1861–2010.* USPG 2010.

944 Bateman was also the Principal of St Andrews College in Kingani. He died in 1897.

which he felt 'almost everyone in the parish could do'. Then another initiative was to join the Parish Missionary Union by subscribing less than ½d a week or 2s 2d a year (£13.60); members got a free ticket for the annual Missionary Tea in January and occasional reports from the Mission. There was a monthly working party to make things for the annual sale of work. The Mission had the full backing of the Church.[945]

In June 1884 a missionary from South Africa who was an Old Boy visited. He was Revd W. M. Cameron from the Society for the Propagation of the Gospel in Foreign Parts (SPG) and he gave a talk on 'Kaffraria'. The SPG established a mission in Umtata which was in northern Natal. Reginald described the talk as 'very jolly'.

To the ends of the earth: Barbados, India, Ceylon, Canada, Australia and Japan

In November 1884 he heard Bishop Minchinson preach – he was the Bishop of Barbados and the Windward Isles in the British West Indies. He was not an Old Boy, like some of Thring's guest speakers, but he came back the next year and conducted the annual confirmation service.

Reginald heard a stirring talk by The Revd Robert Winter[946] in June 1885 about the work of his wife, Priscilla, in Delhi. She founded a medical mission for women called the Delhi Female Medical Mission. Her deep concern was that 'women in India get no relief from suffering … [because] the medicine man takes them in hand and his remedies are the crudest'.[947] The work continues to this day as St. Stephen's Hospital for Women and Children.

Later in the Autumn Term of 1885 the school had another talk by missionaries – this time a Mr Kelly and Mr de Winton[948] (an OU) on Ceylon. 35-year-old Revd Frederic de Winton had been at Uppingham in 1863 and had been in Thring's School House. He left in 1870 to go to the University of Oxford and was the last Missionary Fellow of Jesus College, Oxford.

945 *All Saints Parish Magazine* 31.01.92.

946 Winter was the head of the USPG missionary work in Delhi.

947 https://en.wikipedia.org/wiki/Delhi_Female_Medical_Mission 26.04.19.

948 He was a Fellow of Jesus College, Oxford. This appointment was made by the Admiralty and the Bishop of London to serve in 'His Majesty's fleet at sea and foreign plantations'. De Winton went out to Ceylon as the Chaplain of the Bishop of Colombo. He was eventually appointed Archdeacon of Colombo in 1902. (https://en.wikipedia.org/wiki/Frederic_de_Winton 27.0419.) There is no record available for Mr Kelly.

In October 1886 Reginald heard a talk given about the work of the SPG in Canada.

The following month he heard a talk from Henry Parry, the Bishop of Perth[949] in Western Australia, about missionary work in that continent. Parry had been educated at Rugby School. Three days later at evening chapel, intercessory prayers for missionary work were said.

Finally, Lionel Cholmondeley, an Old Boy from Uppingham, visited his old school in February 1887 before going out to Japan as a missionary for the Society for the Propagation of the Gospel in Foreign Parts (SPG). He was 29 when he left and was to serve under Edward Bickersteth, the first Anglican Bishop of South Tokyo[950] until the 1920s. A special hymn was composed by Skrine for the occasion, which made an impression on Reginald. Cholmondeley went back to his old house at Redgate and after evening prayers spoke about his trip. A missionary hymn was sung after which he spoke movingly about his call. Reginald proposed a rousing 'three cheers and one more'[951] for him at the close of prayer time.

---

[949] The Diocese was established in 1872 only 14 years before Parry visited Uppingham. He championed the building of St George's Cathedral, Perth which was consecrated in 1888.

[950] He was a pupil at Uppingham at Redgate and left in July 1878. After Uppingham he studied at Oriel College, Oxford, and then trained for ordination. He was to remain in Japan until 1921, serving in later years as the Chaplain to the British Legation in Tokyo.

[951] The origin of this custom at Uppingham is traced in Volume 2.

CHAPTER 20

Faith under Fire

'... the age of traditional beliefs is passed.'
Edward Thring[952]

THE BREATH OF THE SPIRIT OF GOD

Lytton Strachey gave a jaundiced and somewhat inaccurate thumbnail sketch of the Church in the early 19th century:

> For many generations the Church of England had slept the sleep of the ... comfortable. The sullen murmurings of dissent, the loud battle-cry of Revolution, had hardly disturbed her slumbers. Portly divines subscribed with a sigh or a smile to the Thirty-nine Articles, sank quietly into easy livings, rode gaily to hounds of a morning as gentlemen should, and, as gentlemen should, carried their two bottles of an evening.
>
> To be in the Church was in fact simply to pursue one of those professions which Nature and Society had decided were proper to gentlemen and gentlemen alone. The fervours of piety, the zeal of Apostolic charity, the enthusiasm of self-renunciation – these things were all very well in their way and in their place – but their place was certainly not the Church of England. Gentlemen were neither fervid nor zealous, and above all they were not enthusiastic. There were, it was true, occasionally to be found within the Church some strait-laced parsons of the high Tory school who looked back with regret to the days of Laud or talked of the Apostolical Succession; and there were groups of square-toed Evangelicals who were earnest over the Atonement, confessed to a personal love of Jesus Christ, and seemed to have arranged the whole of their lives, down to the minutest details of act and speech, with reference to Eternity. But such extremes were the rare exceptions.
>
> The great bulk of the clergy walked calmly along the smooth road of ordinary duty. They kept an eye on the poor of the parish, and they conducted the Sunday Services in a becoming manner; for the rest, they differed neither outwardly nor inwardly from the great bulk of the laity,

[952] Thring, Edward, *Thoughts on Life-Science* (Macmillan and Co., 1869), p. 1.

to whom the Church was a useful organisation for the maintenance of Religion, as by law established.'[953]

Strachey missed the point that, in fact, God was at work breathing new life into the Church through different individuals and movements in the Church of England, the Roman Catholic Church, and in those who were Nonconformists. This was despite, or perhaps because of, the assault on religious beliefs across Europe through the ideas of philosophers like Jean-Jacques Rousseau and Adam Smith, in what became known as the Age of Enlightenment (or Reason) in the late-18th century. This new life brought theological disagreements, which were often heated and sadly acrimonious, in the years before Reginald was born. But God was still working His purposes out.

In Great Britain the Evangelical Revival, fired by the teaching and preaching of George Whitefield and the Wesley brothers, and later by the work of men like William Wilberforce in his anti-slavery crusade, resulted in Christian faith flourishing. The Methodist movement at John Wesley's death in 1791 had c.57,000 adherents, and numbers grew by 1850 to c.489,000, particularly in rural areas. Across the Christian denominations, numerous agencies were formed which promoted Christian work in prisons, relief for the poor, legislation to improve working conditions, and missionary work at home and abroad, as described in the last chapter.

FAITH UNDER FIRE

While the period in which Reginald grew up was distinctly religious, faith was under threat from both agnosticism and secularisation. Less than 20 years before Reginald was born, the Census of Religious Worship[954] put the proportion of those attending a church or chapel in Great Britain at least once on a Sunday at 60%.[955] Of course, many more who did not attend on that particular Sunday had not stopped believing in God. Church and chapel attendance did not fall between 1851 and 1881; in absolute terms

953 Strachey, Lytton, *Eminent Victorians* (Folio Press, 1918), chapter 2.

954 Mann, Horace, *Census of Religious Worship* (1854) George Routledge & Co, London, abridged version.

955 The Census was taken at the end of March 1851. In Huntingdonshire, there were 96 Church of England churches with 25,453 recorded as attending. There were 2074 who worshipped as Independents at 7 chapels, 8,375 Baptists at 30 chapels, 7,642 who were Wesleyan Methodists attending 46 chapels, and 3,636 listed as 'other'.

it actually grew up to the end of the century, although it fell relative to the overall population.[956]

There is no doubt that Christian faith and its values affected the everyday thinking, behaviour and social conventions across society. The stereotypical view of the Victorian period – that of piety and outward observance of religious duties – has much truth in it. Clergy, whether Church of England, Nonconformist or Roman Catholic, were generally respected for their views and had a standing in society far greater than today. Their influence was considerable – from the sermons they preached which were often reported in the local press, to their appointments on various civic bodies. While church- or chapel-going was commonplace, for some this was as much as observing social convention rather than personal conviction.

But the times were changing and the Christian faith came under renewed threat.

This was firstly from some scholars who challenged the authenticity of the Bible. The German scholar, David Strauss, published his *Das Leben Jesu, kritisch bearbeitet* in 1835, which was translated into English by George Eliot (Marian Evans) in 1846 under the title *The Life of Jesus, Critically Examined* in three volumes. Strauss questioned the miracles of Jesus, as well as his divinity. The book was read widely. The evangelical Lord Shaftesbury, well known for his reforming work among the poor, described it as 'the most pestential book ever vomited out of the jaws of hell'.[957]

But it was not only scholars who caused some to doubt through questioning old certainties. In literature, intellectuals actively attacked faith, particularly during the 1870s and '80s. The poet Swinburne is a case in point. His anti-Christian views were evident in his published verse, as he saw Christianity as a fetter on human life. His hatred of Christianity became more apparent when his letters were published after his death.[958] Given the close friendship of Swinburne with Watts-Dunton from St Ives (as explained later in the chapter), it is interesting to speculate on the discussions at the Watts household to which Reginald's father may have been party.

Secondly, the widespread debate about new scientific discoveries began to challenge traditional beliefs. In 1833 Sir Charles Lyell published *Principles of Geology*. In it he stated there was no evidence for the creation

---

[956] Evans, Richard, *The Victorians: Religion and Science* (2011) Gresham Lecture. p. 1.

[957] Ibid.

[958] Chadwick, Owen, *The Victorian Church Part II*, p. 402 and pp. 116–18.

happening in 4004 BC, as was claimed by the 17th-century writer, James Ussher. Lydell also claimed there was no evidence for the story of the Flood in Genesis. The anonymously published *Vestiges of the Natural History of Creation*[959] in 1844 described the emergence of the solar system and mammal life, with humans being just one of many animals. It prepared the public for the scientific theories of evolution by natural selection propounded by Charles Darwin 15 years later.

While there were divisions within the Established Church, this did not weaken the message of the Gospel but enabled it to flourish in differing ways. What became known as the Low and High Church wings held strong and passionately argued differing beliefs, and somewhere in between were those defined as the 'broad Church'. Additionally, the development of Christian Socialism presented a further strand of Christian expression, although its roots lay in Chartism which many believed to be a subversive movement.

Outside the Established Church there were a wide range of flourishing Nonconformist congregations, too, especially in St Ives. East Anglia had been a bastion for Dissenters since the 17th century. Baptists, Independents and Congregationalists,[960] Methodists and Quakers had their own different credos, but coexisted generally with little discord, worshipping in a number of chapel buildings. The Salvation Army emerged during the last 30 years of the 19th century. It grew out of the 'Christian Mission' started by William and Catherine Booth, both from a Methodist background, in the East End of London in 1878. The essence of their belief was summed up: 'We are a salvation people – this is our specialty – getting saved and keeping saved, and then getting somebody else saved.' While The Salvation Army formed congregations during the 1880s and 1890s in nearby Godmanchester, Huntingdon, St Neots and Willingham, none was formed in St Ives.

Roman Catholic congregations grew across the country, especially after removal of discrimination through the passing of the Catholic Emancipation Act in 1829. St Ives was no exception. Many of the cattle drovers bringing cattle to the livestock market in St Ives from Ireland and

---

959 The author was later revealed to be Robert Chambers, a Scottish journalist.

960 Independents traced their origins back to the Puritans of mid-17th century and met in independent congregations. Each congregation appointed its own pastor and members were jointly involved in all aspects of Church life and worship. During the period 1760–1810 the number of independents, or Congregationalists, as they came to be called, increased by approx. 78% and it is estimated they had approx. 800 churches by 1810. This increased to c.3,200 by 1850.

Lancaster were Catholics who wanted to attend Sunday mass; the first Roman Catholic congregation since the Reformation was formed in 1843 In St Ives.[961]

There was a growing questioning of Christianity as new scientific discoveries in geology and animal species challenged belief. But, despite these threats, religion still mattered immensely to the Victorians: God was at work and the Grove family was no exception. This was the religious climate in which Reginald grew up.

SCIENCE VERSUS SCRIPTURE

Atheism and agnosticism began to gain ground and matters of faith were debated publicly,[962] especially by the growing number of those who were educated in public or state schools, those who could be called 'intelligent agnostics'. The question of belief or unbelief became common in public discussions. Scientific discoveries of the natural world challenged the Biblical interpretation of creation and posed a major threat to faith as the fundamental truths of Scripture were challenged. Could someone who did not believe every word of the Bible literally be a Christian? A sermon preached at Uppingham in February 1886 by Revd George Handforth, one of the Assistant Masters at Uppingham, is good example of the debate that raged. Thring encouraged healthy discussion, and Handforth's sermon comparing science and the Bible stimulated this. Listening intently was Reginald who thought the sermon was 'rather good'.

The growing public debate between reason and religion was stoked by the controversy generated by the new scientific discoveries in the fields of biology and geology. Charles Darwin's famous work, *On the Origin of Species,*[963] was published in November 1859, only ten years before

[961] The well-known 19th-century architect, Augustus Pugin, designed their church building dedicated to St Andrew in Union Road (near the junction with Hills Road). It served the expanding Catholic population for over 40 years before being replaced in 1890 by the much larger Church of Our Lady & the English Martyrs at the junction of Lensfield and Hills Roads, St Ives.

[962] An example was the publicity generated by the stand taken by Charles Bradlaugh, the new Member of Parliament elected in 1880 for Northampton. As an atheist, he refused to take his seat in Parliament as he was required to take an oath as a Christian. He was only able to take his seat without swearing on the Bible after a struggle of six years. The issue was a major point of public discussion and debate.

[963] *On the Origin of Species by Means of Natural Selection, or the Preservation of Favoured Races in the Struggle for Life* is now considered to be the foundation of evolutionary biology.

Reginald was born. Interestingly, John King Watts,[964] who was a solicitor in St Ives and living at The Red House[965] in Market Hill,[966] was one of the earliest members of the Geographical Society. He was keenly interested in the findings of Darwin and others. Appointed a Fellow of the Society, he was also one of the founders of the Anthropological Society. His outside interests and erudition were unusual for a solicitor in a small country town. One of his sons, Walter, became a well-known poet, friend of Algernon Swinburne and literary critic besides practising as a solicitor both in St Ives and later in London.[967] He also acted for Dante Gabriel Rossetti, the well-known Pre-Raphaelite painter, as his solicitor.[968]

Besides knowing the explorer and missionary David Livingstone, Watts also knew Darwin and others interested in geology and geography – Sir Roger Murchison,[969] Sir Charles Lyell, Revd Dr William Whewell, Paul Du Chaillu, Alexander Findlay and Dr Norton Shaw. All were well known and respected in their fields. It is possible, but not proven conclusively, that Watts entertained Darwin at his home in St Ives.[970] Inviting Darwin to St Ives would have been quite a coup. Darwin, in later life, despite his

---

[964] John King Watts (1808–84) was 'a naturalist intimately connected with Murchison, Lyell and other geologists, a pre-Darwinian evolutionist of considerable mark in the scientific world of London and the Gilbert White of the Ouse Valley'. *Chambers' Encyclopaedia*, Chapter 4, cited by Douglas, James, in *Theodore Watts-Dunton.*

[965] This house still stands today and has an inscription outside which reads: 'Walter Theodore Watts-Dunton who was born in the town on 12th October 1832 lived for many years in this house'.

[966] The Red House was listed as at 11 Sheep Market in the National Census 1861.

[967] Watt's son Walter Theodore (1832–1914) trained as a solicitor and practised with his father until he went to London sometime after 1881 to practise there. One of his clients was Algernon Swinburne, the poet who was also a chronic drug addict. Watts (later in life he took the name Watts-Dunton using his mother's maiden name) befriended Swinburne in 1872 and later in 1879 lived with him and his wife in Putney, SW London for 30 years where he helped to keep Swinburne out of trouble. Watts was also a friend of Alfred Lord Tennyson and Dante Gabriel Rossetti. The great love of this son of St Ives was literature and for many years he wrote his own poems whose 'exquisite examples of the English sonnet and judicious criticisms in the kindred realms of poetry and art are familiar to lovers of our national literature'. Douglas, James, *Theodore Watts-Dunton* (1904), p. 27.

[968] Hughes, Kathryn, *Victorians Undone* (2017) p. 279.

[969] Murchison was an opponent of the theory of evolution.

[970] Carter, Mary, *A Remarkable Journey* (2005), p. 36. There is no other record I could find of Darwin's visit although Herbert Norris in his *History of St Ives* (1889) mentioned that Dr Latham, a famous ethnologist, was a frequent visit to Watts at St Ives. It is possible that Carter may have made a mistake unless she found another source.

exploits as a traveller for five years on HMS *Beagle* exploring the coast of South America in the early 1830s, preferred to stay at home in Kent writing, and disliked being away. When he did, he never liked to stay as a guest at any of his friends'. According to Dr John Chapman, to whom Darwin sent a list of his medical symptoms in 1865, he suffered for 25 years from an embarrassing and distressing condition – he farted excessively throughout the day and night.[971] He also had similar bouts of vomiting.[972] As a consequence he preferred to stay at a local inn when visiting friends. The Robin Hood Inn was next door to Watts, the Golden Lion Inn a few doors down, and the White Horse Inn opposite the Red House. Darwin was spoiled for choice if he did come to visit his friend Watts.

Darwin was a man honest enough to admit that there were challenges to his theory, and he gave over one chapter of his book to detailing these.[973] Darwin dealt with scientific issues, rather than theological ones. He wrote *Origins* with a scientific, not a theological, intent. He was a deist when he wrote it. 'It seems to me absurd to doubt that a man may be an ardent Theist and an evolutionist', Darwin wrote to John Fordyce in 1879. 'In my most extreme fluctuations', he continued, 'I have never been an atheist in the sense of denying the existence of a God'.[974] But by the time of his death he had become an agnostic. Darwin corresponded for decades with Asa Gray, a Professor of Natural History at Harvard University,[975] about his theory. Besides being a respected academic, Gray was also a devout Christian who described himself as 'one who is scientifically and in his own fashion a Darwinian, philosophically a convinced theist and religiously an acceptor of … the Nicene Creed as an exponent of the Christian faith'.[976] He promoted and defended evolution in 19th-century America. He showed it was possible to accept the theory of evolution, as well as believe in God's role in creation, but it was on the latter point that that he disagreed with Darwin.

---

[971] Chapman prescribed a spinal freezing treatment in the form of bags of ice applied to Darwin's spine. It made no difference to Darwin's condition.

[972] Hughes, Kathryn, *Victorians Undone*, p. 129.

[973] Chapter 6: Difficulties on Theory.

[974] Spencer, Nick, and Alexander, Denis, *Rescuing Darwin* (Theos Think Tank publication, 2009), p. 13.

[975] He was also President of the American Academy of Arts as well as the American Association for the Advancement of Science.

[976] *Rescuing Darwin*, p. 62.

The discussions about Darwin's theories and the role of God would have animated the dinner table at the Watts' if Darwin visited and mirrored the discussions across society. Watts was a friend of the Minister of the Free Church at St Ives, Revd Thomas Lloyd, who was interested in the issues of the day, and encouraged debate within his congregation and with his friends. Discussion over the interpretation of the Creation story in Genesis was frequent and passionate in relation to the new scientific findings. As Watts and Lloyd were well known to Reginald's father, it is inconceivable that Dr Grove was not one of Watts' guests if Darwin did indeed stay at St Ives. While a Dr Ellis of Swavesey attended Watts[977] when he had a heart attack and died in the nearby village of Over,[978] Dr Grove was more likely to be his doctor. The date of a visit by Darwin to St Ives is not known, but as Darwin died in 1882 aged 73, and Watts died in 1884 aged 76, it must have been in the 1870s. George Lloyd was the son of Thomas Lloyd, as well as being a good friend of Reginald's, as previously explored. He studied medicine at Cambridge and later at medical school in London, as Reginald later did. The role of science and the theory of evolution would have been a subject of their discussions, too, as it was for many across society.[979]

---

[977] At his death he had practised since 1840 – for 44 years.

[978] This information was given by James Douglas in Chapter 4 of the biography of his son, Walter Watts.

[979] Discussion about the origin of man was vigorous from top to bottom in society and was not confined to those with education. 'Freak' shows were common in the Victorian period with exhibits aimed at the curious and gullible. Some show business entrepreneurs cashed in once the theory of evolution became well known and a woman called Karo Farini appeared at the Royal Aquarian, Westminster as the missing link between the monkey and human kind. A poster advertising her appearance at the Aquarian, was headlined 'Krao, 'The Missing Link' a living proof of Darwin's Theory of the Descent of Man. The poster then went on to state that 'The usual argument against Darwinian theory that man and monkey had a common ancestor, has always been that no animal has hitherto been discovered in the transmission state between money and man. Krao [is] a perfect specimen of the step between man and monkey discovered in Laos by that distinguished traveller Carl Bock, will be on Exhibition in the New Lecture Room the afternoon and evening'. Bock gave lectures daily at 2.30, 5.30 and 9.30pm. In fact Karo was an American who was born with hypertrichosis, the symptoms of which are excessive body hair. Her name was said to mean 'ape' in Siamese. She was also described as having a number of anatomically unusual features in addition to her body hair including an extra thoracic vertebra, an extra pair of ribs, cheek pouches, hypermobility of her joints, and lacking cartilage in her ears and nose. She arrived in England in 1882 aged 6 and died in New York in 1926. Besides being exhibited in London, she also did tours in Europe and later, in 1899, went to Edinburgh and Cardiff. (https://en.wikipedia.org/wiki/Krao_Farini 27.01.20.) Reginald was at school when she first arrived in England but made no reference to her in his diaries.

Darwin's views were aptly put in a note that he made in one of his notebooks when he wrote: 'Man, in his arrogance thinks himself a great work worthy of the interposition of a deity. More humble, and I believe, true to consider himself created from animals.'[980] Thring was troubled by the impact of Darwin's theories and the growing rejection of creation in the Bible. A rejection of this truth led, he believed, to a rejection of other Scriptural passages. However, some Christian Socialists embraced the scientific evidence presented by the evolutionists.

But Thring did not. He believed it was 'nursery babble'.[981] He dismissed as 'a most consummate donkey' Herbert Spencer, one of the chief protagonists for Darwin's controversial theories.[982] As noted at the beginning of this chapter, Thring observed with sadness that 'the age of traditional beliefs is passed'.[983] While he was a man who embraced scientific study and learning who passionately promoted science in the curriculum at Uppingham, Thring mounted a strong defence of traditional beliefs 11 years after the publication of *Origin of the Species.* He feared that 'Learning and Science are claiming the right of building up and pulling down everything, especially the latter'. In the Preface to his *Thoughts on Life-Science,* published in 1869, he said that 'if these claims are well founded mankind at large are hopeless slaves, totally incapable of getting any sound hold on truth, whether of religion or anything else worth having'. He went on to write that

> I venture to think this is not likely. It certainly is not an agreeable theory at least for the slaves. There must be some broad, solid, unmistakeably ground for the unlearned to stand on; some food more plentiful and more wholesome than those crumbs from the rich man's table. I put forward a few suggestions for others stronger and abler than myself to work out.

And this he did over the course of 13 closely argued chapters based on reason.

Each chapter began with 'The facts of the world show…' and then he built up his argument. In Chapter Three he argued vigorously that

---

980 Darwin, Charles, *Charles Darwin's Notebooks 1836–1844* transcribed and edited by Paul H. Barrett et al (1987), p. 300.

981 Skrine, J. H., *A Memory of Edward Thring* (1890), p. 123.

982 Richardson, p. 160.

983 Thring, Edward, *Thoughts on Life-Science* (Macmillan and Co, 1869), p. 1.

'the facts of the world show that man's powers are very imperfect; that he is put in a world where he can see much and is totally unable to deal with'. In Chapter 12 he argued that embracing the new learning without reference to God was a new idolatry and 'idolatry is from first to last an intellectual revolt against the supremacy of God'. Mankind, he believed, had descended to worshipping 'wood, and stone and animals, so now we are descending to forces and the perfectibility of man and self-development from apes, and philosophy, for our Gods'.[984] Skrine was to muse

> whether or not he contributed by it [Life-Science] anything to the logical armoury of Christian apologetics, he brought something hardly less precious to the defenders of ancient positions – heartiness in his own belief, and iron unimpressibility against the noise and flourishes of an enemy.[985]

The book sold well and he revised it before it was republished two years later. This was the same year that Darwin wrote his second book on evolutionary theory: *The Descent of Man, and Selection in Relation to Sex.* This revitalised the debate. In his first book he had been vague about man's beginnings and hinted that 'light will be thrown on the origin of man and his history'. In *The Descent of Man* Darwin argued his theory of the common descent of man from apes. Thring did not address the science of Darwin's theory in his book; perhaps this was because he did not see science and theology being rivals, as others did. He did not fear new scientific discoveries or contemporary scientific ideas, and believed neither were mutually exclusive. Preaching in 1884 when Reginald was at Uppingham, he spoke against those who tried, Luddite-like, to suppress new discoveries, taking the view that if God did not see anything in His creation as unclean, as the Apostle Peter made clear,[986] then it was not for Man to challenge this. In his Bible, he wrote down that 'God requires us to take His teaching, obey it, test it, thus find it true. Man a pupil, not a judge.'[987]

Thring and Darwin's views were the subject of much discussion over dinner in many middle-class households, and Dr Grove and his friends in St Ives were no exception.

---

[984] Richardson, pp. 179, 182.

[985] Skrine, J. H., *A Memory of Edward Thring*, p. 124.

[986] Acts of the Apostles 10:11: 'The voice spoke from heaven … do not call anything impure that God has made clean.' 11:9.

[987] Richardson, p. 213.

The fierce debate about the theory of evaluation continued throughout the 19th century, as indeed it does to the present day.

DIVISIONS WITHIN THE ESTABLISHED CHURCH OF ENGLAND

The Church in which Reginald was brought up and into which he affirmed his faith aged 14 at his confirmation was sadly divided. Two strands of theology emerged in the 1830s from the Evangelicals and the Tractarians. The terms 'Low Church' and 'High Church' became increasingly in use in the 1880s. A third strand evolved in the 1850s with the growth of Christian Socialists. In their different approaches they had success in winning souls, but acting as one 'Catholic and Apostolic' Church[988] they did not.

Evangelicals (Low Church)

The 'Evangelicals' grew out of the Clapham Sect[989] who were Church of England social reformers based in Clapham, London, at the beginning of the 19th century. Their beliefs were rooted in the Bible and its teaching on repentance and salvation through faith in Jesus. Their faith was overt, demonstrable and generally outworked through social work and campaigning against injustice and inequality in society. They found kindred spirits among many of the Nonconformist groups like the Methodists, Baptists, Congregationalists and the new church of The Salvation Army. The Methodists, of course, under the two Wesley brothers, grew out of the Church of England in the late-18th century, and were successful through open-air preaching and a clear message of repentance and forgiveness, to lead countless working men and women to faith. Small congregations met in rooms and studied the Bible to understand the truths contained in it.

Archibald Tait,[990] who had succeeded Thomas Arnold at Rugby School as Headmaster, was appointed Bishop of London in 1856. His heart was

988 From the Nicene Creed.

989 The Clapham Sect, or Clapham Saints, were active from the 1780s to the 1840s, and shared common political and social views to campaign for the abolition of slavery, the end of the slave trade and the reform of the penal system.

990 Tait (1811–82) was confirmed in 1830 in his first year at Oxford and later was appointed as the successor to Thomas Arnold, the distinguished head of Rugby School. He never favoured the Oxford Movement. He was appointed as Bishop of London in 1856 and then as Archbishop of Canterbury in 1866. During his time in office, Parliament enacted the Public Worship Regulation which sought to curb the use of ritual in the Church.

to reach out to the poor and dispossessed,[991] and he was an enthusiastic evangelist, preaching in the open air in Covent Garden at omnibus depots and ragged schools,[992] and to groups of gypsies in Shepherd's Bush which was then semi-rural. A year after his appointment he founded the Diocesan Home Mission, and arranged services for working people in the East End and North London. At some of these services he spoke himself. The next year, in 1858, popular evening services, designed to attract those who would not generally visit a church, were organised at Westminster Abbey and later at St Paul's Cathedral. He also encouraged the use of theatres and public halls for evangelistic services. In 1868 he was appointed Archbishop of Canterbury.[993] Tait would probably not have called himself an Evangelical, although neither did his sympathies lie with the Tractarians. But if the new rituals opened up the Gospel to the poor by their colour and sense of mystery, he was supportive of them provided they were not excessive.

A group called the East London Special Services Committee was formed in 1865 to co-ordinate the efforts of evangelists and street preaching;[994] their efforts were boosted by the 1874–85 evangelistic visits of the American preacher, Dwight L. Moody, and gospel singer, Ira D. Sankey, holding evangelistic meetings in public halls across England. A clear message of salvation was preached with well-organised after meetings to pray with those responding to the message given.

Evangelical Christians within the Church of England realised that working men and women in large towns and cities would not darken a church door, and so Church-based missions became common. Some bishops appointed 'canon-missioners' who were released from all other duties to focus on evangelistic preaching. A week's preaching was often arranged in a parish with a full evangelical call. This happened at All Saints St Ives, as Reginald noted in his diary.

---

[991] In 1866 during the cholera epidemic he and his wife visited survivors in the East End and spoke at the consecration of St Peter's in the London Docks. (Lowder, C. F., *Twenty-One Years in St George's Mission*, 1877.)

[992] These were schools set up in working-class districts to give a basic education to society's most destitute children.

[993] *Dictionary of National Biography 1885–1900 Volume 55.*

[994] The East London Special Services Committee was a group of Christian businessmen who did evangelistic work in the East End of London. William Booth was soon asked to lead the ministry. It was later called the Christian Mission and became the predecessor of The Salvation Army. (https://archiveshub.jisc.ac.uk/search/archives/abe2076c-5d47-3166-bded-93e5343005d0 13.01.20.)

Tractarians (High Church)[995]

The second strand of belief grew out of the Oxford Movement, whose members produced a series of controversial but influential 'Tracts for Our Times' from 1833 onwards. Tractarians, as they became known, advocated a return to what was seen as the beauty and purity of the Middle Ages before the 16th-century English Reformation. They emphasised salvation by the grace of sacraments administered by ordained clergy and saw the Church of England as part of the ancient Catholic (universal) Church. Much of the theology and thinking behind this movement was based on ideas expounded by John Keble, a renowned scholar from Oriel College in the 1830s, that Roman Catholic practices could be embraced within the Anglican Church.[996] A number of talented and charismatic adherents, besides Keble, included Edward Pusey, a Fellow of Oriel College, John Newman,[997] another Fellow of Oriel, and Henry Manning,[998] who, like Newman, later converted to Roman Catholicism. Interestingly, Manning became drawn to social work among the urban poor and worked closely with The Salvation Army movement.

There was also a desire to return to the ornaments, statutes and rituals of the Medieval Church, including the adoration of Mary, Mother of Jesus. Outward forms of expression such as priests standing facing east at the Communion service (rather than at the north end of the Communion table), lit candles on the Communion table, the wearing of coloured stoles over surplices, or full Eucharistic vestments were their outward symbols. Whether these practices were allowed legally depended on how the Book of Common Prayer was interpreted.

As part of their mission to fight the rise of secularisation and atheism, the Tractarians attracted those with working-class backgrounds who were drawn by the drama and mystery of their services. Interestingly, ritual also reflected the taste of the age in interior design. The middle-class Victorian drawing room was well furnished, even elaborate in many respects, with thick, colourful, embroidered drapes and much ornamentation. The

---

[995] Also known as Ritualists and later as Anglo Catholics as well as High Church.

[996] John Keble's model was the English Church of Archbishop Laud in the 17th century.

[997] John Newman became a Roman Catholic in 1845, was the first Rector of the Catholic University of Ireland, and was appointed a Cardinal in 1879. He was canonised by the Roman Catholic Church in 2019.

[998] Henry Manning was appointed Archbishop of Westminster in 1865 and in 1875 was made a Cardinal.

interiors of High Church buildings were furnished similarly with colourful altar cloths, mosaic floors, rich and elaborate carving and statues. The dress of clergy at services became more flamboyant, too, with purple vestments and the use of pastoral staffs for bishops. As importantly, the sermons and writings of those in the Oxford Movement became widely read and argued; despite some of them turning to Catholicism, their influence on the Church of England was significant.

The Tractarians had adopted customs that raised concerns that the Established Church was moving away from those reforms of the 16th century which set it apart from the Roman Catholic Church. Passions sometimes ran high: in the 1850s a mob gathered outside St Barnabas Church, Pimlico, near where the new Victoria Railway Station was to be built and burst into the building to protest at the form of the 'Romanish' services.[999] Across England a move took place to formally restrict these outward forms of worship. As a result, under pressure from those who felt that 'Popery' was being let in through the back door, under Disraeli's premiership in 1874 the Public Worship Regulation Act was passed.[1000] This forbade certain ritual acts such as the mixing of wine and water in the chalice at Communion, and the wearing of Eucharistic vestments. Five clergymen were imprisoned for refusing to comply with the requirements of the act. None were from the Diocese of Ely in which St Ives lay. In fact, the legislation failed to stop the movement, and ritualist practices became more commonplace as the century drew to a close.

Reginald's boyhood at St Ives was exposed to the controversies that sadly divided the Church of England.

The Vicar of All Saints Church St Ives during most of Reginald's boyhood was Revd Dashwood Goldie,[1001] a Tractarian who brought a level of ritual and ceremony to the parish church which had not existed before. His predecessor, Revd Yate Fosbrooke, held more middle-of-the-road

[999] Wilson, A. N., *The Victorians* (2007), p. 183.

[1000] Interestingly, Gladstone, who had some sympathy with the Ritualists, opposed the Act because he believed that Church and State should be kept separate.

[1001] Goldie was well known for stepping in to play cricket for the University of Cambridge against Oxford in 1846. One of the Cambridge batsman did not appear for the match and the team played one man short for the first innings. Goldie was asked to stand in and bat at number 11 in the second innings. He scored one run. He was well connected. At the 1871 Census, Lord George Young, the Scottish Liberal MP for Wigton Burghs and the Lord Advocate of Scotland, was staying as a guest.

beliefs, but Revd John Hunt,[1002] Fosbrooke's recently appointed curate, held evangelical views. Appointments were decided by the patrons of the Church, and they chose Goldie largely because of his private means rather than his beliefs. It could be said that he had virtually bought the living, and Hunt, who sought the appointment, was in no position to compete.

Shortly after he was installed as Vicar in 1866 Goldie had a disagreement with Hunt.[1003] Hunt, sadly, fell out with Goldie. As Hunt lived in the vicarage with his wife, the breakdown of relationships was particularly awkward. After leaving the parish he published a pamphlet anonymously about a town called 'Ousebank' which clearly was St Ives. In it he wrote that 'We had always passed in Ousebank for being a little high church. But Mr. Goldwing [aka Goldie] surprised us all. He was no Jesuit introducing things by stealth. He was no man of half measures.' Hunt then went on to describe the High Church forms of worship which included much genuflecting before the altar.[1004]

Goldie's immediate actions after this also stirred up controversy. Reginald's father had only just come to St Ives. A local paper reported years later on Goldie's death[1005] that

> the indignation aroused among a large and influential section of the church goers was very great when it was found that the new Vicar held ritualistic views of a pronounced type. So distasteful was the appointment, that many parishioners absented themselves from the services and attended churches in the surrounding villages. The Easter vestry meetings for several years became notorious for disorderly proceedings. These feelings gradually subsided as the years passed. Mr. Goldie, notwithstanding the immense

[1002] Dr John Hunt came to St Ives 1n 1864 after a 5-year curacy in London. He was interested in literature and published 'An Essay on Pantheism' when he was at St Ives which enabled him to move to London after he left to join *The Contemporary Review*. Later he was appointed as the Vicar of Otford in Kent. He married a local lady from St Ives, Miss Thorpe, in 1873. (Norris, p. 77.)

[1003] Dr Hunt wanted to be appointed as Vicar but the patrons of the Church preferred someone with private means, who would spend money maintaining the church. Revd Goldie had private means and was appointed to the living. It was not a good start for their relationship. Within a very short time of Goldie's appointment Hunt was dismissed because he had preached two sermons after Fosbrooke's death, which Goldie found irreconcilable with his own views on Church doctrine.

[1004] A full account of the dispute between Hunt and Goldie is given in *St Ives: Slepe by the Ouse* by Noel Hudson, pp. 96–102.

[1005] Goldie died in January 1886 aged 60 after a long illness, under the medical care of Reginald's father.

> odds against him, very consistently maintained the attitude he had taken up and continued it until his death.[1006]

Besides his High Church practices, he immediately got off to a poor start with the appointment of the churchwardens. In the past, the vicar nominated one for election, and the congregation the other. Goldie wanted to nominate both, and there was considerable opposition to this change of practice. Of course, this was before Reginald was born but Dr Grove was involved. As mentioned earlier in Chapter 10, a meeting was called for the election to be held in the vestry of the church. As 200–300 people arrived it had to be moved to the public institution.[1007] Goldie's plans were thwarted as a Mr Read Adams[1008] was elected as the People's Warden, although he later left the church because of his objections at 'the introduction of sensuous and Romanish hymns, intoning the services, fantastic dresses and gorgeous ceremonies'.[1009]

Goldie's personality worked against him and he was not much liked in the town, even by his parishioners. The same newspaper report stated that 'the Nonconformists of the town were bitterly opposed to his teaching and the methods by which he carried it on'. Given that on one occasion when preaching he warned his congregation against even setting foot in a chapel, this is not surprising! Someone who felt slighted at this message paid the Town Crier of St Ives to walk through the streets clanging his bell and proclaiming: 'This is to give notice that whoever enters a dissenting place of worship commits an offence against God. These are the words spoken in the Parish Church of Ousebank on Sunday morning last and he who said them is a liar and a fool.'[1010]

One focus of the confrontation in the next decade was The Revd Thomas Lloyd, mentioned earlier. He fought for the running of the British Schools, supported and managed by the Nonconformists. The other type of school, the National School, was run by the Church of England. There was also considerable controversy about the setting of the parish rates.[1011]

[1006] Norris Morris Museum newspaper cutting collection dated 16.01.86; newspaper not cited.

[1007] This was a huge turnout representing 8% of the town's population.

[1008] Adams, St Ives' first mayor, owned a grocery shop in the Bullock Market.

[1009] Carter, Mary, *19th Century St Ives*, p. 77.

[1010] Hudson, Noel, *St Ives: Slepe by the Ouse* (1989), p. 101.

[1011] Parish rates were set by the churchwardens together with the parishioners, and were used to pay for running the church. It was personal charge on property owners who, if they were Nonconformists or Roman Catholics, understandably resented this imposition.

In 1868, a year before Reginald's birth, Lloyd opposed the rates that Goldie was proposing – 2d in the pound. It was to be spent on raising the footpath from the Bullock Market across The Waits to the parish church. The improvement mainly benefited those attending the parish church as a new footpath would enable the boots, shoes and clothes of those going to the parish church not to get dirty in the mud. No other improvements were proposed from this rate and Lloyd led the vote against this in the Corn Exchange. By all accounts it was a rowdy meeting, and when put to the vote, Goldie's proposal was rejected.[1012] Lloyd led opposition to Goldie some years later in 1875 in the latter's attempt to get elected to the Board of the British School. This type of school was supported by the Nonconformists who resisted the idea of Goldie trying to ensure the pupils had an Anglican education. Goldie was eventually elected to the Board of the British School, and resisted the ideas of the other members who were Nonconformists.[1013]

Goldie's legacy was continued by his successors. In the middle years of Victoria's reign, photographs of the church show that the nave was quite plain, but by the end of the century, an elaborately carved and painted rood-screen had been erected across the chancel arch, and the empty brackets on the nave pillars had been fitted with the statues of saints.

Christian Socialists

The third vibrant strand stemmed from the failure to improve working and living conditions after the collapse of Chartism in 1848. This was the popular working-class movement 'born out of hunger and political frustration, that demanded universal suffrage and annual parliaments'.[1014] Christian Socialism developed from this movement, emphasising a social gospel to address the poverty and deprivation within society. Proponents within the Church of England believed this was implicit in Christianity and in Jesus' teaching in Matthew 25:31–46.[1015]

Christian Scientists were particularly concerned for the suffering of both the poor in rural areas (whose jobs were at threat from cheap

---

1012 Carter, Mary, *A Remarkable Journey* (2005), p. 37.

1013 Ibid, p. 40.

1014 Hughes, Kathryn, *Victorians Undone* (2017) p. 99.

1015 The parable of the sheep and the goats stressed the importance of feeding the hungry, giving hospitality to strangers, clothing the poor, caring for the sick and visiting those in prison.

food imports and agricultural mechanisation) and the poor working in factories in large metropolitan areas in inhuman conditions. Their concern was not their sole preserve as both the Evangelicals and Tractarians also sought to alleviate their hardships. The writer Charles Kingsley, Thomas Hughes, one-time Headmaster of Rugby School, and F. D. Maurice were prominent Christian Socialists.[1016] Kingsley also happened to be a friend of Charles Darwin's.

In 1851 Kingsley gained national attention in the press through a sermon he preached at St John the Evangelist's Church, Charlotte Street, London, laid on partly to attract visitors to the Great Exhibition. F. D. Maurice had arranged with the Minister, G. S. Drew, for Kingsley to preach six evening sermons on the 'Message of the Anglican Church to the Labouring Man'. The first evening attracted a large audience of workers. In his sermon Kingsley appeared to attack the English clergy, and spoke of the Gospel as being 'liberty' (through freedom in Christ for all believers), 'equality' (through baptism of all confessing their faith irrespective of social status) and 'fraternity' (through sharing the Lord's Supper together). At the end of his address, Drew immediately criticised it and there was nearly a riot by the mainly working-class congregation.[1017]

Thring knew F. D. Maurice, who was the godfather to one of the sons[1018] of Alexander Macmillan, a close friend, who sent his sons to Uppingham. While Thring never met Kingsley, he was friendly with his wife, Frances,[1019] as they corresponded regularly on educational matters, especially for women. Thring respected her husband as a 'true pioneer',[1020] and expressed his interest in the work of her 'distinguished husband'.[1021]

Thring's ideas for reaching out to those on the margins of society, mentioned in the last chapter, had much in common with Christian Socialism in practical terms. But he loathed socialism as a concept and believed that it had been hijacked by those who promoted 'Christian'

[1016] The key figure for Christian Socialism was F. D. Maurice (1805–72) who, from 1840 to 1853, was Professor of English Literature and History at King's College, London, until his controversial and radical writings led to his dismissal from the college.

[1017] Chadwick, Owen, *The Victorian Church (Part II)*, pp. 358–59.

[1018] The boy was named Maurice after his godfather and went to Uppingham in 1866. Maurice became the father of Harold Macmillan, Prime Minister.

[1019] Thring visited her in 1886.

[1020] Richardson, p. 263.

[1021] Parkin, George, *Life and Letters of Edward Thring*, p. 486.

socialism. While he was a fervent believer in the brotherhood of Christians, he was emphatic that

> the term Socialism has nothing Christian in it ... it has been started and preoccupied by a devil's parody of Christian brotherly love, and that it had better be left in the hands of those who started it.[1022]

It was an opinion over which Reginald pondered.

THE NONCONFORMIST CHURCHES

Reginald grew up in a town with a long Dissenting[1023] tradition dating back to the 17th century.[1024] During the English Civil War, St Ives was in Roundhead hands, and by the 19th century there were Presbyterians, Congregationalists, Quakers, Independents, Baptists, Particular Baptists and Methodists,[1025] reflecting the theological differences and worship practices of their Nonconformist congregations.

Generally, Nonconformists came from middle- and working-class backgrounds. Dr John Hunt in his pamphlet about 'Ousebank' mentioned earlier gave his thinly disguised description of St Ives in the mid-1860s: 'It was a quiet, old-fashioned country town. It had no gentry but the trades' people were well-disposed, simple, industrious and perhaps, I may say, with some qualification, intelligent. It was empathically a Dissenting town. There was but one Church,[1026] while there were seven or eight meeting

[1022] Thring, Edward, Diary (07.11.86) and Letter 08.11.86 to a Mr Girdlestone, Uppingham School Archives. Cited by Tozer, Malcolm, *Edward Thring in Educational Research and Perspectives,* Vol 15 No 2 (1988).

[1023] 'Dissenter' was the name given to Christians who were not part of the established Church of England. Under the Toleration Act of 1688 they had freedom of worship, but were discriminated against under other legislation, chiefly the Test Act 1673 and Corporation Act 1661 which effectively barred them from serving in any civil or military office. These acts were eventually repealed in 1828 after considerable pressure had been brought on the government of the day. The remaining areas of discrimination (for instance, the bar to nonconformists going to Oxford and Cambridge) were gradually removed during the next thirty years.

[1024] Carter, Mary, *Not an Easy Church* (1982).

[1025] Also known as Wesleyans after Charles and John Wesley, the founders of Methodism in the 18th century.

[1026] He was referring to the Church of England All Saints Church. There was also the Free Church in Market Hill, built in 1863–64 to hold 750 people. A Baptist congregation merged with an Independent congregation, and with the financial help of a wealthy local Dissenter called Potto Brown the building was erected. Brown owned a milling company and lived in the village of Houghton.

houses, and the meeting houses were not small places which held only a few people but large buildings, with congregations numbering three, four and five hundred.'[1027]

In the small, professional and middle-class St Ives community, the Grove family had many friends who worshipped in the various Nonconformist churches. While differing in some matters of doctrine, and conducting services differently, the basis of their faith was a shared belief in a Trinitarian God of Father, Son and Holy Spirit. These Christians occasionally came together with the congregation of the parish church to share their grief in the death of one of their number. In January 1886 Goldie died after 20 years of service.[1028] He was a controversial and in many respects unpopular man, as well as being derogatory and antagonistic towards Nonconformists in his early years at St Ives. But at the Sunday evening service after his burial Mr Roffe, a previous curate, returned and preached at a memorial. Reginald was there and wrote that the church was 'crammed, a good many dissenters were present including the Mayor [Warren]'. Grace and forgiveness by the Nonconformists prevailed.

Revd Paget, the Vicar appointed after Goldie, said of St Ives that

> there is what is called a good deal of nonconformity. The Minister[1029] of the Congregational Chapel proved a very good friend. He said once that if I were high church, he was high chapel; and he took great pains with his services and eventually joined the Church.[1030] There were also nonconformists of another type whom I learnt to admire and respect. I wish I had come to know more of them. There were genuine Puritans of the Cromwellian type.[1031]

The Ulph and Warren families were Nonconformists who, of course, were friends with the Groves. Both were in business; another respected Nonconformist family were the Days who lived in the Bullock Market. Father and son were solicitors. The Ulphs lived in Cromwell Terrace next to the Groves. Reginald was a good friend of Arnie Ulph's, and his father was prominent in the Free Church in Market Hill. His wife ran a Bible

[1027] Carter, Mary, *19th Century St Ives*, pp. 78–79.

[1028] Revd Charles Dashwood Goldie, Vicar from 1866 to 1886.

[1029] This was Revd Arthur Turberville who was Minister of the Free Church from 1886 to 1890 after Lloyd left.

[1030] Church of England.

[1031] Paget, Emma, *Henry Luke Paget: Portrait and Frame* (Longmans Green, 1939).

class for young people for many years, and held a picnic for them on the lawn in front of Cromwell Terrace annually to which Reginald sometimes went. A newspaper report gave the number of her Bible class (presumably past and present) as nearly 200.[1032] Frederic Warren was another prominent Nonconformist who was in the corn and coal business. The Grove, Coote, Day, Ulph and Warren families were close friends together.

The practices of some Nonconformists drew the attention of crowds on occasions. Public baptisms of adults in the river were not uncommon. An account by Herbert Norris stated that in 1833 'five persons [were] baptised in the river, the 5th January. The next day the river was frozen over.'[1033] A local paper reported one April in 1890 that 'thousand persons[1034] assembled on the Quay at St Ives on Sunday' to witness the public baptism of two young ladies in the river, Miss Nugent of St Ives and Miss Crisp of Swavesey. They were part of the congregation of the Crown Yard Baptist Chapel. The ceremony was carried out by the pastor Revd Samuel Haynes and one of the church deacons, Mr Lowings. The report concluded that Miss Crisp

> went through the ceremony without flinching in the least, although all of them must have been as cold as they were wet when they came out of the water. Both ladies were dressed in black dresses as though they had just come out of the house. The ceremony over, the crowd quickly vanished.[1035]

This was the context in which Reginald's faith was nurtured, taught and challenged at St Ives and Uppingham.

1032 *Ramsey Herald* 27.07.00.

1033 Norris, Herbert *History of St Ives* (1889). p. 79.

1034 Given the population of St Ives (c.3,000) and the space available on the Quayside, this was a huge crowd to be present. The report may well have been an exaggeration.

1035 *Hunts County News* 09.04.90 The baptism was on Sunday 6 April; Reginald mentioned going to Holy Communion at 8.00am and then to the morning service. It is probable that the service was still in progress when the river baptism took place.

Part 4

The Changing World

***

CHAPTER 21

The Age of the Train

'The Queen was dead ... in '37 when she came to the throne...coaches still ran, men wore stocks, shaved their upper lips, ate oysters out of barrels... women said 'lah' and owned no property.'

Soames Forsyte[1036]

As described earlier, in September 1886, when Reginald was 17, a telegram arrived at St Ives to inform the family that his Grandmother Grove, who lived in Southsea, was ill. She was 70 and her health had been worsening. His father immediately took the train to visit her, and as she seemed better he returned late in the afternoon of the following day. The next day a telegram came to say she was worse so his father and mother left by the midday train to see her. His father returned by the 7.15pm train the next day but sadly, shortly afterwards, another telegram arrived to say that she had died at 6.30pm. His mother returned a couple of days later, and soon afterwards, Reginald and his father travelled by train to Southsea for the funeral, meeting Uncle Frank there, who had travelled by train from Brixham in Devon.

Telegraphic and postal communication across the country was surprisingly efficient, and the 145-mile train journey from St Ives to Southsea was easy, quick and convenient. This sad episode illustrates how the train and telegram were so integral to the lives of Victorians.

The 19th century was a period of immense change which affected every area of social life, and the last quarter particularly so. The greatest change was a demographic one as the population grew in leaps and bounds. The first modern Census taken in 1801 put the population at 10.5 million. In 1851, the year of the Great Exhibition,[1037] the size of the population of Great Britain was 21 million. By Queen Victoria's death it was 37 million.

[1036] Galswothy, John, *In Chancery* (1920), Penguin Edition reprinted 1967, Part 3, Chapter 10, p. 267.

[1037] This was the first of what became international World Fairs and showcased British innovation, design and manufacturing.

This growth was similar in other European countries. The main impact was the shift of the population from rural areas to growing urban conurbations besides London – the West Midlands, Tyneside, South East Lancaster, Merseyside and West Yorkshire. The size of rural towns like St Ives and Uppingham[1038] was not significantly impacted and remained relatively stable; the former at c.3,000 and the latter at c.2,500. However, in the countryside around these market towns the numbers of farm workers who left the land in rural areas increased as the century drew to an end. This affected Reginald's many farming uncles and aunts.

By 1902, half the nation's population lived in towns and cities.[1039] This demographic change did not affect Reginald directly, but there were multiple other changes across society that did.

It was indeed an age of immense innovation and technological change which affected the life of Reginald and his family as he grew up.

The author H. G. Wells, looking back in 1902 for a symbol to characterise the Victorian period, wrote that it would be 'almost inevitably … a steam engine running upon a railway'.[1040] The growth of what became a comprehensive network of railway lines, built by a growing number of private railway companies, changed the face of rural Britain beyond recognition. Despite the fact that the building of each line needed an Act of Parliament,[1041] what was termed 'railway mania' took hold.

Food, manufactured goods, people and post were transported quickly, cheaply and efficiently. Not only was the face of Britain changed, but it is also no exaggeration to say that the lives of every inhabitant across Great Britain was revolutionised by the railways. It was certainly true for the Grove family.

It is difficult for us nearly 200 years later to appreciate the impact of someone even seeing a steam locomotive for the first time. It was less than 30 years before Reginald was born that a Wiltshire clergyman, Revd

---

[1038] The population of St Ives in 1851 was 3,572; 1881, 3,002; and 1901, 2,910. In Uppingham in 1851 it was 2,068; 1881, 2,549; and 1901, 2,585.
https://web.archive.org/web/20160215102922/http://www.cambridgeshireinsight.org.uk/file/2001/download (http://www.rutlandhistory.org/pdf/populationrutlandparishes.pdf.)

[1039] Walvin, James, *Victorian Values*, p. 8.

[1040] Wells, H. G., *Anticipations of the Reaction of Mechanical and Scientific Progress upon Human Life and Thought* (Chapman and Hall, 1901), chapter 1.

[1041] A private bill was passed by Parliament in 1846 to build the railway line from March to Wisbech and thence to St Ives. The line was opened in 1847.

Charles Mayne, took his parish clerk called William Hinton to watch the passing of one of the first trains along the Great Western line. Standing on the edge of a newly dug cutting, he records them watching as the train laboured up a very steep gradient belching steam and smoke, and when it reached the top it let out a shrill scream of its whistle from where it then rushed down the incline at 60mph.

> The novelty of the sight, the strangeness of the sounds, the marvellous velocity with which engine, tender, carriages and trucks disappeared, the dense columns of sulphurous smoke were altogether too much for reason of dominie [Hinton] and he fell prostrate on the bank side as if he had been smitten by a thunderstruck. When he had recovered his feet, his brain still reeled, his tongue clove to the roof of his mouth, and he stood aghast, unutterable amazement stamped on his face. It must have been quite five minutes before he could speak, and when he did it was in the tone of a Jeremiah. 'Well, Sir, that was a sight to have seen; but one I never care to see again! How much longer shall knowledge be allowed to go on increasing.'[1042]

Engineering knowledge, skill and experience led to railway lines, viaducts, tunnels, embankments and bridges gouging out the face of the countryside. Railway lines bulldozed into towns and cities to create termini at their very centres. A well-known description of a railway being built in London is given in Charles Dickens' *Dombey and Son*,[1043] which describes how the London and Birmingham Railway drove through Camden Town in North London, causing massive upheaval and destruction.[1044] In Chapter 6 Dickens gives a description of houses knocked down, streets broken through and stopped, deep pits and trenches dug, enormous heaps of earth and clay thrown up … a chaos of carts, overthrown and jumbled together… He concluded:

> in short, the yet unfinished and unopened Railroad was in progress and from the very core of all this dire disorder, trailed smoothly away upon its mighty course of civilization and improvement.

In St Ives, the railway and station had been built in 1848 and its location was

---

[1042] Young, J. C., *Memoirs of Charles Mayne Young* (2nd edition 1871), pp. 296–7, cited by Jack Simmons – *The Victorian Railway* (1995), p. 378

[1043] Published in instalments between 1846 and 1848.

[1044] Dickens, Charles, *Dombey and Son,* chapters 5 and 16.

in open fields on the outskirts of the town. The inhabitants, as a result, did not experience any of the construction disruption that occurred elsewhere. By the 1870s, when Reginald was a young boy, the once-thriving river port was in gradual decline and the new railway network began to take the bulk of freight traffic and drew passengers. An ugly iron railway bridge, built in 1882, was visible from the quayside, a constant reminder of the railway engineering that criss-crossed the country. Built across the Ouse to the east, it carried the branch railway line to Huntingdon across the beautiful meadow to the south of the town.[1045] A stark, utilitarian structure, it changed the view from the old, medieval bridge dramatically until it was taken down in the late-20th century when the line was discontinued.

This line running from St Ives to Huntingdon had a number of weak, wooden bridges which crossed and recrossed the Ouse near Godmanchester. On numerous boating trips upstream Reginald and his friends passed under these bridges. Victorian engineering was not always of the grand design or constructed in brick, stone or iron. None of the wooden bridges have survived to this day. The bridges which Reginald rowed or sailed under (or over which he travelled to Uppingham and back) were a constant fire hazard from sparks in dry weather. The line had a speed limit of 40mph, but over some of the bridges it was reduced to 10mph which restricted its attractiveness for passengers.[1046] Sometimes, on returning from school at the end of term, he got a lift in a pony and trap with the Warren brothers from Huntingdon to St Ives, as it was quicker.

In Rutland the feats of railway engineering were impressive. On his walks around Uppingham Reginald often saw the stunning Seaton Viaduct just three miles from the town. It spanned the River Welland and was built in 1876–77 by the London and North Western Railway Company a few years before Reginald went to Uppingham. Still in use today, it is 1,280 yards long with 82 spectacular arches.[1047] Another impressive feat of railway engineering was the railway tunnel built at Manton by the Midland Railway. It was reported that 1,000 navvies arrived to work on

---

[1045] The iron work was supplied by the Stockport Engineering and Iron Company. Not one train 'was stopped or delayed during the whole time occupied by its construction', according to Norris in his *History of St Ives*, p. 32.

[1046] http://www.disused-stations.org.uk/g/godmanchester/ 03.06.10.

[1047] It was designed by William Henry Barlow and his son Crawford was the resident engineer. Crawford described the viaduct as being one of the grandest and most perfect pieces of workmanship to be seen in the United Kingdom.

the tunnel in July 1846.[1048] 749 yards long, the tunnelling work was finally finished in 1850. The tunnel is still in use today and passes under the village of Manton. Another tunnel with which Reginald was familiar was the Glaston Tunnel on the line that ran from Wing to Seaton. Built in 1878, it was an incredible 1,842 yards long. He walked there specifically in April 1884[1049] to look at it with his friends Blois and Evans.

Besides the dramatic engineering feats that littered the countryside, the impact of railways on Victorian society itself was immense. Initially the railways carried freight, rather than passengers. An interesting aside is that horses were transported by train for hunt meets in other counties. The Fitzwilliam Hunt, based in Cambridge, arranged regular hunts each week on Wednesdays around Huntingdon where foxes were more plentiful. Special rates were available from the railway company for huntsmen to transport their horses.[1050] None of the Groves hunted, but Reginald enjoyed following the local hunt around Uppingham when he was at school.

Besides bulk freight and manufactured goods from the growing industrial centres of the Midlands and the North, railways enabled foodstuffs to be transported quickly and cheaply from the source of their production to wholesale markets in London and elsewhere. A good example is how fish were loaded overnight from coastal ports and freighted to metropolitan wholesale markets to feed the growing urban population. Inland, the cattle market at St Ives was a hub for livestock sales which were boosted by the railway network. Cattle reared in Ireland and the North of England were transported easily for sale at the St Ives livestock auction.

Fresh foodstuffs, which in the past were considered luxury items for the rich, became readily available for the middle classes, like the Groves, who could afford them. When Reginald was lying sick in bed with German measles at King's School in March 1883, his mother visited him. She brought some oranges to cheer him up. She would have bought them at the local greengrocers, probably William Burgess who sold fruit as well as fish in the Bullock Market. Prior to going on sale, they had been transported by train, probably from Covent Garden Market in London. The Post Office service delivering parcels began in 1883 via the train network, meant

---

1048 Rutland History Society vol 3, *Railways in Rutland* (1980) Spiel Press. p. 5.

1049 Diary 08.04.84.

1050 *Baily's Sports and Pastimes* March 1881 Volume 37 https://archive.org/details/bailysmagazineof37gilbuoft/page/34

that gifts and presents for birthdays became commonplace.[1051] Reginald frequently mentioned gifts he sent or received. Local newspapers from St Ives and Cambridge were sent to him at school by his mother, and small gifts such as flowers[1052] all came courtesy of the General Post Office and the railway companies.

But it was the potential for passenger transport which really changed the work and social habits of the population. The *Stamford Mercury* newspaper reported in 1845 that a lady went from Wansford (15 miles from Uppingham)

> by the seven o'clock train, spent four hours in London, engaged a governess and returned to her home by the evening train with much less fatigue than lately attended a day's travelling by horse coach up to London.[1053]

As travel of this distance at the beginning of the 19th century could only be done by horse and stagecoach, this development was revolutionary.

Before the coming of railways, each town set its own time – shown on town hall or church clock. One of the by-products of train travel that affected everyone, in every part of Great Britain, was the necessity of moving to 'universal time' so that timetables could be aligned across the country with the different train lines run by numerous train companies. In fact, the term 'timetable' entered the language and was first used by the London and Birmingham Railway in 1838.[1054] The Great Western Railway was the first to standardise its timetable on Greenwich Mean Time, in November 1840. The Midland Railway adopted London Time at all of its stations on 1 January 1846, but it was not until August 1880, when the Statutes (Definition of Time) Act was passed, that a unified standard time for the whole of Great Britain achieved legal status. Reginald had been travelling to school in Cambridge for two years by then. Every church and town clock now showed the same time. Reginald was 11, and it was just six months before he wrote his first diary entry.

The famous *Railway Time Table*, first published by George Bradshaw in Manchester in 1839, was by now well established. His *Railway Guide*

1051 In February 1883 at King's he received a letter from his brother Ernest with 2s enclosed.

1052 In May 1886 Reginald received a box of lilies of the valley from his mother to decorate his study.

1053 Ibid.

1054 Simmons, Jack, *The Victorian Railway* (1991), p. 183.

was published under different titles every month for 120 years.[1055] But, like today, trains did not always run to their scheduled times. Reginald in October 1886 left school with special permission to attend a funeral of a relative.[1056] He waited at Seaton station and the train to Peterborough was 20 minutes late. He planned to travel via March rather than Huntingdon, and he then missed his connection and had a two-hour wait at the town of March. Having left at 1.00pm he got back at 6.00.

While railway travel was quick, it was not initially comfortable. Only first-class carriages had upholstered seats, and second-class had bare wooden ones. Reginald never mentioned whether he went by first- or second-class. The cost of his train journey from home to Uppingham was around £3s 8s (£375), so it is likely that this was first-class. The trap from the station to his house at Redgate was 1s 6d (£9.60).

Passengers were encouraged to bring their own 'air cushions' to sit on for long journeys; with the average speed being 30mph, train travel for longer journeys could take some time.[1057] As there were no lavatories on trains, it was wise to use whatever facilities were provided at stations.[1058] The best seat to avoid the ash and smoke from the engine was one in the corner facing away from the engine; apparently it also protected the passenger from the jolting of the train. Train tickets had to be bought on the day of travel and were valid only for specific railway companies. Reginald's visits to his uncle and aunt on their farm at Shippea Hill involved travel on the St Ives to Cambridge line run by the Eastern Counties Company on one ticket, and then another ticket to take him on the Norfolk line via Ely and on to Mildenhall Road station for a short trip via horse and trap to the farm.

Some of Reginald's journeys back to school were left until as late as possible, as was the case with many schoolboys keen to stay on holiday as long as possible. Consequently, during the winter months it was dark for

---

[1055] Simmons, Jack, *The Victorian Railway*, p. 183.

[1056] It is not clear who the relative was or when the funeral took place. He got to St Ives late on Saturday afternoon and left on Monday afternoon to return to school. There were two church services that he went to on the Sunday, but no mention of a funeral service was made in his diary.

[1057] Goodman, Ruth, *How To Be a Victorian*, p. 179.

[1058] The Great Northern Railway began to introduce a few carriages with lavatories for first-class passengers in 1882, and the Midland Railway for third-class passengers in 1883. By the 1890s they became more common but the reduction of carriage space and thus less revenue was an initial caveat for railway companies.

most of his journey. There was no lighting in the carriages until the 1890s, although fishtailed gas burners (named because of the shape of the flame they produced) were used to give some light at stations. They offered only very dim lighting and were replaced by electricity in the 1890s.[1059] This innovation was a huge improvement. *The English Illustrated Magazine* described the 1890s station in this way:

> At night, standing under the bridge just where the steps come down from Bishop's Road station and looking outwards, the scene is most impressive and weird. High in the air gleam two great electric lights, the apexes of two ghostly pyramids of light, around swirls the streams of passing engines, beneath all is rush, swish, and darkness and innumerable coloured lights twinkling and blurred.[1060]

Reginald's family used the railway extensively. His father went for the day to London on medical matters or for social visits. Reginald made a number of day visits to see specialists about his eyesight in London. A visit in March 1886 saw 17-year-old Reginald leave with his father on a train from St Ives at 8.50am, arriving in London at 11.15. Having seen Charles Higgins, a well-known occulist, about his eyesight, they had lunch at the Pimms Restaurant[1061], meeting an uncle (Tom Williams). They had time to pay a visit to Mercers' Hall and then took a train from Liverpool Street station to get home by 7.15pm. And of course, it was by train that he went to and from school at King's and then at Uppingham.

From the 1860s, when his father arrived to set up practice in St Ives, the town had become something of a railway hub, as it could be reached from four directions. The first line was built by the Eastern Counties Company between St Ives and Cambridge which was opened in 1847. This line was then continued on to Godmanchester, one mile outside Huntingdon itself; confusingly it was called Huntington station. The Great Northern Railway line, snaking northward from King's Cross, reached Huntingdon in 1850, and this station was called Huntington, too. In July 1882 the line from St Ives to 'Huntingdon' was transferred to the Great Northern and Great Eastern Joint Railway, and this station was then renamed

---

[1059] Although the London, Brighton & South Coast Company used electricity for the first time in 1881, most rail companies found it too expensive to introduce. The Midland Company which Reginald used often to get to Uppingham did not install electricity until 1921.

[1060] Goodman, Ruth, *How To Be a Victorian*, p. 185.

[1061] The location of this restaurant is not known.

Godmanchester.[1062]

The section of line from Cambridge to March was opened in 1848, giving St Ives a direct link with the North.[1063] A link was made to St Ives by the Midland Railway Company in 1866 from Kettering to Huntingdon through St Ives to Cambridge, which carried both freight and passengers. In 1887 St Ives station had seven 'good waiting rooms', according to Herbert Norris who wrote a *History of St Ives*, 'being more than any other station in England'. This seems rather far-fetched and it is not possible to verify the claim.

The route from St Ives to Huntingdon and thence northwards became one of the routes Reginald used to get to Uppingham at the beginning of each term. While different railway companies built their own track, they shared the use of stations. At Huntingdon station, for instance, in 1887, there were three stationmasters – one for the Great Eastern Railway, one for the Great Northern Railway, and one for the Midland Railway.[1064] Passengers changed at a station not only for a different direction of travel, but also for a different railway company. It was not until the rail network was nationalised in 1948 that this changed.

A growing desire of prosperous middle-class parents seeking an education for their sons was a major factor in the growth of public schools in the last half of the 19th century. As Thring said, 'hundreds go to schools now who thirty years ago would have not thought of doing so'.[1065] But this was only made possible by the expanding railway network and the new prosperity of the middle classes. Reginald's father and uncle were educated at a local grammar school near where they lived in Staffordshire. It would not have been practical or possible for them in the 1840s and 1850s to travel to a boarding school. What was once a protracted journey from home to a boarding school like Rugby now became quick, easy and cheap for prospective parents and pupils.

Schools like Marlborough, Cheltenham and Rossall (where Reginald tried for a scholarship before going to Uppingham) promoted their accessibility by train; Uppingham did the same. When he first came to

---

1062 Godmanchester station was closed to passengers in June 1959, to freight in June 1962, and then later demolished.

1063 Little, Bryan, and Werba, Herbert, *St Ives in Huntingdonshire* (1974), p. 29.

1064 *Harrod's Directory of Huntingdonshire 1887.*

1065 Richardson, p. 27.

Uppingham, Thring realised the potential that improved transport gave:

> We stand on the threshold of a new world. Railways and steamships, and telegraphs have made this earth of ours to all and intents and purposes another planet ... all nations are suddenly being poured together into one great tumultuous sea of stormy life.[1066]

Reginald (and his parents when they visited) always travelled by train to Uppingham, and the journey generally took about three hours,[1067] depending on which route was taken. As often as not, he and his parents took the train westwards to Huntingdon station (actually Godmanchester). The journey from St Ives took just over 20 minutes.[1068] Having taken a fly[1069] from Godmanchester station to the station at Huntingdon, there was easy access to the north, stopping at St Neots and Peterborough. The train service north provided by the Midland Railway ran from St Pancras and King's Cross stations in London and stopped at Manton station.[1070] Trains north from London Euston station run by the London and North Western Railway stopped at Huntingdon and then at Peterborough. There he changed onto the Stamford and Peterborough branch line which took him either to Manton station (on the line north to Oakham and Melton Mowbray) or south to Seaton station.[1071] This station had been opened in 1850.

Uppingham was therefore served by two stations – Seaton and Manton. Manton was four miles and Seaton three miles from Uppingham and, depending on his route, Reginald made use of one or the other. Whichever

---

1066 Richardson, p. 27.

1067 Travelling back for the Summer Term 1885 he took the 4.50pm train from St Ives and arrived in Uppingham at about 8.00 (diary 07.05.85). Also returning for the Autumn Term he caught the same train and arrived at Uppingham around 8.00pm (diary 24.09.85). Returning to school in January 1886, he took the same train, via Huntingdon, but arrived at about 9.00pm. There were nearly two inches of snow at Uppingham when he arrived so this may have accounted for a longer journey.

1068 For example, leaving St Ives at 9.05am passengers arrived at Huntingdon at 9.24. (*Hunts County Guardian* train timetable, February 1887.)

1069 A light, two-wheeled, horse-drawn public carriage.

1070 Manton station was opened in 1848.

1071 Seaton station was opened in 1850 and was originally a minor stop on the London and North Western Railway line from Rugby and to Stamford which opened in 1850. In 1873 it became a junction when the LNWR double-tracked the line from Rugby to Seaton and opened a new double-track line to Wansford. The route from Rugby to Peterborough was then operated as the main line, and Seaton to Stamford as a branch line.

station was used, it was necessary to take either the omnibus service or a pony and trap, especially as invariably he had a trunk with him. In his early days as Headmaster, when the numbers in the school were much smaller, Thring would often walk to Seaton station with his old English sheepdog called 'Queer' to meet parents off the train who were considering sending their boy to the school. He then walked back with them with their luggage loaded onto a horse-drawn cart (see Volume 2).

A horse-drawn omnibus service left the Falcon Hotel in Market Place in the town three times a day, except on Sundays, to Manton station at 8.00am, 11.50am and 4.20pm. A similar omnibus service ran to Seaton station from the White Heart Inn at 8.50am, 12.15pm and 5.50pm.[1072]

The omnibus was really just a long cart about 12 feet long with a single bench seat along each side – 6 feet wide. For use in cities, the omnibus was often roofed over, and on the top a further two benches were placed back to back along the centre, a low railing running around the outside to stop people falling off. A ladder was used to get to the roof from the rear. Reginald used an omnibus when he visited London in September 1886.

It is not known whether a double-decker was used at Uppingham, but, given the steep hills which had to be negotiated to get to either station, it is unlikely. There were also drivers with a horse and trap at the stations who waited for the arrival of trains, much like modern taxis and cabs. Arriving back from the Christmas holidays, for instance, in January 1887, he and his friend Berry arrived at Redgate just before 9.00pm, being the 'only two fellows who came by this train and there was only one trap at the station'. Thankfully, there was one, otherwise it was a long walk to school. That evening there was a good deal of snow on the ground, too.

On one occasion returning to school in January 1885 he overpaid the cabman by mistake, giving him a sovereign[1073] instead of the usual fare. The next day he walked back the three and a half miles to Manton station with another boy, Arthur Heald.[1074] Heald had joined in the same term as Reginald and was in the same house. Reginald got his sovereign back, giving the cabman the 2s 6d (£15.72). This amount was part tip, as it was more than the normal fare.

1072 *Kelly's Directory of Leicester and Rutland 1881.*

1073 A sovereign was a gold coin worth £1.00 (£126).

1074 Sadly, Arthur Heald drowned in 1892 in a shipwreck a few years after leaving Uppingham.

On some occasions he did use Seaton station, and while the distance was shorter than from Manton, the route was hillier. At the end of term in April 1885, he took the 8.27am train from Seaton station, travelling back with the two Warren brothers who were at school with him and also lived at St Ives. They gave him a lift in their trap from Huntingdon station back to St Ives, thus avoiding having to cross the town to catch the train to St Ives from the Godmanchester (Huntingdon) station. There were other times when he travelled with the Warrens. At the beginning of term in May 1884 he went back to school with them and another school friend called Blois[1075] (Charles Blois lived at Felsham, near Bury St Edmunds, Suffolk). In all probability Blois spent some of the holiday with Reginald at St Ives, as he and Blois were good friends; between January and May 1884 they went on walks around Uppingham on ten different occasions.

The Falcon Hotel, besides being a hostelry offering travellers rooms for the night, and an omnibus depot, was used for a number of other activities. By Reginald's time the stagecoach service, which had been well known in the past, had ceased, and in his time was used as a county court once a month, an auction venue, and the Inland Revenue and Excise for their offices. It was popular for parents visiting boys at the school, as indeed it is to this day.

Thring pushed for Uppingham to have its own train link and station, as did others who lived in the town. Ten years before Reginald started at the school a proposal was drawn up by the Midland Railway Company to bring a line to Uppingham in 1871:

> The general wish of the inhabitants was that the line should run close to the town and so remove the present inconvenience arising from the division of passenger and goods traffic for the town from Manton and Seaton and Rockingham on the LNWR.[1076]

But it was not to be, and the three-mile-long line from Seaton to

[1075] Charles Blois was the son of Sir J. R. Blois of Cockfield Hall, Felsham. The Blois family were landowners in Suffolk. Charles joined Uppingham in January 1883 and was a boarder like Reginald at Redgate. Sadly, he died on a voyage out to Australia in December 1900 when he was 33.

[1076] *Stamford Mercury* September 1871.

Uppingham was not finally built until 1894,[1077] well after Reginald had left. It took three years to build and had a steep gradient of 1 in 60 for half a mile from the new junction, rising afterwards to 1 in 60 again for the rest of the track.[1078] A new road was built to the new station.

Before general passengers could use the line, there were three special trains laid on to bring boys back from their summer holidays. The reality, however, was that the passenger traffic of the line was light even before the advent of the car and bus changed passenger travel. And before that it was still quicker to take the train to Manton station and hire a 'fly' to get to the town, which the parents of boys at the school often did. Often the normal train had only one coach. The line was finally closed in 1960.[1079]

Travel for Reginald and his family from St Ives to Cambridge and vice versa was quick and frequent by train; it took just 31 minutes.[1080] It was easy to travel to Cambridge and return in comfort the same day. The 18-mile journey by pony and trap took an hour and a quarter at least. His father used the railway network sometimes to get about his practice. After all, it took only a matter of minutes to walk to the station from Slepe House, and if he caught the right train, the trip to one of the villages up the line was easy and quick. So, a trip to visit patients or on errands for his father or one of his Medical Assistants to Swavesey, was just one stop away. On other occasions Reginald went by train to Bluntisham and Earith on the single-track line from St Ives to Ely which was built in 1866 by the Ely, Haddenham and Sutton Railway Company (later taken over by the Great Eastern Company). Bluntisham was the first stop, and Earith Bridge the second.[1081] Travelling to Bluntisham by train to go skating on the flooded, frozen meadow called Bury Fen was easy for the Groves.

The railways revolutionised work and social life for Victorians and the

---

[1077] A Mr Joe Love was 10 years old when he travelled on the first passenger train that ran; 66 years later in 1960 he was to travel on the last public passenger train to run (*By God's Grace*, Bryan Matthews, p. 127.)

[1078] Very unusually, when the Uppingham branch line was completed, gravity shunting was used at Seaton. Detailed information is given in *Railways in Rutland*, published by the Rutland Historical Society Vol 3 1980, p. 63.

[1079] *Railways in Rutland* Vol 3 (Rutland Local History Society, 1980), pp. 62–3.

[1080] For example, leaving Cambridge at 9.57 in the morning passengers arrived at St Ives station at 10.28 (*Hunts County Guardian* train timetable February 1887).

[1081] Bluntisham station was closed for passengers in 1931, as was Earith Bridge (which had been opened in 1878). The line closed for freight in 1964, although Earith Bridge closed before this in 1958.

Grove family was no exception. In the year of Reginald's birth Robert Smiles wrote a biography of a well-known businessman called Henry Booth. Booth had played an important role in developing railway companies[1082] in the early part of Victoria's reign. Smiles wrote:

> We, who accept with as little gratitude as wonder the marvellous results of our railway system, who complain of the slightest delay or inconvenience, and in whose estimate the slightest casual annoyance outweighs a thousand continuous and unspeakable benefits – find it difficult, if we even try, to realise the enormous difficulties of the first beginning and early progress.[1083]

Truly it was the age of steam. By the time Reginald was growing up the railways were firmly established as a normal part of everyday life on which so much depended. But within a few years all this was to change with the age of the motor car. Reginald became one of the early motoring pioneers in Huntingdonshire, registering the sixth motor car in the county: EW6. The impact of the motor car on his life is described in Volume 3.

[1082] In particular the Liverpool and Manchester Railway Company.

[1083] Smiles, R., *Memoirs of the Late Henry Booth* (Wyman & Sons London, 1869), p. 113.

CHAPTER 22

A New World of Communications

'For this is eminently a novelty loving age. We have lived in such a whirl of inventions, and discoveries that a new idea, a new plan, a new theory commends itself to us on the first blush because it is new.'[1084]

Edward Thring

THE POSTAL SERVICE

The penny postal system had been introduced in 1840 with the 'Penny Black' stamp which enabled letters to be sent for exactly the same cost anywhere on the mainland. From their very first entries, Reginald's diaries are full of the details of letters and cards that he wrote, as well as those he received. The day after his twelfth birthday,[1085] he wrote to his Grandmother Grove, perhaps a thankyou letter for his birthday.

Letter writing was an integral part of middle-class life in the Victorian era – the equivalent of today's email and social media postings. During the course of a typically average week in February 1885, Reginald received four letters, and in addition a copy of his *St Nicholas* magazine from home. During that week he wrote four letters. Similarly, two years later in February 1887 Reginald wrote four letters, two of which were to his father and mother, and he sent a copy of the School Magazine to his Uncle Frank. He received five letters, one of which was from his mother. He spent a lot of his allowance at school on postage stamps – in January 1885 1d, February 7d and March 7d, totalling 15d (£7.80). As the postage for letters was just a penny (52p) this represented 15 letters over the three-month period. Over the same period two years later, it had increased to 3s (£56), largely due to his letter writing to Mary, his sweetheart.[1086]

Sending letters became extremely popular, especially as the railway network ensured swift, often overnight delivery. Mail was sorted en

[1084] *Contemporary Review* January 1866, p. 81, commenting on Thring's *Education and School.*

[1085] 13 January 1881.

[1086] These figures are assessed on his monthly accounts in 1885 and 1886 which were kept at the back of his diaries.

route in specially designed carriages early on, and then it became a legal requirement for all railway companies to provide a separate carriage for sorting letters[1087] or to send mail by ordinary trains.[1088]

The Victorians kept in touch with each other by writing to a degree we can scarcely envisage today.[1089] In the 1890s there were 12 deliveries *a day* in the City of London. A letter could arrive, if addressed correctly, within four hours of being sent.[1090] Letters in St Ives arrived at 7.30am and 12.45pm each day. They were despatched daily at 8.30pm with London mail leaving at 12.00 noon. The Post Office and Telegraph Office[1091] was in Bridge Street until a new and more central one[1092] was built in the Jubilee Year 1887 with its imposing façade in Market Hill.[1093] At Uppingham letters arrived from London and elsewhere via Oakham at 5.40am and from Manton at 2.30pm; the collection was despatched via Manton at 11.35am via Oakham and at 7.10pm and 7.35pm. An extra stamp ensured a collection at 4.15pm on Sundays from the Post Office.[1094]

From 1880 postmen began to use bicycles to deliver the mail and there were increasing numbers of the familiar red pillar boxes erected, although those mounted in walls were also favoured. The first boxes were painted green before red as a colour became universal by 1879.[1095] The efficiency

---

[1087] Travelling post offices were special carriages dedicated to sorting mail in transit with their own clerks and sorters. They operated between major cities and towns. A specially designed device was invented to allow mailbags to be snatched by a mechanism beside the track from the train as it passed. No stopping was required.

[1088] The Mails on Railways Bill (2 Vic. Cap. 98) became law in 1838.

[1089] In 1863 the annual ratio of letters written per person was 22 (First Report of the Postmaster General on the Post Office) cited by Fava-Verde article, Royal Society Journal of the History of Science 2018, page 277.

[1090] Walvin, James, *Victorian Values* (André Deutsch, 1987), p. 82.

[1091] *Harrod's Directory of Huntingdonshire 1887.*

[1092] Little, Bryan, and Werba, Herbert, *St Ives in Huntingdonshire,* p. 42.

[1093] I remember working as a temporary postman over Christmas 1965 in this building. It is now used as a shop, since the Post Office moved back to Bridge Street towards the end of the 20th century.

[1094] *Kelly's Directory of Leicester and Rutland 1881.*

[1095] In 1853 the first pillar box was erected in Carlisle. Roadside wall boxes first appeared in 1857 as a cheaper alternative to pillar boxes, especially in rural districts. An ornate pillar box for use in London and other large cities was designed and once this design had been modified in 1859 it became the first National Standard pillar box. Between 1866 and 1879 the hexagonal Penfold post box became the standard design for pillar boxes and it was during this period that red was first adopted as the standard colour.

of the postal system enabled letters and cards to arrive at their destination the following day.

Today, besides a postcode, most addressees have a designated house number given them. Post codes are a 20th century innovation of course, but until the end of the 19th century, no streets had house numbers. In a small town like St Ives, the post office staff knew the houses where the professional and tradespeople lived who were most likely to receive correspondence. None of the houses in the Bullock Market, where Reginald grew up until he was 12, for instance, had house numbers at the time. This makes identifying the houses where people lived from Census returns difficult, although by a process of elimination and deduction the Grove family house has been identified as Number 33. By the time of the 1891 National Census the terraced houses opposite Slepe House in Cromwell Place, as well as in Cromwell Terrace, were all numbered.

It is estimated that in 1839 67 million letters were delivered in England and Wales;[1096] four years before Reginald was born this had increased to 741 million.[1097] This figure does not include any postcards, which were cheap, easy to use and increasingly popular. The Post Office first issued plain cards with a preprinted stamp in 1870, but other companies were not allowed to print or issue cards, with the Post Office having a complete monopoly. Reginald occasionally sent postcards – he sent one, for instance, to Dr Reynell, his old Headmaster at King's, in December 1886 and another a few days later before Christmas to his friend George Lloyd. The postal rate was 1/2d (26p). Picture postcards were only allowed in 1894,[1098] well after Reginald had left school. As soon as issuing them stopped being a Post Office monopoly, their use became commonplace.

As mentioned earlier, the railway network enabled the Post Office to deliver packages as well as letters. The parcel post service was introduced in 1883 just before Reginald went to Uppingham and he and the other boys at boarding school benefited from the packages, often of food, that were sent, besides newspapers and magazines. In April 1886 some Devonshire cream, primroses and violets were sent by his Uncle Frank from Brixham

---

[1096] The Royal Mail delivered 11.7 billion letters in 2016. Ofcom Annual Report 2016. https://www.ofcom.org.uk/__data/assets/pdf_file/0019/108082/postal-annual-monitoring-report-2016-2017.pdf.

[1097] Fava-Verde, Jean-François, 'Victorian Telegrams: the early development of the telegraphic despatch and its interplay with the letter post' (2019), *Royal Society Journal of the History of Science*.

[1098] Hart-Adams, *What the Victorians Did for Us* (2001), p. 130.

in Devon for example. Later in May that year, his mother sent him a box of lily of the valley as previously mentioned and in June she sent him some cream cheese. Besides fresh food or flowers he also received other items in the post like the parcel he was sent enclosing an umbrella, boots, cake and 'brass' from home. What the latter was is uncertain.

TELEGRAPHIC COMMUNICATION

The electric telegraph was developed in 1837 by William Cooke and Charles Wheatstone. Cooke's vision was 'a new system of railway communication, at once safe, economical and efficient'.[1099] They realised that telegraph wires could be laid alongside railway lines and messages could be sent from one station to another to a signalling point which was used to prevent a head-on collision on single-track lines. The first use was on a short track of the London to Birmingham Railway between Euston and Camden. Originally the lines were housed on tubes beside the railway lines, but later it was found to be easier and cheaper to use a single wire slung off the ground between 'telegraph poles'. The telegraph service was initially offered by the Electric Telegraph Company, which was established by an Act of Parliament in 1846, and by the 1850s telegrams were being used by businesses; for instance, in Norwich in 1846 the London stock market prices were sent by telegraph along the Norfolk Railway.[1100]

A few years before Reginald's father came to St Ives, most major cities had been linked. The network was eventually taken over by the General Post Office in 1870 and nationalised. Posting a letter or sending a telegram was a matter of personal choice, but just prior to the national telegraph being launched, the overall number of telegrams sent was less than 1% of the total number of letters sent.[1101] Initially, telegraph offices were located at railway stations,[1102] but gradually offices were opened in city and town centres, which made them much more accessible. The telegraph office at St

[1099] Cooke, William Fothergill, *Telegraphic Railways; or, the single way recommended by safety, economy and efficiency under the safeguard and control of the electric telegraph* (Simpkin, Marshall & Co. London, 1842).

[1100] Simmons, Jack, *The Victorian Railway* (Thames & Hudson, 1991), p. 227.

[1101] Fava-Verde, Jean-François, *Victorian Telegrams*, p. 276.

[1102] The 1868 edition of *Bradshaw's Descriptive Railway Handbook* stated that there was a 'telegraph station' at St Ives station, as well as at Ely, Huntingdon and Cambridge. Only main stations had them. At Somersham, with a population only of 1,600, the nearest telegraph station was six miles away at St Ives with its population that was three times larger.

Ives was located in the Post Office, and later in the new Post Office building in Market Hill. At the time Reginald was born in 1868, it is estimated there were 1,289 telegraph offices.[1103] The use of telegrams increased, especially by domestic, rather than commercial, customers. The process of sending a message was quick and easy – customers took their written messages to telegraph offices to be transcoded and transmitted usually within five minutes or so after being handed in at the counter. At the other end, the transcribed telegrams would be delivered within a three-mile radius of the telegram office by uniformed messengers who were generally boys paid piece rate, one penny (52p) per message delivered.

Undersea cables began to be laid between continents – the first being from Europe to the USA in 1866. By 1875 cables had been laid across the world to India, the Far East, Australia and South America.

Interestingly, telegrams were first used in May 1864 for commercial marketing, rather like junk email today. A number of Members of Parliament, as well as former ones, whose names and addresses were well known, received a telegram from the London and District Telegraph Office delivered by a delivery boy. The telegram did not give them news of a family bereavement or a financial loss or some other disaster. Each telegram read: 'Messrs Gabriel, dentists, Harley Street, Cavendish Square. Until October, Messrs Gabriels professional attendance at 27, Harley Street, will be 10 to 5.' The telegrams caused some consternation – not because Gabriels were not qualified dentists, but because of the cheek of their self-advertising! They sold their own branded dental products, such as toothpaste and dental powder, too. Later that year, the National Provincial Clothing Depot in Bristol followed suit and sent an advertising telegram to potential customers.[1104]

At Uppingham, telegrams played an important role in making sure that the scores of a School First XI or XV, when playing away, were sent back to the boys eagerly awaiting the first word of the outcome. A cricket match against Repton School in the Summer Term 1886 resulted on the first day with the Uppingham team being all out for 96 – our 'spirits fell', Reginald wrote. The second match resulted in Repton scoring 154 all out and their spirits fell even lower. In the second innings, which began on the same day, Uppingham scored 154 for 4 wickets: 'a tremendous rise in spirits through

1103 Fava-Verde, Jean-François, *Victorian Telegrams*, p. 283.

1104 Sweet, Matthew, *Inventing the Victorians* (Faber and Faber, 2001), pp. 38–39.

the school'. The next day a further telegram arrived from the Uppingham Team to report that they had got 167 in Uppingham's second innings, and then a later telegram came to report that Uppingham had won by 9 runs! 'Close', Reginald wrote, 'but good enough to win!'

For the Grove family, telegrams were used mainly for emergencies or urgent matters, as illustrated when Grandmother Grove became ill in Southsea. On another occasion, the month after this, Reginald telegraphed his father to ask that he contact his Headmaster Thring to get special permission to attend the funeral of his Great-Uncle Edward Long.

A telegram was used the following year in April 1887 to inform the wife of a patient of Reginald's father of her husband's death when he was away on a short business trip. He had had a heart attack on the platform of Bletchley railway station and the stationmaster there telegraphed his counterpart at St Ives so that the widow could be informed. As previously described, Dr Grove had the sad duty of having to inform her.

TELEPHONE COMMUNICATION

Telephone patents were taken out by Alexander Graham Bell in 1876, and two years later the first commercial telephone enterprise was set up in Chislehurst, Kent, with The Telephone Company (Bell's Patents) opening Britain's first public telephone exchange at 36 Coleman St, London, in 1879. Another two exchanges were opened by the end of the year in London, and the number of subscribers was 200. Elsewhere across the country, exchanges were opened later in the year in Glasgow, Manchester, Liverpool, Sheffield, Edinburgh, Birmingham and Bristol.

The railway companies began to experiment with connecting stations via telephone. The Great Northern Railway in 1879, for example, connected King's Cross with Finchley a few miles away in North London. By Reginald's last year at Uppingham one of the first free-standing phone booths (later to be known as 'kiosks') was introduced in Bristol by the United Telephone Company. This was a small, wooden hut where a three-minute call could be made for 2d (£1.04).

The use of telephones grew by leaps and bounds as new technical improvements made calls easier, cheaper and more widespread. The earliest reference to telephones being used by the Grove family was in June 1890 when Reginald described an incident at Slepe House when a drunk broke some of their windows in the middle of the night; after he and his father confronted the man, Dr Grove 'went off and rung the police'. The St Ives police station was less than half a mile away so the use of the surgery phone was more of a convenience, than a necessity. The impact on Reginald's life of telephone usage on practice life when he returned to St Ives to take over from his father is covered in Volume 3.

By 1912, when the Postmaster General took over the system of the National Telephone Company for £12,515,264, 9,000 people were employed, there were 1,500,000 miles of wire, and 1,565 exchanges, of which 231 had more than 300 subscribers each. The National Telephone Company provided for 561,738 subscribers altogether. Communication has never looked back.[1105]

THE PRINTED WORD

The second half of the 19th century saw an explosion in written communication. As described in an earlier chapter, the 1870 Education Act extended the educational provision for most children and created a huge reading public. The rapid advances in printing techniques for the mass market were the other reason for the revolution in printed communication.

With technological improvements, print could be produced more quickly, more cheaply and in volume, with illustrations (initially engravings and towards the end of the era photographs) making publications more marketable. The *Illustrated London News* was first published in 1842 on a weekly basis priced at 6d (£3) and relied heavily on lavish engravings to sell its copy. It covered topical stories ranging from presidential elections in the United States, foreign conflicts, disasters, court cases and other human-interest stories. The text could be 'wrapped around' the illustrations so the style of newspapers and periodicals changed.

With newspaper journalism, reporters were able to travel easily by public transport to report on news quickly and then telegraph stories to be wired for publication within hours. Uppingham was agog in Reginald's last year when the news broke in the nationals about the trial of his Science Master, Hinton, for bigamy, as described in Volume 2. The event showed clearly how before the day was out, the evening London papers carried the story – followed up by the national ones the following morning which Reginald and his friends avidly read, as did everyone else in the school and town.

By 1894, when the *Evening News* was bought by Alfred Harmsworth

---

1105 https://www.britishtelephones.com/histuk.htm (29.05.20).

who launched *The Daily Mail* two years later, the paper's motto was 'all the news in the smallest space', and his popular style of journalism was concise, gossipy and, in a sense, trivial. Not all publications were in this genre: there were a range of weekly periodicals which were more serious. Some, such as those published specifically for the edification and wholesomeness of their readership, and which had a religious content, achieved this end.

With national papers, Reginald borrowed copies from other boys until the Sixth Form when they were available in the Sixth Form Common Room. Big national events printed in the papers were discussed among the boys, even at King's; the assassination of the Tsar Alexander the Second (or 'Czar', as Reginald wrote) in St Petersburg in March 1881, mentioned earlier, when Reginald was 12, is one example. He also made a diary note about the death of Benjamin Disraeli the next month. The death of General Gordon in the Sudan in January 1885 was another landmark noted in his diary.

These events were national talking points, even among young boys of 12. The results of parliamentary elections were also eagerly read about in the papers, as described elsewhere.

On a personal note, he first learnt about the death of his friend Bensly in the *Standard* in February 1887, which came as a huge shock to him, rather than a note from Bensly's parents.

Reginald also enjoyed reading the local papers, which his mother sent him regularly at school. There were a number published, such as the *Cambridge Chronicle*, the *Hunts County News*, *The St Ives Chronicle* and *The Hunts Guardian*. One story which amused him which he noted in his diary was about a fracas in the town between some soldiers from Huntingdon who had been drinking and who had a fight with some local lads, and the sentence for the soldiers was three weeks' hard labour.

Besides newspapers, magazines proliferated for different target readers and encouraged readers to write in. The influence of home magazines on the ideas and the readership of middle-class wives has been described earlier. The correspondence section of magazines almost always had comments by readers about articles published previously. Entrepreneurs made more and more use of newspapers and magazines to market their products and services – Reginald bought stamps for his collection in this way.

Books became more available, too, because reduced production costs made them cheaper and more widely available, but the pages still had to be cut with a small knife by each reader. The growth of public libraries as the century progressed also helped the readership expand beyond those who could afford books, as did reading rooms set up by the temperance movement as an alternative to public houses. St Ives had its own Literary Institute which Reginald visited occasionally. With the growth of the railway network, besides enabling national papers to be transported daily across the country, passengers were tempted to buy reading material for their train journeys. W. H. Smith, already a bookseller, expanded into newspaper distribution, but also station bookstalls; the first was at Euston station in 1848, and by 1878 when Reginald was nine, the number had grown to over 400.

CHAPTER 23

The Agricultural Revolution

'Farming will become a commercial speculation carried on by large joint stock concerns occupying from three to ten thousand acres.'
Richard Jefferies, *Fraser's Magazine*, 1873[1106]

FARM WORK IN VICTORIAN TIMES

Reginald's mother's parents, grandparents, brothers and sisters were all involved in farming in Cambridgeshire. His uncles were tenant farmers concentrating on arable rather than livestock production. The acreage of their farms was large – Uncle Hanslip farmed 1,600 acres,[1107] Uncle Daniel 1,700, Uncle Lawsell 1,200, and Uncle Arthur 1,700. Farming was labour-intensive in the mid-19th century but this was to change significantly by the time of the First World War.

In 1852 46% of the population lived in rural communities, with the majority of working children in Victorian times engaged in agriculture. The last 30 years of the 19th century have been termed the 'Great Depression[1108]' by historians, and Reginald's farming relatives were faced with huge economic challenges beyond their control. With mechanisation, cheap corn imports from Russia and North America, and in the 1890s poor weather conditions, there was a huge move of the rural population to towns and cities. It is estimated that the number of agricultural labourers dropped from about a million to 600,000 by 1901.[1109]

It was common for children to carry out farm work, either paid work or helping their parents. The Long farmers all used child labour – generally young boys, according to the Census records, rather than girls, although at harvest time every available helping hand was brought in.

Many boys became employed from 12 onwards by a farmer and lived

---

1106 Richard Jefferies, *Fraser's Magazine* (Longmans, Green & Co, 1873).

1107 He owned, as opposed to rented, 51 acres and 3 rods in 1873 which had an estimated rental value of £127 18s per annum (Return of Owners Land Vol 1 1873).

1108 This term has also been used to describe the world wide economic slump in the 1930's of course.

1109 Cook, Chris, *Britain in the Nineteenth Century 1815–1914* (2005), p. 198.

on his farm away from home. Agriculture (unlike mining or manufacture) was unregulated by any legislation at this time. Life was tough, abuse common, the diet was often poor and, of course, the work was carried on outdoors throughout the year. Crow scaring and wood cutting were done by boys, plus cleaning out stables and farmyards, and building dung heaps. Crow scaring was a lonely, all-day occupation, throwing stones at birds that landed from dawn to dusk. William Arnold, born in 1860 at Everdon, a village about 13 miles from Northampton, who later became a Methodist preacher, was one such lad. His father, Matthew, was a shoemaker. William was one of 14 children, and family life was a struggle. William recalled that in his childhood he always felt hungry. He started work when he was six years old scaring crows. He earned 18d (£9.30) a week and dinner on Sundays was thrown in by the farmer.[1110] Reginald scared off crows when he stayed on his Uncle George's farm at Carleton Grange, but it is one thing to spend a little time on a task like this and quite another to work for a living as young William Arnold did.

Harvest time saw the biggest demand for child labour (which is why schools were closed over the summer). Gathering the cut stems of wheat, tying them into sheaves, stooking the sheaves,[1111] gleaning the fields for fallen grain and carrying in the harvest were all jobs children did. Or with other crops, there was pea picking, digging potatoes, hop picking or pulling flax. Weeding the fields could be done by children, too, as small hands were useful for the task. As unwaged workers, children helped their parents make ends meet by collecting water and foodstuffs from hedgerows, as well as working smallholdings or cottage gardens.

Farming was a way of life for Reginald's Long uncles, aunts and cousins; as already seen, he spent holidays staying on these farms, and many of his father's patients were farm workers, too. This was the rural environment in which he grew up, but it underwent massive change.

[1110] https://www.myprimitivemethodists.org.uk/content/people-2/lay-people/surnames-beginning-with-a/james_william_arnold_known_as_william 02.06.19.

[1111] A stook, (also known as a shock or stack), was an arrangement of sheaves of cut grain stalks placed so as to keep the grain-heads off the ground while still in the field and prior to collection for threshing. Stooked grain sheaves were typically wheat, barley and oats.

IMPROVED FARMING METHODS

The world that Reginald grew up in was one of extensive scientific discovery, as well as technical innovation.

Fertilisation

From the 1840s onwards, chemical fertilisers were produced and became available; the use of dissolved animal bones in a sulphuric acid solution produced phosphates which in turn produced superphosphate manure.[1112] This was sold to landowners, as well as tenant farmers who could afford it to produce better yields. By 1870 it is estimated that with over 1,200 manufacturers of artificial manure in England and Wales, an average of £3 (£380) per acre was being spent on artificial manure.[1113] The centuries-old practice of crop rotation was no longer needed, as farmers were able to restore vitality to the land, which could be fertilised with the relevant chemicals for the crops they wanted to grow. A public health benefit was that the use of human excrement from the earth toilets to manure fields became less.

Animal feed

The commercial production of animal feed meant, too, that farmers were not dependent on home-grown feed; feed cakes became available for livestock made out of rapeseed, cottonseed and linseed, which were biproducts of other industries.

Mechanisation

This played a huge role in changing the face of farming, as more and more machines became available, although largely powered by horses. Small machines which originally were hand-powered became horse-powered through a horse 'gin' or 'gear'. This device enabled a horse to be used as a stationary power source for chaff cutters, root slicers and kibblers.[1114] A special building, generally circular or pentagonal, was built for the horse gin. Reginald did not mention these on his visits to his uncles' farms, but it is likely they had them.

Initially horse-powered, steam became used towards the end of the period for threshing machines which replaced the use of much labour during the

[1112] John Bennet Lawes was a pioneer of this product who began commercial manufacture in 1842.

[1113] Langlands, A., Ginn, P., and Goodman, R., *Victorian Farm* (Pavilion Books, 2008), p. 22.

[1114] A type of heavy-duty mill.

winter months when thrashing a pile of grain with flails[1115] had been the method for centuries. They were portable so could carry out the work in the field itself and were often hired out to farmers. The machine could beat the grain from the husks, as well as winnow it by cleaning off the husk, chaff and straw and then deposit it in a sack ready for transport. Steam was also used for ploughing through a pulley system – the steam engine stationary in a corner of the field with a system of cables and pulleys moving the plough back and across the field. Reginald made no mention of his uncles using these machines. But it is interesting to note that one of the local manufacturers of traction engines for farm use was a local family in St Ives at a workshop a few hundred yards from Reginald's home at Slepe House.

George Fowell set up a workshop in the New Road, St Ives, in 1876 after being a draughtsman with the well-known Norfolk traction engine business run by the Burrell family in Thetford.[1116] Burrells had started with a simple portable steam engine in 1846 towed to its worksite by a horse, and this evolved by 1856 to the Burrell-Boydell heavy traction engine fitted with an 'endless railway' system of boards which provided a smooth surface for the wheels to run on, and at the same time spread the load, especially important on soft ground. After Fowell left the Thetford business his father and brother, who also worked for Burrells, later joined him. The business was called Joseph Fowell and Sons, and the main engineering workshop was 100 feet long and 30 feet wide, and had a yard at its side.

Although there were two other foundries in St Ives, Fowell, who lived for the first few years at 7 Cromwell Place opposite where the Groves lived at Slepe House, was able to set up his business without much competition. His main focus was making and maintaining agricultural machinery. Traction engines were made to give the workers employment during slack periods.

A catalogue printed in 1883 for prospective buyers described their seven-horsepower machine as

> the lightest and most compact engine in the trade. These engines, though specially designed for threshing purposes are equally available on the round-about system, driving circular saws or any fixed machinery and hauling loads on common roads. They are fitted with two speeds, steam jacketed cylinder, link motion reversing gear, water lifter with 25ft of suction hose, two lamps, waterproof cover, firing tools and anchors for

[1115] A flail was two wooden sticks hinged together with iron loops.

[1116] Burn-Murdoch, Bob, *Victorian St Ives* (Witley Press, 2007).

soft ground. Each wheel is driven separately by strong internal gear rings and pinions from a steel counter which gives extreme lightness combined with strength. A winding drum is fitted if required.

These machines were examples of precision mechanical engineering. An account of the business was given in 1893 by Mr S. G. Jarman in his *Trades and Industries of St Ives*: 'One of the most important industries of St Ives is that described by the above headline, insomuch as some forty persons find constant employment at Messrs Fowell's works in the Station Road and New Road adjoining'.[1117] Reginald's eldest daughter was to marry one of the Jarman family, as detailed in Volume 3.

Writing in 1873[1118] in *Fraser's Magazine*,[1119] Richard Jefferies said in his article 'The Future of Farming', that all the facts of the hour point irresistibly to the conclusion that the era of development has just commenced'. Farming in the late-19th century was in a state of considerable change, and in the last quarter farming experienced serious economic depression.[1120]

THE GREAT DEPRESSION AND THE RURAL ECONOMY

Depressed conditions could be a result of national or local circumstances, or both.

Disease

A local example occurred when rinderpest was found around St Ives and the weekly cattle market was closed in 1868. This had a considerable impact on local farmers whose income depended on their fields being used to graze livestock awaiting sale in the market. The closure hit shopkeepers, innkeepers, tradesmen and others who relied on the market business. The visible impact could be seen daily as the grass grew between the cobblestones in the Bullock Market, outside the newly wedded Dr and Mrs Groves' new home.

Such was the concern and desperation by the local farmers and tradesmen that they stormed the Quarter Sessions which had closed the market, to demand that it reopen. It did shortly afterwards.[1121]

1117 http://www.rgreen.org.uk/ff1.html 07.06.19.

1118 Jefferies, Richard, 'The Future of Farming', *Fraser's Magazine* Vol VIII (July–December 1873), published by Longmans, Green & Co. pp. 688–89.

1119 This was a monthly magazine first published in 1830.

1120 Fletcher, T. W. *The Great Depression of English Agriculture 1873–1896* (1961).

1121 Carter, Mary, *A Remarkable Journey* (2005), p. 39.

Poor harvests and cheap imports

While agricultural practices were improved with mechanised machinery which resulted in less labour being used, periods of poor harvests affected farm workers and their dependants savagely. In five poor yield years in the 1850s and 1860s wheat prices fell directly as a result of the increasing cheap foreign wheat imports. This was partly due to the repeal of the Corn Laws in 1846 which reduced import tariffs on grain grown overseas, as well as improving farming production methods across the Atlantic.

Then the period 1873–96 was one of general economic depression which particularly hit rural areas. In the 1870s imports from the virgin plains of North America and Russia, coupled with ease of transport via newly laid railways and more effective ocean travel, saw imported wheat rise from 50% of British consumption in the '70s to nearly 80% in the '90s.[1122] The widespread building of the railway network in North America saw a massive change in the way in which farm produce could be transported abroad. In 1860 the USA had 30,800 miles of railway; by 1870 this had increased to 53,200 miles, and by 1880 it was 94,200 miles. It meant that farmers in the great prairies of North America could send their grain to Europe cheaply and quickly. The cost of sending a ton of grain from Chicago to Liverpool in 1873 was £3 3s (£400). This had fallen by 1884 to as little as £1 4s (£150).[1123] By the 1880s Britain was importing 65% of its grain, and millions of agricultural workers had left the land to move to the cities for industrial work or to emigrate.

Land drainage

While Huntingdonshire was less dependent on grain production, local conditions, especially flooding, affected not just houses in St Ives abutting the Ouse, but the whole of the economy. Land drainage was of particular importance for the use of artificial fertilisers. There was no point in applying expensive fertilisers if water logging or flooding washed away nitrates, phosphates and potassium from the soil.[1124] In 1877 the St Ives

---

[1122] Webb, Robert, *Modern England* (1968), pp. 367–69.

[1123] Wilson, A. N., *The Victorians* (2007), p. 213.

[1124] The invention of machines to manufacture cylindrical drainpipes, the Drainage Act 1845, and the abolition of tax on clap pipes (through which water was pumped) led to cheap ways of draining boggy land. It has been estimated that 2 million acres were drained between 1846 and 1870. (Alex Langlands, Peter Ginn and Ruth Goodman, *The Victorian Farm*, Pavilion, 2009, p. 24.)

Town Council sent the Home Secretary a 'memorial'[1125] about the floods which had affected property as well as the health of residents (although Reginald's father had noted an improvement in his Medical Officer's report as described in Volume 3), and 18 months later they asked for legislation to reduce flooding which was becoming more frequent. This was due to better drainage being introduced upstream which increased the river flow, particularly when it rained heavily. The summer of 1879 was particularly bad as it rained incessantly and the Huntingdon/Cambridgeshire border was badly affected. The Prime Minister, Mr Gladstone, was petitioned himself in 1880 as around St Ives some 30,000 acres (which yielded a good crop of corn in normal circumstances) frequently had their yield destroyed by flooding. This affected market gardening and livestock production too. The Mayor was included in a deputation which met with the Prime Minister, but nothing resulted from this visit. Flood losses continued to depress the local rural economy and a further memorial sent a year later stated that the flooding 'caused a steady and serious decline in livestock production'. This had a direct impact on the livelihood of agricultural labourers who were thrown out of work, many ending up in the St Ives Workhouse. Over a period of 30 years the rural area around St Ives experienced a dramatic depopulation. In 12 parishes in Huntingdonshire and Fen Drayton in Cambridgeshire, the loss by 1901 was over 20% of the population.[1126]

THE IMPACT ON REGINALD'S FAMILY

Farming was indeed a precarious business, and not just for farm workers. Farmers themselves were at risk. As ever, the weather played a significant role in the difference between prosperity and penury. It is estimated that during the 1880s one in 20 farmers in the St Ives area went bankrupt. The impact on the local economy can be seen on the life of Revd Thomas Lloyd, the Minister of the Free Church. The offerings in the church diminished and he offered to take a voluntary reduction of his annual salary of £50 (£6,340).[1127] Thankfully, this was not found necessary in the end.[1128]

1125 Effectively, a petition.

1126 Little, Bryan, and Werba, Herbert, *St Ives in Huntingdonshire* (1974), pp. 41–42.

1127 Carter, Mary, *A Remarkable Journey* (2005), p. 40.

1128 Lloyd was a keen supporter of the St Ives Temperance Society and they offered to increase the rent they paid for the church schoolroom which they used for meetings. A ladies' bazaar was helped also to raise funds for him.

Tragically, two of Reginald's farming uncles in North Cambridgeshire and Suffolk lost their farms, homes and livelihoods, as well as those of their farm workers in the years up to the end of the century. The first was Uncle James Gosling, the husband of one of his mother's sisters, Louise. Married in 1858, they lived in the village of Elveden on the Suffolk/Cambridge border at Chalk Hill Farm. In the 1861 Census he was listed as farming 300 acres and employing 10 men and 4 boys. They were still there 20 years later, and his acreage had increased to 1,200 and he employed 19 men and 2 boys.[1129] Within a couple of years he had lost everything. The exact cause is not known, but maybe he overextended himself and, with the downturn in agriculture, his business collapsed.

Like so many who lost their livelihoods in agriculture, Uncle James, Aunt Louise and their three children were forced to find employment in a city. For them it was a 75-mile journey to north of London's East End in Walthamstow which was to the east of the River Lea that flowed into the Thames at Bow Creek. Walthamstow was an area that saw huge urban development in the 1880s with long terraces of two-storeyed, slate-roofed houses being built. It was in one of these that the family lived. There were also three other families living on the farm in tied cottages and employed by him: two as labourers and one as a shepherd. What happened to them is unknown.

We know about the collapse of the Gosling family fortunes from the 1891 Census when they were shown as living at 230 Bromley Road in the parish of St Leonard's, in Bow and Bromley, Middlesex. It was a stone's throw from Walthamstow railway station, with Epping Forest a few miles away. It was at this address that Reginald and his cousins stayed in September 1886 when they visited London. The Gosling family now lived in very modest circumstances. Using his livestock experience he found work as a stable manager. Where he worked is not recorded, but perhaps at a tram or bus depot as they were drawn by horses at this time. One omnibus used ten horses a day, so the stabling required was considerable. When Reginald and his cousins stayed with his uncle and aunt they travelled on the omnibus to the centre of London, so Walthamstow was on one of the tram and omnibus routes.[1130]

1129 National Census 1881.

1130 By 1853 there were 3,000 omnibuses in London carrying an estimated million passengers a day. Each route had its own name and colour – Nelsons, Royal Blues and Paddingtons painted in their own distinctive colours. (Flanders p. 363.)

But it was a huge change of fortune for a man in his fifties, and, not unnaturally, he clung to the past. By the 1911 Census, aged 79, he listed himself as a 'retired farmer'.[1131] Farming had been his life.

Reginald noted in his last term at school in July 1887 the severity of the drought that year during a long, hot summer:[1132] 'Still very hot all day but a night looked like a bit like rain which is sadly wanted: the waterworks here have almost shut up altogether. Other parts of England are also in great drought.' The late Victorian period climate extremes were not dissimilar to those of the early 21st century.

The impact of the agricultural revolution on Reginald's other uncle, Lawsell Long, who farmed at Carleton in North Cambridgeshire, was devastating. As explained earlier, aged 51 he went bankrupt in 1903 after a succession of bad harvests. It was not for nothing that the 20 years prior to 1910 became to be known as the 'Long Drought' despite some very wet winters; this was not the case during the winter of 1903 when rainfall was minimal.[1133]

When Lawsell took over the farm it was valued at £7,000 (£887,670) and comprised 1,200 acres, which was comparable to his brothers Hanslip, Dan and Arthur. Less than 30 years later his liabilities were £3,975 0s 9d (£504,000) and his assets were £1,843 13s 2d £233,719), leaving a deficit of £2,131 7s 7d (£270,232). His stock was sold off at auction at the farm – livestock and equipment.[1134] It was a sad day.

He found himself in difficulties after the 1893 harvest, with successive poor ones driving down his profits. In the three years prior to his bankruptcy he had made no profit, 'nor did any farmer that he knew'. But at a court

---

1131 He and Louise were living then at 162 Humber Road, Westcombe Park, Blackheath, south of the Thames.

1132 During the late winter and summer of 1887 there was a severe, five-month drought across Great Britain. Major Droughts in England and Wales 1800–2006 (https://rmets.onlinelibrary.wiley.com/doi/pdf/10.1002/wea.67).

1133 Marsh, Terry, Cole, Gwyneth, and Wilby, Rob, *Major droughts in England and Wales, 1800–2006*. Published by Weather April 2007, Vol 162 No 4.

1134 The newspaper advertisement stated: 'The whole of the Valuable Live and Dead Farming Stock, Comprising 31 HORSES, Viz.: 20 Cart Horses and Mares, 4 two-year-olds, 2 Yearlings, 2 Nags, a Thoroughbred Yearling Filly, a Pony and a Cart Foal. 12 HEAD OF CATTLE, Including 6 Cows, 2 Heifers, 2 Steers, and 2 Calves. 40 Head of SWINE and 11 SHEEP, Also 12 Carts, 2 Waggons, 2 Dogcarts, Hooded Wagonette, 4 Drills, 3 Binders by Hornsby, 8 hp. Portable Engine by Burrell. Threshing Drum, 2 Elevators, 5-knife Chaff Cutter by Maynard, Seed Drawer, and the usual Implements for the Cultivation of 800 Acres'. (*Cambridge Independent Press*, 25 December 1903.)

hearing in 1905 when he applied for a discharge of his bankruptcy the judge felt that he had lived above his means prior to his business failure. While Long admitted that his expenditure was £300 (£38,000) per year, during the last three years it had been only £100 (£12,681). Challenged by the judge about the account of £105 (£13,315) for beer and wines, he said that only £30 (£3,804) was wine. He drank only a bottle or two of this, the rest being available for the creditors 'for whose benefit it had been realised. As to beer, farmers generally paid their men at harvest and threshing times partly in beer and partly in money.'[1135]

The court proceedings continued, as reported in the local press:

> The Bankrupt gave evidence bearing out his solicitor's statement. He said that the bad harvest of 1903 meant a loss to him of £1,400 or £1,500. The Official Receiver pointed out that even if he had made £1,400 he would still have had £1,400 he could not pay. Mr. Lyon said the bankrupt had a contingent interest in an estate at Swavesey,[1136] which, if he outlived his sister, would be worth about £400 a year to him. Mr. Cox said that many bankrupts in the neighbourhood of Newmarket expected to come into a few thousands [sic] next time the Derby was run. (Laughter). His Honour granted the application, the discharge to be suspended for two years.[1137]

It was an ignominious end to his farming business which cast gloom among his relatives and friends.

In 1910 his son Charles Lawsell Long was farming at Church Farm. Perhaps he was able to make the farm pay, unlike his father. Charles[1138] died in 1952 in Newmarket.[1139]

As Jefferies said in 1873, 'the old methods handed down are proved incapable of putting the strain put upon them [for greater productivity] and have to be relinquished for machinery and procedures founded on theories rather than tradition'. His article described that farming had become more businesslike to survive, and was confronted with the voracious appetite

---

[1135] *Cambridge Independent Press* 20.06.1905.

[1136] This was his actually his sister-in-law Elizabeth Long whose husband, George Long, Lawsell's brother, had died the year before in 1902. George and Elizabeth had no children so on her death in 1917 part of the estate may well have been left to him.

[1137] Ibid.

[1138] In 1913 in Brentford, Middlesex, Charles married Daisy Helen de A Lima, who was born in Brazil. https://gw.geneanet.org/kidman?lang=en&p=daisy+helen+de+a&n=lima 02.06.19.

[1139] https://www.thegazette.co.uk/London/issue/39578/page/3435/data.pdf 02.06.19

of a growing population and the 'almost unaccountable increase in the appetite for meat. This is a singular phenomenon,' Jefferies said. 'In one year, the amount consumed increased per head of the population from 98 pounds to 102 pounds'. Livestock production was therefore extremely important but 'wheat itself has been rendered unprofitable. As a crop it does not pay for the cost of production except in isolated instances.'

With uncanny accuracy Jefferies predicted the demise of tenant farmers and the rise of industrial farming methods:

> Farming will become a commercial speculation carried on by large joint stock concerns occupying from three to ten thousand acres.

Maps of St Ives and Surrounds

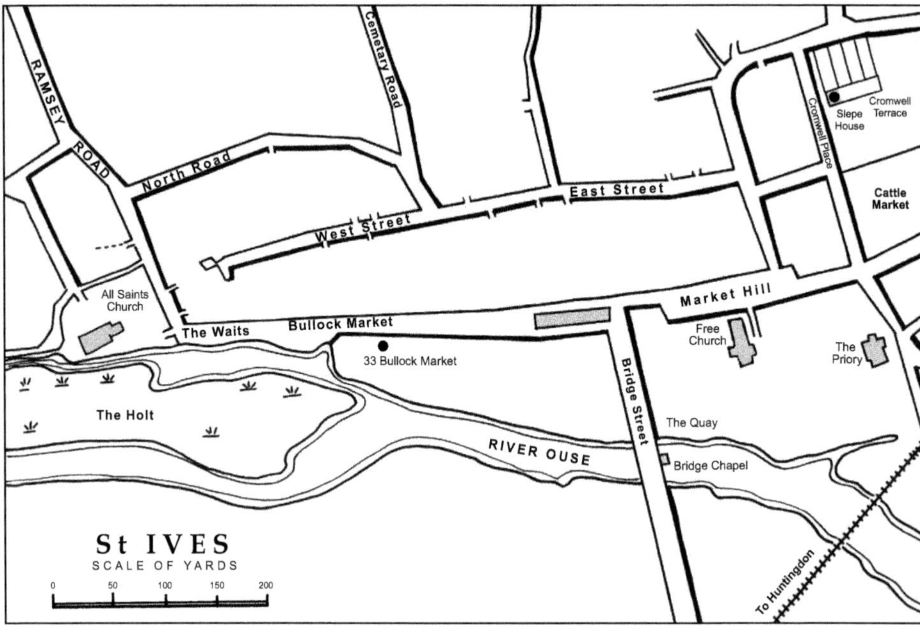

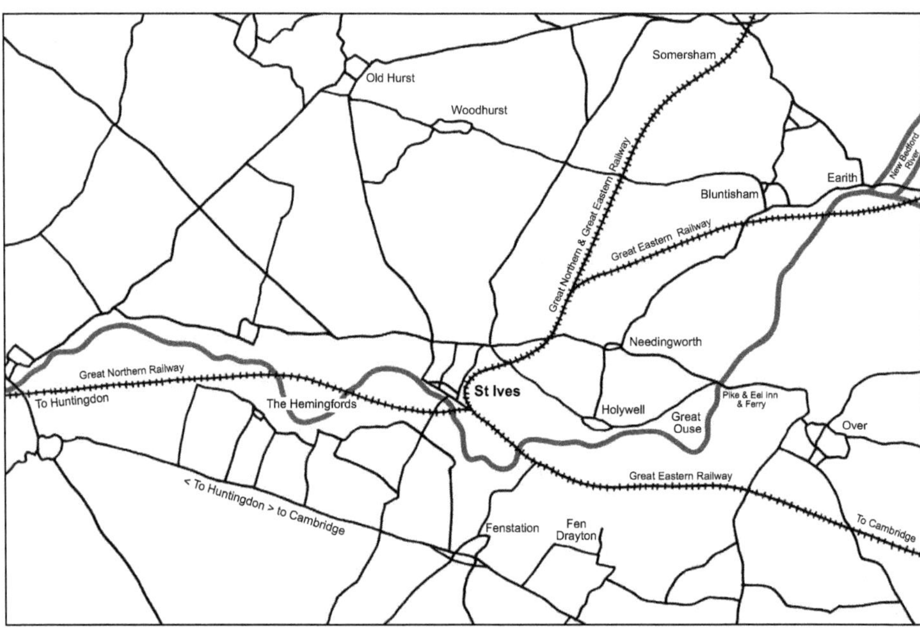

APPENDIX 1

Introduction to Reginald's Diaries 1881–1887

'If a man keeps no diary, the path crumbles away behind him as his feet leave it; and days gone by are little more than a blank broken by a few distorted shadows.'
Lord Bacon[1140]

BACKGROUND

Reginald left a unique set of seven handwritten diaries dating from 1881 to 1887 when he was a boy aged 12–18 living at home and at boarding school. He also kept diaries when he went to Sidney Sussex College, University of Cambridge, and then to study at Guy's Hospital, London. These diaries are for 1890–93. Those for 1888 and 1889 are missing.

The diaries from 1881 to 1887 form the basis for the first two volumes, and those from 1890 to 1893 for the third volume.

On the death of his wife Hilda in 1952, the diaries were passed to one of his daughters, Jane (Janet) who, together with Hilda, was the executor of his will. Jane had read History at the University of London, and became a History teacher at a grammar school in East Dereham. She understood their historical and family value. The early diaries were eventually passed to one of her nephews, Reginald's grandson, William (Baird) Grove, and the later ones to another grandson, John Flower.

A typed transcript of each of the school diaries was made by Jane's brother, David Stephenson Grove, during his retirement years in the 1970s. They were typed on an old ribbon typewriter, when he sat in his conservatory at his retirement home at 'Riverside', Hemingford Abbots, Huntingdonshire. The lawn of his house went down to part of the River Ouse where Reginald had spent many a happy hour rowing in his holidays.

David Grove's meticulous work in transcribing the diaries has been of great help in writing this book.

1140 Cited on the first page of Reginald's first diary 1882 published by Letts, Son and Co, London EC.

RESEARCH USE

The diaries have been made available for historical research on three occasions. Firstly, Jane Grove lent them to W. David Smith for his book *Stretching their Bodies: The History of Physical Education*, published in 1974. Reginald's experiences at Uppingham School were featured on pages 28–30.

A little later, Robert Henderson, a master at King's College Choir School, contacted Jane Grove to use the early diaries for his research. Published in 1981, his *History of King's College Choir School, Cambridge* contained material from Reginald's diaries. Henderson's book has been used in my own research.

Thirdly, they were used by Malcolm Tozer, who taught at Uppingham School from 1966 to 1989. He had published a number of books[1141] on Uppingham School and Edward Thring's headmastership. He approached the author in 2018 to use the diaries in his *Edward Thring's Theory, Practice and Legacy* published in 2019.

A photocopy of the 1883–87 diaries for the Uppingham years is now kept in the archives of Uppingham School.

HIS FIRST DIARY ENTRY

His first entry[1142] on Saturday 1 January 1881 read: 'Had three walkers to tea from Mrs Honeybournes'. Reginald and his family were living in their first family home in the Bullock Market in St Ives.

Who were the three walkers who came to tea at the Grove household from Mrs Honeybourne on that New Year's Day, and what were they doing in St Ives at that time of year?

Twenty-six-year-old Mrs Virginia Honeybourne was the wife of the Headmaster of the small grammar school in St Ives. The school was situated at Manchester House, a large, imposing house in front of the parish church a few minutes' walk from where the Groves lived. The house was built in the 18th century and still stands today. The blue plaque at the front of the house states that it was used as a grammar school from 1858 to 1939.

Ten years earlier the school was owned by James and Sarah Thomas,

---

1141 Notably Tozer, Malcolm, *The Ideal of Manliness: the Legacy of Thring's Uppingham* (2015).

1142 Diary 01.01.81.

and there were 29 pupils boarding at the Academy.[1143] Thirty-year-old John Honeybourne bought the school from them, but the number of pupils fell drastically to eight in 1881. As the boarders went home over the Christmas period the Honeybournes used the large premises as a guest house to bring in extra income.

As Reginald's diaries reveal, guests, relatives and local friends and acquaintances frequently were invited for tea or dinner, or stayed for a few days in their home in the Grove household. While a walking holiday was more popular in warmer weather, St Ives was on the edge of the bleak Fen country which had a beauty of its own in winter. This may have been the attraction for the three walkers who stayed with the Honeybournes.

But two weeks later on 18 January England was struck by a massive snowstorm, subsequently called the 'Blizzard of January 1881'. It lasted for ten days and about seven inches of snow fell in Huntingdonshire. Across Southern England transport and communication links were paralysed; three-foot snowdrifts were seen in London, and the press reported that about 100 people had died nationwide. Reginald had gone back to school at King's on 13 January, thankfully. It was cold enough to go skating and he wrote that it was so windy that he and other boys were blown along on the ice. That night and the following day it snowed very hard. He may have caught a chill skating, as he ended up a few days later in the school sickroom together with three other boys with colds. Confined to bed, he did not recover until the thaw came on 27 January 1881.

What happened to the three walkers after their teatime visit to the Groves remains a mystery.

[1143] National Census 1871.

APPENDIX 2

The Grove Family Tree

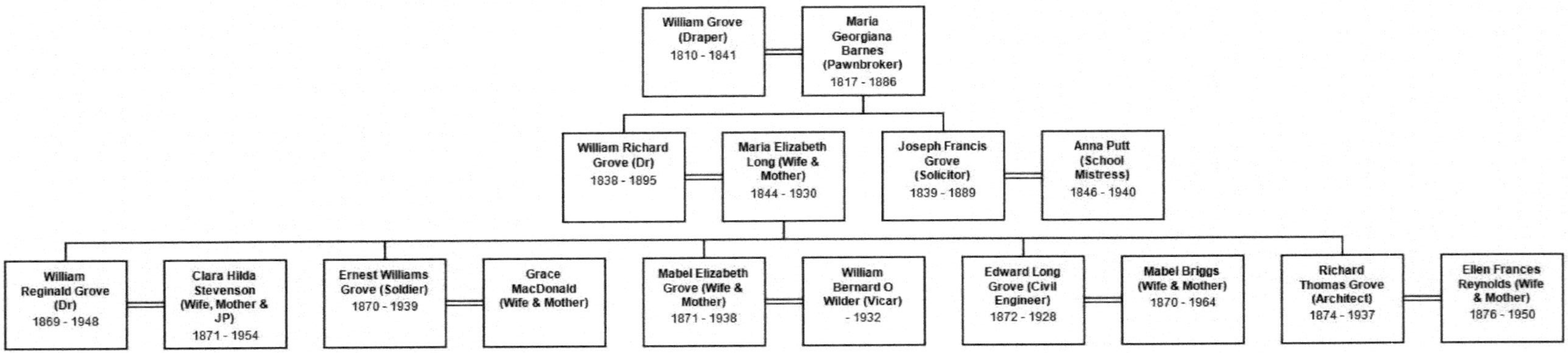

APPENDIX 3

Our Concert

Uppingham School Magazine,[1144] 5 February 1887[1145]

Written by Reginald Grove under the pseudonym M.M.

'I tell you what we'll do,' said the Pater, on Sunday morning after church, 'we'll have a concert in the village. All the proceeds shall go towards the Church Roof; it is beginning to get awfully bad. A concert will give you girls something to think about and you boys too, for that matter.' (We all smiled).

The Church Roof was getting bad, a great many of the tiles had come off, and all the others looked as if they were tired of life and would like to commit suicide by dashing themselves down on the gravestones. This state of things had already been noticed, and a subscription list had been started, but the money did not come in very briskly. Everyone wanted to know how much his neighbour was going to give. This morning, when we drew the blinds, it was raining hard, and when we went to church it was still raining in church there were little pools dotting the stone floor like lakes on a 5th Fr, but in our pew everything seemed dry. All went well till the sermon. The Pater sat thinking when he was going to let *that* farm. I had inwardly called half time (all our Rector's sermons were as near as possible eleven minutes long; one did duty more than once; I often recognise an old friend) when suddenly the Pater's head went a little forward and an extra big drop, which almost seemed to have been waiting an opportunity, dropped neatly down his neck. The Pater started back, shivered all over, grew very red and moved his place: for the remainder of the sermon he stared with a very stern expression up at the roof, which had now quite drawn out all thoughts of the sermon and even *that* farm. I don't know why it was but everyone in church seemed to have seen that drop, a titter went all round, even the Rector must have seen it, for the sermon was a full

---

1144 Reginald noted in his diary that despite reading the proofs prior to going to print, the magazine omitted to include an engraving of Uppingham from the south by his Art Master, Rossiter.

1145 Printed and published on 4 February 1887 by John Hawthorn, who owned a bookshop in Uppingham.

minute longer than normal.

The first thing we had to do was to fix a date; it proved rather a difficult matter to do this, as the dates which suited our chief lady performer were the very days the fiddle could not possibly put in an appearance. However, the fiddle very kindly promised to shift a very pressing engagement, and come to us. We then fixed a great day for J----10th,[1146] giving ourselves about a fortnight to get ready. When all our friends and neighbours heard we were intending to give a concert, they all came in crowds to call on us, each with a different suggestion as to what they would do in our case. One very gushing lady was very anxious we should have a young tradesman from the next town, who sang tenor divinely. We, therefore, told our next visitor (NB – All the visitors were ladies) we thought of getting Jones over at which she looked very wise and said she knew plenty of others we should like much better than Jones, who was really getting terribly conceited and didn't at all know his place, you know. So poor Jones went to the wall. Several, however, recommended Johnson, a tailor who also lived in the next town; we were told he had a deep and heavy bass and would be a great favourite with the back seats and he sang really well. Accordingly, a note was dispatched to Johnson, and a few days later a folded note was brought by the errand women, who daily walked from our village to the town and back; it ran somewhat as follows –

MEMORANDUM

From	To
W. B. Johnson Cheap Tailor, etc, Slowton (Suits from 45/-)	Mrs Blank Wylington

Mr William Johnson presents his compliments to Mrs Blank, and will be very happy to assist at your charity event. I feel very much flattered by your kind invitation. My *repertoire* consists of The Village Blacksmith, Nancy Lee and many others. Have you any choice? I shall be ready on the 10th when you like to send for me [sic].

Your obedient servant,

WILL B. JOHNSON

NB – if you have any comics[1147] I shall not sing.

[1146] It is unclear why Reginald wanted to disguise the date.

[1147] Reginald means comical songs.

The word *repertoire* had been underlined twice, as though he wished us to note his French! Although the note greatly amused us it was resolved that it ought to be kept as a curiosity.

We determined not to have any comic songs not because we should have Mr Will B. Johnson's services, but because we were simply flooded with offers and at the most we couldn't have taken more than two of these: so the broad comic element was left to the readings, which part was to be sustained by the Rector and the Pater. All the rest of the performance was to be taken from our own party and our friends, with the exception of the light haired young man, who played the organ in church on Sunday; he spent the week drawing hideous noises from the flute and cello, both of which instruments he told us he meant one day to be master of. I hoped the day would not be far off.

After we had made out our programme, the next thing was to get it printed and then we had to fix the price of seats. We couldn't possibly charge more than a shilling for front seats; the next seats must then be sixpence and we had quite made up our minds to charge threepence for back seats. But when the woman at *the* shop heard of our intention, she was sure it ought to be tuppence: as there'd be a lot come for tuppence who couldn't pay thrippencee [sic]. She knew for sartin [sic] the Smiths wouldn't pay thrippence. So tuppence was determined on. The room, of course, the village school room, so there was no trouble about that.

The great evening came round at last. All day the girls had been trying to make themselves nervous and they had succeeded. Tea was, therefore, a very gloomy proceeding. Some tried very hard, but hardly succeeded in putting on a cheerful look; others wholly gave themselves up to groans, and 'sure they'd break down' and other phrases of a like nature. We walked down to the school room at seven, half an hour before we were announced to begin. The room was already half full, and it was rapidly filling. The stage had been put up at the far end of the room and covered with red curtains instead of baize. On the right of the stage there was a door leading into what in the usual course of events was a class room, for 'this night only', had a warming fire and was intended for the use of the performers. This was immediately dubbed the 'Green Room'[1148] by a gentleman who had very much wanted us to have private theatricals instead of a concert.

[1148] This expression dated back to Tudor times to describe a room behind the scenes where actors waited to go onstage.

There was, of course, the usual late arrival, who was wanted in the second piece, and as it approached 7.31 he turned up, full of apologies and excuses. At once someone very valiantly offered to go and light the piano candles. From the clapping which ensued we presumed the audience was in good temper. Then two of the girls went on and performed a hammer and tongs[1149] duett [sic]. At its close there was a feeble display of clapping. Then after a song and a reading by the Rector came the chief thing of the concert; the Mater had got a lady friend of hers, with a splendid soprano voice, to come and stay with us for the concert. She went up smiling sweetly, and sang a very plantive [sic] ditty about a sailor who went to sea and returned never......never......ah never! There was no increase at all in clapping. The lady came down snappish and cross; she had expected an encore at least. She knew she had a good voice, and had sung well and this was very humiliating. The audience was an awful lot of country bumpkins. The Mater saw this would never do, so she called me and gave me instructions what to do. Before the great lady was to sing again, I strolled down to the end of the room, took a seat, and I am afraid there was a good deal of whispering from our quarter during her song, but at the end there arose such a yell, as the old room had never heard before. The word encore was not used but variations of it as *'core, co----a*, were very frequent: some of the more learned got a step further and yelled *hencore* (the first syllable pronounced like the English word hen); a good many contented themselves with plain English – *Fetch 'er back, Git'oop*, and other similar phrases. She graciously consented to be fetched back. The audience were at last roused they henceforward encored everything to the end of the programme. Only two incidents need to be mentioned: two sisters played Mozart's Gloria in Excelsis as a duett [sic] on two violins; as an encore they played Hypatia Walz![1150] However, very few noticed it, so it did not matter much. Mr Johnson was perhaps the favourite of the evening, he delighted the audience by descending, on every possible occasion, deep down with the depths of his voice; the poor letter *h* was neither 'whispered in Heaven, nor mutter'd in Hell'.[1151] Just before 'God save the Queen' a fat little gentleman made a rush for the platform. After thanking the performers, he wished to remind them about the Church Roof; he would

[1149] This is not a musical term. Reginald must be meaning they played with great enthusiasm.

[1150] This was a waltz composed by May Ostlere for the piano.

[1151] From the first line of Lord Byron's poem 'Enigma'.

give his five guineas,[1152] and hoped others would follow suit.

So ended our grand village concert. Though the proceeds from the concert were not much, money from other sources came in plentifully.

The builders are now busy at work on the roof.

M.M.

(MM stood for the initials of Reginald's sweetheart and cousin, Margaret Mary Long.)

[1152] 21 shillings (£133.11).

APPENDIX 4

Monumental Brasses

Uppingham School Magazine, 6 June 1887

Written by Reginald Grove

These seem to have come into use in the 13th century, and their popularity appears to have continued for the next four centuries. The oldest known monumental brass is said to be that of Simon de Beauchamp, Earl of Bedford, 1208, which is stated to have been in St Paul's, Bedford. The oldest existing brass, however, is that of Sir John D'Aubernoun, at Stoke D'Abernon in Surrey, 1277.

Brass was not made in England until the 16th century, but was imported from the Continent; the engraving, however, was done in England. There are nevertheless some brasses in England which were made wholly on the Continent: these are Flemish brasses and, in common with all foreign ones, consist of one large sheet of metal, on which the figure as well as inscriptions and canopies are engraved; while in English ones the figure is cut out, and the background of the design is formed by a marble or hard stone slab (called the matrix) on which the brass is laid, the canopy, inscription, and other parts consisting of separate pieces. They were about the most appropriate and durable memorials, as far as material is concerned, that could be adopted. When first adopted laid down lines were filled with some sort of black substance, and the effect was heightened by gilding and enamel.

They are most useful and interesting to us for the costumes of ladies, the vestments of ecclesiastics, and the various parts of the armour and dress of the men during the four centuries of a most exciting part of English history. In addition to the great variety of costume, many curious customs and usages of those times are directly or indirectly very often illustrated. The destruction of them at one time or another has been immense, and though objects of archaeological interest are better preserved than formally, many have disappeared recently. England, in this respect, has not suffered so much as the Continent: there, where they were first used, there must have been many thousands, but revolutions and wars have done their work and there are now about 400, while in England there are about 4,000.

On the destruction of the monasteries the brasses on the tombs were frequently sold with the church plate, and churchwardens when in want of money did not hesitate to sell the metal and enter the fat in their accounts. Yarmouth, in 1551, recast its brasses into weights and measures for the use of the town. To this subject belong those brasses to which the term 'palimpsest' has been given. These are brasses that have been used a second time: either engraved again on the back, or the original figure altered to suit another person of a later date and costume, or the original figure remains unaltered, but a fresh inscription, shield etc is introduced. In Burwell Church, Cambridgeshire, there is a curious palimpsest; as you see it, it is a brass of an ecclesiastic soon after the Reformation, with nothing very particular about the vestments; you unscrew and turn over the lower part of the figure and there you see the lower part of another priest in a great and fine variety of vestments.[1153] Also, if you turn over a good-sized piece of the canopy in this same brass, you will find the lower part of a figure of a lady with a dog at her feet. There are other curious palimpsests known, and probably others unknown, but this is perhaps the most curious of all.

After Sir John D'Aubernoun, the next oldest brass is that of Sir Roger de Trumpington, in Trumpington Church, Cambridge, 1289.[1154] He became a Crusader in 1280 and went to Palestine with Prince Edward and consequently has his legs crossed, though this does not necessarily mean he was a Crusader. It used to be supposed that only Templars had their legs crossed, but this idea has been altogether explored. Some authorities say that cross-legged effigies were Crusaders who had vowed to accomplish, or had accomplished, a pilgrimage to the Holy Land, and had either died without fulfilling it or compromised by payment of money or by finding a substitute. Others consider it a mere fashion in monumental sculpture, which prevailed during the latter half of the 13th and beginning of the

[1153] On his various excursions to collect rubbings during the Easter holidays 1887 in Cambridgeshire, he did not visit Burwell so this information must have been taken from another article that he had read.

[1154] While Reginald did not visit this church and take a rubbing, he was given one of Sir Roger in the Easter holidays by a Mr Streeten. He met him by chance on the train coming back from Cambridge to St Ives and got chatting to him. It is possible he was a friend of Revd Pollock's, who was encouraging Reginald in this hobby. (Diary 21.04.87.)

14th centuries, indicating that the deceased possessed judicial authority.[1155]

The finest engraving of a knight is at Acton, in Suffolk, of Sir Robert de Bures, 1302. There is also another very fine one at Chatham, Kent, of Sir Robert de Septvans, 1306. Of Flemish brasses there are fine examples in St Margaret's, King's Lynn, 1864, on which is depicted the Peacock Frest,[1156] and also at St Albans Abbey, one of an abbot, 1360. But these are only fine examples; almost every neighbourhood has its brasses, all of which are worth rubbing to anyone who is interested, or wishes to be, in costumes and other things ancient and historical; and in most neighbourhoods you will usually find at least one fine brass.

In our own neighbourhood there are brasses in the chancel of Lyddington church of a lady with a very fine example of a butterfly headdress, 1486, and also of a Knight (J.P.) and wife, 1530. The brass plate that figures below, between the children, is in memory of another worthy, one Edward Watson.[1157] At Braunston[1158] (six miles through Ridlington and Brooke) there is one to Kenelm Cheseldyne and his wife, of Vpingham [sic], 1590; and at Manton there is a very good inscription on the north wall. At Stockerston there are two, a knight and wife, 1467, and another knight and wife, 1490. But the latter is almost entirely covered by a tomb, and the former is very loose and very little care is evidently taken of it.[1159] The collector will experience great difficulty in taking this as the loose metal will tear through his paper. At Deene (eight miles) there

1155 The cross-legged attitude of many brass effigies and stone figures of knights was long supposed to imply that they had served in the Crusades and had taken crusading vows, or more specifically had been a Knights Templar; but these theories are generally now rejected by modern historians who consider crossed legs as merely a stylistic convention. http://journals.cambridge.org/action/displayAbstract?fromPage=online&aid=7884801&fulltextType=RA&fileId=S0003581510000053.

1156 There are three figures and below their feet a strange scene known as The Peacock Feast (not Frest). It is uncertain what this scene represents. One theory is that it shows a feast given by Braunche to Edward III when he was Mayor of King's Lynn. Another theory is that it depicts a scene from a medieval legend.

1157 Reginald took rubbings when he visited the church on 27.01.87.

1158 He visited this church on 10.03.87 and took a rubbing and also the church at Manton on the same day.

1159 He visited Stockerston Church on 26.02.87 and took two rubbings; this was not his first visit as on this occasion he noted how new pews had been put in since his earlier visit.

are three:[1160] the date of one is 1585, but the others I have not been able to find anything.[1161] There is also at North Luffenham a brass inscription on the chancel wall, to our founder, Archdeacon Johnson[1162] – a rubbing of which is in the school library.[1163] At Little Casterton (two miles from Stamford and therefore out of range of anyone while at school) there is a fine example of a knight and a lady, in the beginning of the 15th century. In All Saints, Stamford,[1164] there are half a dozen or more, most of them civilians, 1442–89.

In writing this paper I wish to interest the School in these ancient monuments, from which a great deal more is to be learnt on account of their durability, than from the stone monuments and tombs, which are often so rubbed away as to be scarcely discernible: I hope that now most of the School will look upon brasses with different eyes than of yore and consider them of some use and not merely sheets of metal. Undoubtedly the only way to really study brasses is to take exact copies of them, and the best way to do this is to 'rub' them: in this way nothing can escape you, for you can always keep your copy.[1165] It is too much to expect too many fellows in the School to become collectors, but I hope that some few, who do not play cricket for some reason or other may, this term, and

[1160] He visited the church in the afternoon of 21.05.87 after Thring had given him and his friend Evans special permission. It rained during the day (encountering 'two tremendous heavy showers of rain and hail') so they took umbrellas and were pleased that the Vicar, Revd Sylvester, invited them in to his home for sherry and biscuits. Reginald described the rubbing as 'the best I have ever taken'. Evans took one brass and also made sketches of the church. Sylvester sent 'us on our way rejoicing'.

[1161] It is interesting to note from this example that brass monuments continued to be erected after the Reformation.

[1162] Robert Johnson was the Rector of North Luffenham in the mid-16th century who later became Archdeacon of Leicester and founded two grammar schools, one at Oakham and one at Uppingham in 1584. The old schoolroom built then near the parish church at Uppingham is still in use by the school today.

[1163] In fact, this was the only brass rubbing at the school and was in a poor condition according to Reginald.

[1164] Reginald was able to visit the church on 09.07.87 a few weeks before he left Uppingham, and with his friend Evans. He took two brass rubbings, a large one of a man and a woman, as well as a small one of a girl – both c.1480, he thought. The visit took place was after he wrote the article so he must have taken the information about the brasses from a book.

[1165] Despite the ability to photograph monuments, the Monumental Brass Society still recommends rubbing instead. This is because it is important to ensure that the brass is evenly lit, preferably using photoflood sources. The Society does not advocate using camera-mounted flashes, as the reflections often mar part of the photograph.

others in the holidays, at least try to rub one brass. I am certain that a very small percentage of those who once begin will make their first the last. It is a source of enjoyment to the collector and interesting both to himself and his friends. To these as well as others, who may perhaps want to rub some curious brass to which they have taken a fancy, I give a few hints as to rubbing.

Your apparatus will consist of common lining paper sold by paper hangers for about a penny a yard: this is sold in two widths, one twenty-one inches wide,[1166] the other about thirty, both of these are wanted by the regular collector: you will also want a duster, a box of wafers,[1167] and two or three pieces of heelball:[1168] the latter can be obtained at any shoemakers at a penny a piece, the quality sold as medium being the best for your purpose: the duster for your cleaning the brass of dirt, mortar etc (often sadly needed) and the wafers are only used when the brass is mural, when they are used for fixing the paper. Having 'caught' your brass, clean it with your duster of all small stones, dirt etc, and if on the ground, fix your paper (taking care to get it as free from wrinkles as possible) with big prayer books or hymn books you will find about the church: hassocks[1169] will also do, but sometimes these leave a dirty mark. Begin from the top and rub it in parts finishing off each part before you go on to the next, so that if your paper slips you may not spoil the whole rubbing. Taking first the head and shoulders, rub it lightly to get the outline and to make sure you have got no small stones underneath: then rub it to the degree of blackness you like best, only if you wish it to look well, let the colour be on evenly. Do the rest in exactly the same way. Those who are skilful – and skill comes with practice – can heighten the effect immensely by making a difference in the intensity of the black in the various parts of armour or garments of the figure. If you wish to take great care of your copy, cut out the figure, the canopy and whatever remains that is brass, and paste them onto calico but of course they can be kept rolled up in the same state as when you first took them.

[1166] Wallpaper and lining paper are still sold in rolls which are 21 inches wide (533mm).

[1167] It is not clear what these are, or their use, but it is likely that they held the paper in place when the brass was positioned on a wall rather than the floor of a church.

[1168] A mixture of wax and lampblack used to polish shoes.

[1169] A heavy cushion used for kneeling when praying.

If anyone is sufficiently interested in these to wish to take some rubbings, I shall only be too happy to do my best to answer any questions, set him right in the few things he will want and show him some rubbings.[1170]

W. R. Grove

[1170] Sadly, his diary records that no one contacted him for his help.

APPENDIX 5

Grove Family Chronology 1837–1954

Year	*Details*	*Notes*
1837	William Grove married	Georgiana née Barnes (d.1886)
1838	William Richard Grove born	Reginald's father
1839	Joseph Francis Grove born	Reginald's Uncle Frank
1844	Maria Elizabeth Long born	Reginald's mother
1862	William Richard Grove qualified as a doctor	Awarded a degree by St Andrews University in medicine
1862	William Richard Grove moved to Huntingdon	Worked as a junior doctor at Huntingdon Hospital
1863	William Richard Grove moved to St Ives, Huntingdonshire	Worked as an assistant to Dr Girling whose surgery was in the Bullock Market
1866	William Richard appointed Medical Officer of Health for St Ives	First appointment to this new role
1868	William Richard Grove married Maria Long	Lived at 33, The Bullock Market, St Ives
1869	**Reginald born**	
1869	Reginald baptised	All Saints Parish Church
1870	Ernest Grove born	Served in SA War (DSO) then Indian Army
1871	Mabel Grove born	Married Revd Bernard Wilder 1894
1872	Edward Grove born	Became civil engineer
1874	Richard Thomas Grove born	Became an architect
1877	William Richard appointed Vicar's Warden	All Saints Church, St Ives
1877	William Richard appointed Assistant Surgeon (volunteer)	1st Cambridge Battalion Suffolk Regiment
1878	**Reginald started at King's College Choir School, Cambridge**	A boarder in the school
1881	Reginald started his first diary	Aged 12. Diary given by his father

1881	Grove family moved to Slepe House	At Cromwell Terrace, St Ives
1883	Reginald caught scarlet fever	
1883	**Reginald started at Uppingham School, Rutland**	A boarder in Redgate
1886	Mary Georgiana Grove died	His grandmother
1887	Joseph Francis Grove married	To Anna Pratt in Totnes, Devon
1887	**Reginald left Uppingham**	
1887	Reginald went up to Cambridge University	Sidney Sussex reading Natural Science
1889	William Richard appointed a Surgeon Major – Medical Reserves	
1889	Joseph Francis Grove died	Aged 50
1890	Reginald went down from Cambridge	Awarded a BA degree
1891	Reginald began medical training as a surgical ward clerk	Guy's Hospital, London
1892	Met Clara Hilda Stevenson at a dance at Guy's Hospital	Hilda was a daughter of Sir Thomas Stevenson who worked at Guy's Hospital
1893	Reginald part-qualified	Royal College of Surgeons – licensed. MRCS and LRCP
1894	Reginald returned to St Ives to help run the practice	William Richard Grove's illness restricted his work
1894	Reginald appointed St Ives Deputy Medical Officer	No salary, standing in for his father who was ill
1894	Reginald appointed Medical Officer to St Ives Corporation and Sanitary Authority	
1895	William Richard resigned as St Ives Medical Officer of Health	Due to chronic ill health
1895	William Richard died.	Aged 57
1896	Reginald reappointed St Ives Medical Officer of Health	Salary £21 per year
1897	Reginald Grove married Clara Hilda Stevenson	Married at St John's Church, Brixton, London
	The couple moved in to Slepe House	Reginald's mother continued living there for a short period

1899	Veronica Grove born	Became a nurse; in later life hospitalized due to mental health
1902	William Stevenson Grove born	Trained as a doctor: Sidney Sussex, Cambridge. Guy's Hospital
1903	Hilda Mary Grove born	Became a teacher
1904	Reginald bought Slepe House	From his mother who later lived in Station Road, Cambridge
1904	Agnes Norah Grove born	Became a dress designer
1905	David Stevenson Grove	Became an electrical engineer
1907	Sylvia Grove	Became a pharmacist
1909	Janet Elizabeth Grove born	Became a teacher
1910	Frances Geraldine Grove born	Became a teacher
1911	Lettuce Grove born	Became (ultimately) a nun
1913	John George Grove born	Died 1932 aged 19
1916	Reginald appointed St Ives Rural District Medical Officer of Health	
1925	Elected President of the Stereoscopic Society	President until his death
1929	Reginald appointed Assistant Surgeon of Huntingdon County Hospital	
1930	Death of Reginald's mother	Aged 86
1937	Reginald and Hilda Grove moved from Slepe House	Moved to Tenterleas House which they built in Tenterleas, St Ives
1938	William (Bill) Grove joined the practice	Lived at Slepe House
1942	St Ives Practice now called Grove, Grove and Sweeting	
1948	Reginald retired as Medical Officer of Health of St Ives	After 55 years
1948	Reginald Grove died	Aged 79
1948	William (Bill) Grove moved to Norwich and Slepe House sold to Dr Dansie and Dr Musson	Ill with TB
1954	Clara Hilda Grove died	

Acknowledgements

I am indebted to the countless, unnamed people who have provided research material available through Wikipedia's online encyclopaedia and the Project Gutenberg's library of e-books.

Copyright permission

Every effort has been made to identify and obtain permission from copyright holders. If any have been overlooked, I will be happy to make corrections in any subsequent editions of the book. All Scripture quotations, unless indicated, are taken from the Holy Bible New International Version (Anglicised edition), © 1979, 1984 by the International Bible Society, and are used by permission of Hodder & Stoughton Publishers, a Hatchards UK company. Extracts from *Period Piece, a Cambridge Childhood* by Gwen Raverat, © Faber and Faber Ltd, Bloomsbury House, 74–77 Great Russell Street, London WC1B 3DA are used by kind permission of her publishers. Extracts from *A Victorian Family* by Molly Hughes, abridged edition 1990, are used with the permission of Pan Macmillan Publishers (Sidgwick & Jackson Ltd), 20, New Wharf Road, London N1 9RR.

Photographs

Other photographs are from the Grove Family Archive.

Thanks

I have been encouraged in writing this biography by Reginald's surviving grandchildren: John Grove, William Grove, Margret Macnab and John Flower. All have helped in my research; documents have been lent, and photographs given me. These I have called the 'Grove Family Archive'.

I owe an immense debt of thanks to my wife Sandra who has been my research assistant in accessing material online from the National Archives, Kew. These range from National Census returns, probate documents, parish records, bishops' transcripts and electoral records. Her patience in overlooking the files, books and other papers which have cluttered various rooms in our house has been a great blessing.

For this volume my thanks to Marilyn Long and Louise Waller, Practice

Managers at the medical practice in Cromwell Place for allowing me to be shown the interior where my family lived from 1881 to 1948; and Dr Geoff Ferreira, partner in the Cromwell Place practice from 1975 to 2006. Also to Mick Napier and Richard Carter from the Norris Museum, St Ives, for their patient help in my research; Colin Leach from the St Ives Angling Cub; Mike Stevenson from the St Ives Boat Club; Fr Alexander Shannon, Assistant Curate, All Saints, St Ives; and Charles Beresford, fellow local St Ives historian.

Elizabeth Stazicker, the Archivist of the King's School, Ely kindly supplied copies of the *Elean*, the School Magazine, which provided information about Reginald's two brothers, Ernest and Edward, who were pupils there. My thanks as well to Jerry Rudman, Uppingham School Archivist and Malcolm Tozer, author *of Edward Thring's Theory, Practice and Legacy* (2019) and other papers for their help with this volume. Also, to Nigel Richardson, author of *Thring of Uppingham – Victorian Educator* (2014).

Thanks to Revd Dr Mark Smith, Dean & Director of Studies in Theology, Clare College, Cambridge, for reading my draft chapter on 'Faith under fire'. And for his skilled work in enhancing old family photographs, thank you, Tuomas Pirinen, my son-in-law.

I am very grateful as well to Douglas Walker and Frances Prior-Reeves of The Self-Publishing Partnership for their patience and guidance in enabling this biography to be published

The painstaking work carried out by my uncle, the late David Grove, in typing up the diaries during his retirement years, has been a huge blessing. Without this, my research would have taken much longer. A copy of his transcript for the diaries from 1883 to 1887 has now been placed in the Uppingham School Archives.

Finally, thanks to my dear aunt, the late Jane Grove, for her inspiration and encouragement to me as a young historian.

Bibliography

PRIMARY SOURCES

FAMILY DOCUMENTS

Bensly, Robert, Letters to W. R. Grove 1885–1887

Grove D. S. and Grove J. E. *E.W.6 1904–1969 Sixty Five years in one family* (East Anglican Magazine, Ipswich, 1970)

Grove, W. R., Diaries 1881–1887

Grove, W. R., Diaries 1890–1893

Grove, W. R., Miscellaneous letters and documents

Grove, W. R., Letters to and from his fiancée Clara Hilda Stevenson

ARCHIVE MATERIAL

Norris Museum, St Ives:
- Newspaper Cuttings Archive

Huntingdon Library and Archives:
- Rural Sanitary Authority Minutes April 1889
- Minute Book St Ives Borough Council 1891–1897
- Inventory and Valuation of Surgery (Slepe House) October 1947 (No 3266)
- All Saints St Ives Parish Records 1847–1937

King's College Cambridge Archives

Uppingham School Archives

St Ives Angling Club Minutes 1894–1911

OTHER

Anderson-Morshead, A. E. M., *The History of the Universities' Mission to Central Africa, 1859–1898* (Office of the Universities Mission to Central Africa, 1899)

Beeton, Isabella, *The Book of Household Management*, 1861 (ISO-8859-1 www.gutenberg.net)

Douglas, James, *Theodore Watts-Dunton* (Hodder & Stoughton, 1904)

Eastlake, Charles, *Hints on Household Taste in Furniture and Upholstery* (1869) 2nd Edition Longmans, Green and Co.

Gatty, Horatia Katharine Frances, *Juliana Horatia Ewing and Her Books*

(Society for Promoting Christian Knowledge, 1885). The Project Gutenberg eBook of The Works of Whittier, Volume IV (of VII), by John Greenleaf Whittier

Glover, William, *The Memoirs of a Cambridge Chorister* Vol 2 (Hurst and Blackett, London, 1885)

Goodman, Neville, and Goodman, Albert, *Handbook of Fen Skating* (Sampson Low, Marston, Searle and Rivington, London E.C., 1882)

Graham, John, *Forty Years of Uppingham* (Macmillan & Co., London, 1932)

Norris, Herbert E., *History of St Ives* (1889, republished by Friends of the Norris Museum, 1980)

Parkin, George, *Edward Thring, Headmaster of Uppingham School. Life, Diary and Letters*, Vol 1 (Macmillan & Co., 1898), Vol 1 & 2 (Macmillan & Co., 1910

Paget, Stephen, *Memoirs and Letters of Sir James Paget* (Longmans, Green and Co, 1902) (Grove Family Archive)

Raverat, Gwen, *Period Piece, a Cambridge Childhood* (Faber and Faber, 1952)

Skrine, John Huntley, *A Memory of Edward Thring* (Macmillan and Co., 1889)

Walker, Henry, *Memoirs* Book 1 and Book 2 (handwritten) (Uppingham School Archives, 1957)

DIRECTORIES AND MAPS

Bradshaw's Descriptive Railway Hand-book of Great Britain and Ireland Section III and IV (first published 1868, reprinted by Old House Books, 2012)

Craven & Co's Directory of the County of Huntingdonshire (1862)

A History of the County of Huntingdon: Volume 2. Originally published by Victoria County History, London, 1932

History, Topography and Directory of Huntingdonshire (Paul Edward Cassey & Co., 1862)

J. G. Harrod & Co.'s Postal and Commercial Directory of Derbyshire, Leicestershire, Rutland, and Staffordshire (J. G. Harrod & Co., London and Norwich, 1870)

Jackson, H.L., *A Handbook for Visitors and Residents: Huntingdon and the Great Ouse with St Neots and St Ives Editor* (Homeland Handbook, 1905)

Kelly's Directory 1883 (Cambridgeshire)
Kelly's Directory 1885 (Beds, Hunts and Northants)
Kelly's Directory 1889 (Devon)
Kelly's Directory 1899 (Leicester and Rutland)
Kelly's Directory 1894 (Huntingdonshire)
Ordnance Survey, *Reprint of the First Edition of the one-inch Ordnance Survey of England and Wales*, Bedford (Sheet 53), Cambridge & Ely (Sheet 54), (David & Charles, 1970)
St Ives Business Register 1885, https://stives100yearsago.blogspot.com/1985/01/st-ives-business-register-1885.html
Return of Owners of Land Vol 1 (Eyre and Spottiswoode, 1873)
Royal County Directory of Huntingdonshire (1877)

SECONDARY SOURCES

GENERAL BACKGROUND

Cook, Chris, *The Routledge Companion to Britain in the Nineteenth Century, 1815–1914* (Routledge Companions to History, 2005)
Bédarida, François, *A Social History of England 1851–1990* (Methuen & Co Ltd, 1990)
Calder, Jenni, *The Victorian Home* (B.T. Batsford, London, 1997)
Chadwick, Owen, *The Victorian Church Part 11* (Adam & Charles Black, 1970)
Ensor, Robert, *England 1870–1914,* Oxford History of England (Clarendon Press, 1936)
Evans, Richard, *The Victorians: Life and Death* (2010), Gresham Lectures https://www.gresham.ac.uk/lectures-and-events/the-victorians-life-and-death.
Evans, Richard – *The Victorians: Religion and Science* (2011) Gresham Lectures https://www.gresham.ac.uk/lectures-and-events/the-victorians-religion-and-science.
Fava-Verde, Jean-François, *Victorian Telegrams: the early development of the telegraphic despatch and its interplay with the letter post* (2018), Notes and Records: Royal Society Journal of the History of Science.
Flanders, Judith, *The Victorian House* (Harper Perennial, 2004)
Goodman, Ruth, *How to be a Victorian* (Viking Press/Penguin Group, 2013)
Guild, Robin, *The Victorian House Book* (Sidgwick & Jackson, 2002)

Hart-Davis, Adam, *What the Victorians Did for Us* (Headline, 2001)
Hughes, Kathryn, *Victorians Undone* (HarperCollins, 4th Edition paperback, 2018)
Hughes, Molly, *Victorian Family 1870–1900* (Sidgwick & Jackson, abridged edition, 1990)
Langlands, Alex; Ginn, Peter; Goodman, Ruth, *Victorian Farm* (Pavilion Books, 2008)
Marshall, John, and Willox, Ian, *The Victorian House* (Sidgwick & Jackson, London, 1986)
Oxford Dictionary of National Biography (online edition, Oxford University Press)
Paterson, Michael, *Life in Victorian Britain* (Running Press, 2008)
Richardson, Nigel, *Thring of Uppingham, Victorian Educator* (University of Buckingham Press, 2014)
Reader, W. J., *Professional Men* (Weidenfeld and Nicolson, 1966)
Rees-Mogg, Jacob, *The Victorians* (W. H. Allen, 2019)
Rutland Local History Society Vol 3: Railways in Rutland (Spiegal Press, 1980)
Sheets, Diana E., *British Conservatism and the Primrose League: The changing character of popular politics, 1883–1901* (Columbia University, 1986)
Simmons, Jack, *The Victorian Railway* (Thames & Hudson, 1991)
Spencer, Nick and Alexander, Denis, *Rescuing Darwin* (Theos, 2009)
Spours, Judy, *Cakes and Ale: The Golden Age of British Feasting* (2006) National Archives, Kew, London
Sweet, Matthew, *Inventing the Victorians* (Faber and Faber, 2001)
Tosh, John, *A Man's Place* (Hobbs the Printers Ltd, 2007)
Tozer, Malcolm, *Edward Thring's Theory, Practice and Legacy: Physical Education in Britain since 1800* (Cambridge Scholars Publishing, 2019)
Uppingham School Roll 1824–1905 (3rd Issue, Edward Stanford, 1906, via Internet Archive, University of Harvard)
Venn, John, *Alumni Cantabrigienses* (Cambridge University Press), Part 11 Volumes I (1940), II (1944), V (1927) and VI (1954)
Walvin, James, *A Child's World, a social history of English Childhood 1800–1914* (Penguin, 1982)
Walvin, James, *Victorian Values* (André Deutsch, London, 1987)
Webb, R. K., *Modern England* (Dodd, Mead & Co., 1968)

Wilson, A. N., *The Victorians* (Hutchinson, London, 2007)

NEWSPAPERS
Cambridge Chronicle
Hunts County News
The Hunts Guardian
The Hunts Post
The St Ives Chronicle

ST IVES, HUNTINGDONSHIRE
Burn-Murdoch, Bob, *Victorian St Ives* (Witley Press, 2007)
Burn-Murdoch, Bob, *The Shaping of St Ives* (Blueprint, Cambridge, 2009)
Butterfield, Elizabeth, *Growth of Hemingford Grey* (Hemingford Local History Society, 2017)
Carter, Mary, *A Remarkable Journey: The history of the Free Church in St Ives* (Westmeare Publications, 2005)
Carter, Mary, *19th Century St Ives* (CLE Print, St Ives, 2010)
Dady, Jack, *Beyond Yesterday: A History of Fenstanton* (King's Music, 1987)
Day, J. Wentworth, *History of the Fens* (1954), republished by S.R. Publishers, 1970
Dring, W.E., *The Fenland Story* (Cambridgeshire and Isle of Ely Education Committee,1967)
Flanagan, Bridget, *Artists along the Ouse* (Burlington Press, 2010)
Flanagan, Bridget, *The St Ives Problem* (Parrot Print, 2013)
Haughton Threlfall, John, *The Story of Huntingdon County Hospital* (East Anglian Regional Health Authority, 1980)
Hudson, Noel, *St Ives: Slepe by the Ouse* (Black Bear Press, 1989)
Little, Bryan, and Werba, Herbert, *St Ives in Huntingdonshire* (The Pitman Press, 1974)
The Lost Pubs of St Ives: 02.04.2018. http://www.closedpubs.co.uk/huntingdonshire/stives.html.
A social history of St Ives and its people (https://stives100yearsago.blogspot.com)
Westlake, Ray, *Tracing the Rifle Volunteers 1859–1908* (Pen and Sword Family History, 2010)

Index

References to captions are in italic